THE TRUTH ABOUT BEAUTY

FULLY UPDATED FEATURED RE-RELEASE

THE TRUTH ABOUT BEAUTY

TRANSFORM YOUR LOOKS AND YOUR LIFE FROM THE INSIDE OUT

KAT JAMES

ATRIA BOOKS
New York London Toronto Sydney

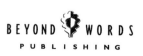
BEYOND WORDS
PUBLISHING

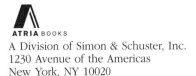

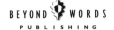

A Division of Simon & Schuster, Inc.
1230 Avenue of the Americas
New York, NY 10020

20827 N.W. Cornell Road, Suite 500
Hillsboro, Oregon 97124-9808
503-531-8700 / 503-531-8773 fax
www.beyondword.com

The information contained in this book is intended to be educational.
The author and publishers are in no way liable for any misuse of the information.

The author and the publisher gratefully acknowledge and thank the following for permission to reprint previously published material quoted in this book:

Excerpts from "The Makeup-less Makeover," by Kat James, edited by Jerry Shaver, *Better Nutrition*, October 2002. Copyright © 2002 by Sabot Publishing, Inc. Reprinted by permission of *Better Nutrition*.

Excerpts from "Kat's 6-Day JumpStart Menu and Recipes for Transformation" and "Transformation Profiles" by Kat James from the website of InformedBeauty.com, reprinted by permission of Informed Beauty, LLC.

Managing editor: Lindsay S. Brown
Copy editor: Gretchen Stelter
Proofreader: Meadowlark Communications, Inc.
Interior design: Sara E. Blum
Compositions: William H. Brunson Typography Services

First Atria Books/Beyond Words trade paperback edition December 2007

ATRIA BOOKS and colophon are trademarks of Simon & Schuster, Inc.
Beyond Words Publishing is a division of Simon & Schuster, Inc.

For more information about special discounts for bulk purchases, please contact Simon & Schuster Special Sales at 1-800-456-6798 or business@simonandschuster.com.

Manufactured in the United States of America

10 9 8 7 6 5 4 3

Library of Congress Cataloging-in-Publication Data

James, Kat.
    The truth about beauty : transform your looks and your life from the inside out /
Kat James. — 2nd ed., fully updated and expanded.
        p.   cm.
Includes bibliographical references and index.
1. Beauty, Personal.   2. Women—Health and hygiene.   3. Holistic medicine.   I. Title.
RA778.J274   2007
613'.04244—dc22

                                                                                        2007023742

ISBN-13: 978-1-58270-195-0
ISBN-10:   1-58270-195-4

The corporate mission of Beyond Words Publishing, Inc.: *Inspire to Integrity*

DEDICATION

*To the woman I was—for whom this book would
have been a godsend—and to all women and men
who seek to regain radiance and
mastery over their own physical destinies*

In memory of Allyn Farmer

CONTENTS

PART III: THE MAKEUP-LESS MAKEOVER

AUTHOR NOTE

Dear Reader:

Please understand that the information, scientific studies, specific solutions, and opinions discussed in this book, while carefully researched, are offered for educational purposes only and may contain errors. They are not intended as diagnoses or treatments for specific ailments or replacements for the expertise of your qualified healthcare provider. If you feel that certain information applies to a health-related issue of your own, it is crucial that you bring it to the attention of your healthcare provider for confirmation and treatment. The use of any of this information without consulting a physician may be dangerous. Neither the publisher nor the author accepts responsibility for any effects that may arise from the correct or incorrect use of information in this book.

My goal is to awaken your excitement, skepticism, curiosity, and hunger for more information, so that you may grab the reins and direct your own path to your true, vital health and beauty potential.

Legal notice: The health-related statements in this book have not been evaluated by the U.S. Food and Drug Administration.

FOREWORD

The Truth About Beauty presents a timely and powerful departure from standard health and diet practices. I find that too many beauty and health experts—including some of my colleagues in the nutrition field—are disconnected from what really makes or breaks people's ability to look their best and treat themselves in the most caring and healthful way. Kat James not only uncovers these missing pieces; she gives us the physical tools to look and live better than ever—no matter where we start from.

Kat and I share a connection because we both bring a personal story of transformation to our work. Kat sees the potential in everyday people that most cannot envision for themselves. This book will help readers uncover that physical potential and avoid the extreme, tedious—even dangerous—measures we've been programmed to believe are necessary. Anyone who takes an interest in his or her health and beauty will find powerful inspiration in these pages, in addition to well-honed, practical strategies that yield marked improvements in health and appearance.

Because Kat is not a beauty or diet "spokesmodel" or a product of fantastic genes, a Hollywood upbringing, or personal trainers, she represents the real possibility for any woman to transform herself without obsession and without committing herself to drastic skin or diet regimens or a commando's workout program. Kat understands all of the points of resistance: what it's like to lack motivation, to prefer certain tastes, to be skeptical or leery of suggestions that are unappealing or ineffective, or to live in a geographical location without easy access to good food and products. Kat deftly navigates all of these and turns them all in the reader's favor.

Kat James's approach challenges several basic notions that many in my field rely on when they run out of answers. She provides a much-needed wake-up call for the millions of people who could benefit from her message. In addition, I strongly recommend Kat's teachings to therapists, doctors, weight loss professionals, fitness trainers, and other nutritionists looking to increase their insights into health, beauty, and wellness, and to dramatically improve success with their clients. With *The Truth About Beauty*, Kat James raises the bar for other books in the field by closing the chapter on outmoded, standard diet and skin advice and opening a new way of achieving the beauty that is everyone's birthright.

Oz Garcia
Multiple winner, *New York* magazine Nutritionist of the Year

ACKNOWLEDGMENTS

There are many people without whom this book would not have been "born" and to whom I wish to extend my deepest gratitude:

To Julie Steigerwaldt, my managing editor, for guiding and delivering my "baby" true to form. To Jenefer Angell, for helping me shape it. To Cynthia Black and Richard Cohn at Beyond Words, as well as Jan Miller, for letting me do the book I was born to do. And to Lindsay Brown, Gretchen Stelter, Sara Blum, Bill Brunson, Meadowlark, Rachel Berry, Marie Hix, Marvin Moore, Jade Chan, Angela Lavespere, Sylvia Hayse, Beth Hoyt, and Dorral Lukas, as well as Holly Taylor, for their hours of work and expertise.

A very special thanks to the amazing Oz Garcia, BS, MA, for writing the foreword. To Dr. Nicholas Perricone, Dr. Susan Lark, Dr. Michael B. Schachter, Dr. David Edelson, and Dr. Deborah Jaliman, Dr. Jeffrey Miller, Dr. Bipin Solanki, MD, FRCS, for their compelling interviews and pioneering insights. And to John Monahan, Danny Vincent, Patrycja Towns, and Jerry Shaver at *Better Nutrition* magazine, for giving me incredible support and a voice through such a great magazine and for use of Jerry's deft edit of my personal story for part I of this book.

Many thanks to the pioneering authors, researchers, and journalists whose work has helped shape my overall perspective and has contributed to this book, including Dr. Ron Rosedale, Dr. Barry Sears, Dr. Samuel S. Epstein, David Steinman, Annemarie Colbin, Dr. Julian Whitaker, Dr. Stephen Cherniske, Dr. Rudy Rivera, Burton Goldberg, Dr. Aubrey Hampton, Dr. James A. Duke,

Michael T. Murray, ND, Dr. Alan Gaby, Udo Erasmus, Dr. Russell L. Blaylock, Nicolas J. Smeh, MS, Ruth Winter, Kim Erikson, Judi Vance, Lindsey Berkson, Michael Pollan, Gary Taubes, and the Life Extension Foundation, as well as the many researchers who've spent countless hours in labs contributing to the published science that supports this book. And to the late Dr. Robert Atkins, without whom the conventional American dietary paradigm might still be frozen in time.

To the people whose stories I share in this book, and especially Courtney Holden, who has, since her own transformation, assisted me greatly, including her help with testing and fine-tuning some of my recipes for this book.

To Stephen Churchill Downes, for the very special cover photo. And to Barry Yee, for shooting the author photo.

To the following individuals who have gone out of their way to mentor or support my journey to publishing: Gina Molinari, Christine Shahin, Linda Troeller, Corinna Benoit Belizzi, Jim Indorato, Maureen O'Brien, Jory Des Jardin, Kate White, Andrea Clark, Mary Rose Almasi, Janet Parker, Neal Hirschfeld, Suzanne Grimes, Jill White, Liz Smith, Ryan Kuhn, Bruce Marcus, Pratima Raichur, ND, Susan Hussey, Stephanie Von Hirshberg, Roger Itkor, Lois Johnson, Annika Hayes, Alexis Luce, Doug Bolin, John and Kristin Armstrong, Lois Greenfield, Jennifer Greenwald, Linda Roemer, Tori Rowan, Cameron Wolbert, Lawrence Rosen, Kristina Sachs, Dennis Tarr, Nancy Trent, Linda Bryer, Caroline MacDougall, Jane Iredale, Cheryl Roth, Mara Engel, Marilyn Dale, Cindy Connelly, Wanda Daniels, Walter Seigordner, Kim Sayer, Karin Miksche, Mary Cooper, Kristen Knowles, Kristy Dellinger, and James Hammel.

To my mother, Suzanne Farmer, for encouraging every road I've taken and for giving me her writing "genes." To Jon Farmer, for his encouragement and review of material. To Lance Rieck, Joseph Bongiourno, Bruce Crossland, Scott Allerding, Cynthia Faye, Lyle Hurd, and especially Robert Morningstar, for watching over me. And finally to Peter Verlander, PhD, for endless research help, for playing the ultimate devil's advocate, for showing me my strength, and without whose material support and companionship this book would not have been possible.

INTRODUCTION AND 2008 AUTHOR UPDATE

*Beauty is the product of enlightened self-cultivation.
Our beauty reflects our self-confidence and
self-knowledge. How we choose to cultivate it reflects
our wisdom . . . and our self-respect.*

—Kat James

BEAUTY NEEDS A SANCTUARY

The Truth About Beauty is about recovering the unique vital essence in each of us. It's not about striving for ideals dictated by culture. Our impulse is to impose our own visions and ideals on our physical selves; however, we have the ability to create something even more stunning, if we get out of its way and allow it to emerge. Our beauty never forgets its essence, even if we—and the world around us—have.

The most precious and elusive beauty attribute of all is vitality. Untold vital potential lies within each of us. To connect with it, we must find sanctuary far from the constant physical and sensory bombardments that challenge inner and outer beauty. Only in that sacred space can we rethink and reprogram the mind-sets and choices that have kept us from thriving. Armed with healthier motivations, exceptional information, and new strategies, we possess the needed tools to rehone our beauty instincts, recover our glowing potential, and deftly navigate the modern beauty labyrinth.

My motivation for writing this book runs deep. As a teen, I developed a compulsive eating disorder that dominated my life for twelve years. That bleak period included the first few years of my career as a makeup artist in New York City, where I worked with celebrities such as Sarah Jessica Parker and Martha Stewart, would eventually act as a spokesperson for cosmetic brands such as Maybelline and Revlon, and enjoyed the spotlight as a TV makeover guru. But despite my deftness at making others beautiful on the outside, it wasn't until I was twenty-four that a physical crisis forced me to face my own ultimate beauty challenge: my compulsive war against my body and my self that had robbed me of my self-respect, my looks, and nearly my life. It took this wake-up call for me to transcend the hair and makeup cover-ups I had depended on for so long and change everything I thought I knew about beauty.

Ironically, my real beauty story began when I finally let go of my superficial beauty goals. Motivated in an entirely new way, I stumbled upon a world of powerful information and options that not only freed me from my eating disorder but from my deadly "denatured" lifestyle and the chronic skin and physical complaints that came with it. Shedding ten dress sizes was the most physically obvious sign of my breakthrough, but it was a mere side effect of a greater victory: getting my health back and discovering my true beauty potential for the first time in my late twenties.

Today I am unrecognizable compared to the woman I was. And my metamorphosis had nothing to do with the kind of hard work, sweat, surgery, or deprivation you see on makeover reality shows. My escape from the physical fate nature never intended for me resulted from a complete reprogramming of my concepts of beauty, how to get a great body, and how to live life to the fullest. I learned in a very powerful way that we are all meant to be beautiful.

My formal training is in aesthetics, cosmetology, and health journalism, not healthcare. I'm not a doctor or dermatologist, and this book is not intended as a prescription or treatment but as a source of information. I encourage healthy skepticism, and I present the scientific research to validate each area of my approach. I hope to help you as I have helped others: by inspiring you with my own transformation and giving you the incentive and tools with which to take control of your own life.

EVOLVING *THE TRUTH*: IN THIS UPDATED AND EXPANDED EDITION

In the years since the first publication of this book in 2003, I've had the opportunity to work with hundreds of women (and many men) through my programs, and have reached many more via my public television special, columns, lectures, and website. To see the succession of lives (and bodies) that have been transformed as a result of this information has been deeply gratifying. My observations and the feedback I've received over the years have led to several exciting expansions in this book. Though much is changing in terms of people's awareness, lifestyle options, and new beauty technologies (some positive, some downright risky), the core beauty truths that guided my own transformation—especially the biological ones—remain unchanged. Most exciting to me since 2003 has been the accelerated rate of research in support of key principles introduced in my first edition. In 2007 alone, several ongoing debates were unequivocally settled, confirming such things as the long-dismissed potential dangers of genetically modified foods, the safety and health benefits of low-glycemic diets, and the serious risks from certain chemicals in cosmetics. It was finally even confirmed that organic foods are nutritionally superior and safer than their conventionally grown counterparts.

Each of the detailed charts throughout this edition has been painstakingly expanded to reflect new research and incorporate new strategies I have honed over the last five years. Here is a quick preview of the journey ahead and what's new in this expanded edition:

In part I, "Uncovering Your True Radiant Potential," I'll share my own journey from my compulsive, denatured past to the crisis that led me to the tools that finally freed and propelled me through the effortless metamorphosis to how I look and live today. Then I'll introduce the Process of Shedding, a systematic uncovering of one's true potential by lifting away the mind-sets and physical burdens that prevent it from surfacing. Finally, I'll outline the critical transformational tools to use throughout your own process, which could have saved me over a decade of struggle had I known about them from the start!

In part II, "Feeding and Cultivating Beauty," I'll help you jump-start your physical journey with a deceptively powerful game plan for upgrading a make-or-break beauty choice: your beverages. Next, I'll challenge the most stubborn food myths and beliefs about a succession of so-called "unhealthy foods." Then, I'll take you through a series of strategic kitchen cabinet upgrades to eliminate the harm and maximize the transforming potential in all of your favorite food categories. What follows is one of the most important new components to this edition. By popular demand, I've included a powerful 6-Day JumpStart Menu with my core Transformation Recipes fine-tuned over nearly a decade of conducting my Total Transformation® programs. I'll then delve into the often-ignored factors behind food obsession that were critical to my freedom, and how to starve negative food issues of their emotional and biochemical support—without starving yourself. You'll then learn how nutritional supplements can transform not only your relationship with food, but every aspect of your beauty. What follows are five compelling, real-life stories of dramatic transformations that were facilitated by my principles and program.

In part III, "The Makeup-less Makeover," you'll learn how to restore your skin's critical self-protective functions by reversing "regimen overkill" and phasing out red flag skin care ingredients. In a series of unprecedented charts mapping out proven natural alternatives to harmful synthetic skin approaches, you will see for the first time a bird's-eye view of the inside-out health connections to an A-to-Z array of common skin challenges. The same at-a-glance reference format is applied in the Bathroom Cabinet Makeover chart that follows. Finally, you'll learn how to minimize the modern-day beauty "wild cards" that challenge all of us, and how to make authentic personal choices that ripple outward to create a more hopeful and beautiful world.

Finally, because of how much searching it took for me to finally find foods, beverages, personal care products, and information sources that met my own informed criterion, and because I don't believe in putting up with low-end products in order to live well and stay beautiful, I couldn't have created this book without an extensive, descriptive, and personally tested resource collection. The Living Beauty Resources feature award-winning and hard-to-find products and educational tools to expand your horizons.

MY PROMISE: VITALITY HAS UNTOLD REWARDS FOR EACH OF US

Each phase of my approach applies an aspect of what I call the Process of Shedding—a rethinking, removal, and recovery (on many levels) from harmful beliefs and choices that simply frees up the radiance waiting within you. This process, when guided by special motivational and informational tools in this book, is so powerful that one can expect to see the return of an essence we think of as looking younger, which is in fact just the result of being healthier. Some of the common short- and long-term rewards include a reemergence of your healthiest glow (without blush or foundation), revitalized skin (without acids or procedures), the end of dry skin (without heavy lotions), reduced under-eye circles, shrunken varicose veins, glossier hair, youthful energy, freedom from cravings, and—best of all—an energetic, comfortable new body that adjusts to your ideal weight without drugs, diets, or formal workouts. In some cases (as in my case), this allows the emergence of something—or someone—you've never seen in yourself before.

Most surprising is how painless some of the most powerfully transforming lifestyle adjustments can be and how quickly the benefits can be seen and felt. You will find that these lifestyle changes are equally rewarding to your spirit as the process begins to perpetuate and inspire itself. Even your taste buds and sensibilities will become enlightened as you begin to crave the very choices that truly revitalize you, increasing your quality of life and allowing an ageless radiance to emerge.

My tools for transformation can be used with great success by people of any age, size, or shape—and, yes, gender. In fact, the more challenged you are at the start, the more dramatic your rewards will be. Think about where I started. Think where you can go.

PART I

UNCOVERING YOUR TRUE RADIANT POTENTIAL

CHAPTER 1

THE ULTIMATE BEAUTY LESSON

THE ULTIMATE BEAUTY LESSON

I was twenty-four, living in New York City, and lying in bed after my usual binge. I tried to breathe deeply and make my heart calm down, but the pounding wouldn't stop. "What makes you do this?" I thought. "What are you afraid of?" I opened my diary, as I so often did in the "aftermath," to escape the reality of the moment with the hope of starting fresh.

On any other night I would write passages from self-help books, lists of positive things about my life, or tally the calories, with the help of my own style of creative accounting, to rationalize that I might make up for what I'd just consumed by eating a couple of hundred calories a day for the next week. I was addicted to starting over. But on this night, I was beyond writing about emotional triggers that could have made me do it or planning a new diet. None of those exercises had ever really worked, and that night I realized that despite everything I knew and all the progress I'd made, whatever was still holding on would probably hold on forever. This was a huge admission to myself.

I flipped back through the pages of my journal, through all my lists of when-I-get-thin dreams ... the dancer ... the singer, the Broadway performer ... the person who would "show" those who had rejected her because of her weight. I had so many plans for *when I got thin*. They had, in fact, sustained me at the darkest times.

As I stared at a blank new page, I suddenly pondered who I might be if I achieved *none* of those things, if I let myself off the hook ... and still loved myself. What if I gave myself the kind of insulation and padding from the world, my challenges, and the pain of failure that my food addiction had provided—literally and figuratively? What if nothing had to change at all "when I got thin"? I would stop judging myself, stop spending so much of my energy "making up for" my physical shortcomings. I could even be antisocial if I wanted ... and love myself anyway. It was such a wild concept, since every day I engaged in a loathable compulsion that "proved" my unlovableness. I remember sitting there trying to wrap my brain around this unconditional self-love thing. Layers of accumulated lofty self-expectations embedded in my subconscious started to float into my mind for their ceremonious dismissal, one by one. I started to feel a kind of comfort, not unlike the way you felt as a kid when you learned the next day was a "snow day." I fell asleep with the kind of limp peace you feel after a good cry. I had no idea that the next morning would be different from the ones before, or that I had just solved the final click of a Rubik's cube that I had struggled with desperately for twelve years.

In the morning I still felt that strange sense of peace, where usually the normal, low-grade agitation foreshadowed the inevitable fix I would give in to later in the day. When I looked in the mirror, instead of feeling the flash of shame and self-loathing my reflection normally evoked, I felt and saw something very different. It was like I was a mother seeing her battered child at the front door after a terrible journey. I didn't judge myself, but instead was suddenly struck by the magnitude of abuse and distortion that that innocent body had endured again and again over the years. I felt an outpouring of sadness and love toward my body that was unlike anything I'd ever felt toward myself. I did not make any new pledges or plans or eat or start anything new. But the "snow day" feeling stayed with me as that day turned into weeks, then months. It has been over ten years, and I have never binged again nor ever even had the thought to. Whatever that destructive thing in me was—which I thought was just who (and what) I was—had *fled*.

EARLY SIGNS

When I was thirteen, I started a string of diets. It was during these first attempts at calorie restriction that I began to binge. By high school, I was a fan of tunics and wore a thick mask of painstakingly applied makeup to distract from my conspicuously pear-shaped body. I'd been a singer and dancer since childhood, but my talent couldn't land me the roles or scholarships I wanted—until my senior year, when I discovered speed pills and began purging. I lost more than twenty pounds. I got the lead in the school play, the boyfriend, the choir scholarship, the dance solo. It was like a dream—until the school cracked down on the supplier of my magic pills. It wasn't easy to watch the weight pile back on. The taste of glory I'd enjoyed made the years that followed all the more painful.

In college, my weight yo-yoed between 140 and 185 pounds. By the time I was twenty years old, I'd become a physically distorted beauty statistic for our times—heavy, but well coiffed, meticulously made up, manicured, perfumed, powdered, and groomed, yet riddled with uncomfortable skin rashes, digestive troubles, allergies, and an unbelievably powerful addiction to food which I was sure was all in my head.

I began to look for books that addressed the emotional causes for my self-destructive behavior. I collected resounding pieces of wisdom from various self-help books. I read about the healing power of self-expression, the destructive power of guilt, the inner child, the fact that feelings aren't debatable, and the rewards of vulnerability. Perhaps the most important theory I learned was the self-defeating trap of indefinite blame. At the dawn of my twenties, I carried years and layers of heavy resentment toward my mother and had become emotionally paralyzed by the weight of that burden, waiting for apologies and becoming more and more resentful each day I didn't get them. In her, I'd found an eternal excuse not to fully address my eating problem myself. Then I finally realized that even if, by some miracle, I were to receive the apologies that I craved, I still would be stuck in a quagmire from which only I could free myself. I began to hone in on the subtle emotional triggers, and I felt a great weight being lifted as I began to deprogram my responses to the old baggage bit by bit. It was a painstaking but amazing process for me that extended through my junior year. Many emotional issues began to heal, especially my vulnerability to having my "buttons pushed." I thought for the first time that I was on the path to freedom from my compulsion. But to my frustration, my torturous daily battle with food remained strong. Feeling I could no longer rationalize a career that required me to look good, I gave up my performing arts scholarship, dropped out of college, and enrolled in beauty school. I later joined my sister in New York City and became a makeup artist, since I'd always been good at making *others* look beautiful.

In late 1988 I arrived in New York City with looks that certainly attracted attention, thanks to the "stunning"—if not shocking—makeup and antigravity hair imported from Michigan and a backside that won the elusive New York City double take. For someone with my body and my background to pursue a career in beauty and fashion was a bit naïve, even masochistic. Everything about me was wrong for the world I was trying to penetrate. I didn't look, dress, or act like any of the top makeup artists who worked with supermodels and celebrities. I wasn't skinny, artsy, or eccentric, and I didn't have an "attitude." On the bright side, my sister's connections eventually led to an interview with Frederic Fekkai, one of the world's top celebrity hairdressers. When I think of what I wore to that interview—even the cab driver asked if I was "from around here"—I can't believe I was hired.

Working with models wasn't so bad. I regarded them as an alien species. I felt no resentment toward them once I adjusted to my place in that world. Next to the models, I was like "Pat" from *Saturday Night Live*, a kind of asexual presence on the set. I suffered moments of extreme mortification, especially on location shoots when everyone was dying to jump into the ocean in their string bikinis after a hot day shooting on the beach, and I was merely dying to escape the situation, get back to my hotel room, and binge yet again.

MY FIRST TASTE OF REAL FOOD

There were some unexpected upsides to big city living and working in fashion. The catered food on photo shoots was a revelation. Who knew that while I was growing up eating instant noodles and iceberg salads, other humans regularly dined on grainy pilafs, grilled vegetables, goat cheese, and herb-encrusted fish? I grew up in the fruit belt, which was really the Hamburger Helper and Shake 'N Bake belt. I had never seen deep green lettuce or drunk mineral water (*without* ice) with meals. I soon learned that not all vegetables needed to be cooked senseless and smothered beyond recognition in order to be edible. I'd always been leery of "health food," but these delicately cooked, aromatic dishes began to change my palate and my views. I began to judge a good salad based on new criteria, not because it was covered with Thousand Island dressing, croutons, and artificial bacon bits. Had I not moved to New

York City, I might never have developed a taste for what I have come to call "real food."

I soon came to realize that eating this way all the time would be the ultimate luxury, though one I could not afford without giving up some of my other splurges. And so, after giving up a few lipsticks and manicures, I was eating—and bingeing on—real food. While changing my palate didn't change my need to use food as a drug, I was becoming a convert to quality vegetables and whole grains; yet I also ordered two or three desserts when I called for delivery. I continued to binge daily, both alone and on the job. I was good at sneaking several portions while other crew members socialized, and I *owned* the dessert tray, generously leaving one of each kind of pastry for the rest of the crew to nibble on. (That's what models do: nibble a *corner* off a brownie, which drove me crazy.) After days or weeks of bingeing, I would muster up epic willpower and eat nearly nothing or binge on fat-free foods, such as frozen yogurt or soup, for a few days or sometimes even weeks. A handful of times, I was able to starve myself down to near-normal size, functioning on loads of diet soda and fat-free frozen yogurt, thinking about food every waking moment.

I didn't have much of a social life. I much preferred the company of food to that of people. I would even leave friends' gatherings early to go home and eat. My journal writing continued to get me through the lows when my outlook was so bleak that I would occasionally stay in bed for days. Sometimes I would write down the reasons I had to live and remind myself of all these things I would do once I became thin. Then, of course, I would plan a new diet, set a new weight goal and deadline, and plan yet another drastic strategy.

Eventually, I decided to look into liposuction. The first two doctors I consulted refused to perform the procedure, saying it would be too dangerous unless I lost at least twenty pounds. The third doctor I saw agreed to do it and even offered a discount if he threw in a knee and abdomen suction. I started to save my money for the procedure, but I never went through with it.

MY WAKE-UP CALL

At twenty-four, my body began to break down. It started with fatigue and heart palpitations. The heart-pounding trudge up the subway stairs had become dreaded misery. Then came the blurry vision on mornings after a binge. But when I finally began passing undigested material (I was actually happy because I wasn't absorbing those calories), I decided to see a doctor. From a liver specialist, I learned that in addition to pre-diabetic symptoms, I had a severely inflamed liver that could "become life-threatening without warning" if I didn't begin taking immunosuppressant drugs right away. It wasn't like me to question a doctor, but I asked him about the drug and what I heard seemed to be more of a dodge than an answer. I asked him if I could put off starting on them for a couple of weeks. When I learned about their notorious psychiatric and immune system side effects—and in light of my own problems with depression and autoimmune issues—I realized that at twenty-four I was looking at a steep downward slope I'd never recover from. The "thin" dreams that I suddenly realized had kept me going all those years were now under threat of never materializing. This revelation jolted me, and from that moment I forgot about the scale, my diet, and the size 10 jeans I wanted to fit into. My decade-long obsession with weight completely vanished, as my vision narrowed on my only beacon of hope: regaining my health.

Interestingly, I wasn't compelled to head to the gym or deprive myself of food this time. I wanted information. I started to read everything I could find about my specific health issue. It was the early nineties, so my search for information beyond my doctor's protocol would require a visit to health food store bookshelves. I looked up "liver" in the back of each health book, and came across the same herb (milk thistle) each time. Overseas studies (the only research I could find back then on such a thing) had found that it regenerated liver cells. I had always figured that herbology was the product of flowery imaginations, but because of my situation I was willing to take the milk thistle and a leap of faith. At my next liver test two weeks later, my enzymes were down more than two hundred points (still a few hundred too high). My doctor was impressed, but said I still wasn't out of the woods. I bought two more weeks during which I consulted with another MD who was also an ND (naturopathic doctor), who congratulated me for taking milk thistle and added fish oil and alpha-lipoic acid to my regimen. My next liver enzyme test was *normal* (around 35), down over five hundred points from the original levels. The liver specialist asked what I had done. As I began to tell him, he started tapping his pencil and looking around. Like him, I too thought it might have been a fluke. But I was certainly intrigued. I began to read about the other symptoms I had.

I wondered what these books might have to say about my other issues—the cravings and the druglike effect I got from food, or my cold hands and feet, my moods, and my skin issues. Until I read these books, I had never imagined that I could possibly have been deficient in anything, since I was always recovering from having eaten too much.

Several weeks after my liver problem was resolved came another physical change I could not ignore. Since high school, I'd depended on hydrocortisone ointment for my flaking red chin and eyelids and "extra, extra dry" skin creams for my painfully parched legs and torso. I thought my skin problems were the hand I'd been dealt for the long haul. But one day, as I reached for my lotion, I realized that my skin wasn't screaming. There was no itch. In fact, there was no need for lotion at all. And I realized then that I hadn't had a rash since I started the supplement regimen. This stunned me, and from that day on, my belief in natural substances was galvanized.

My growing respect for nature led me to begin reading about the ingredients in body care products, which, as a beauty professional, I had never considered from a health standpoint. I was shocked to learn how we absorb and accumulate many topically applied chemicals, and I became determined to eliminate as many external as well as internal irritants as I could from my life. I wanted to thrive, not just react to my choices. And I realized that that was what my body had primarily been doing all my life: reeling and reacting to assaults.

SOLVING MY "INSANITY"

Anyone with an eating disorder occasionally doubts his or her own sanity. If you're compulsive, you literally can't stop thinking about food, and you don't care if your stomach is stretching. There's an uncontrollable force inside demanding that you eat. Doctors never told me that it wasn't my fault (and they didn't know). Instead, they gave me diets to stick to and told me about the great rewards of self-control. So when I started reading about nutrients proven to improve mood, cravings, and blood sugar issues (nutrients most people are deficient in), I began to question some of my harsh self-judgment. Though I continued to be at the mercy of binges, after a little more than a week on these supplements, my "black hole" cravings and even the sedative effect that followed them began to noticeably diminish. I added nutrients to improve my metabolism, thyroid, and hormonal issues, and each made a noticeable difference. When I should have gained weight, I stayed the same, and when I should have stayed the same, I lost weight. My hands and feet were less cold. I even noticed I'd become firmer without changing my activity. Experiencing such incredible physical improvement without struggle was amazing to me. Taking these steps never made me feel guilty, inadequate, or resentful. My sense of self-advocacy for learning and applying this powerful knowledge began to overshadow my negative self-doubt. I was being lifted out of my twelve-year downward spiral, one informed choice at a time.

For the first time since college, I felt that I would soon overcome my disease again. I had long since replaced all of the junk foods with real foods and uncovered my emotional triggers, and it hadn't been enough. But because of these supplements, my binges—and physical reactions to them—as well as my moods were becoming less and less severe. Though I was incredibly frustrated to still be compelled to binge at all, at least I was beating myself up with boxing gloves on and minimizing the consequences, I thought. I knew I had added years to my life, even if I never overcame my disease. But then came that "eve of synchronicity" when I gave up my thin dreams and gave myself that eternal "snow day" of self-love . . . and the demon let go, never to return.

THE TRANSFORMATION

Without exercising more or changing my diet, I started to lose weight. I can't tell you how many pounds I lost each week since I never looked at a scale, but the loss was steady. The change was even more evident to my colleagues in the fashion world and to my own family.

"How are you doing this?" everyone asked. "It must take discipline and willpower." It was almost impossible to explain that I wasn't following any rules and that I was eating what I wanted. I was no longer compelled to eat when I wasn't hungry, and if I was busy, I could even forget to eat, which never could have happened before. At the same time, I was truly tasting and enjoying food more than I ever had before.

A slow and sustained weight loss continued for the next three years. My body stopped shrinking at a size 4—down from my former size 18. I had no idea where I was going or what I could look or feel like. Still focused on my health, looking beautiful was the last thing on my mind. Ironically, that's when the phone started ringing off my makeup agent's hook and the on-camera cosmetic company spokesperson offers started rolling in.

It hit me at one point during that shrinking phase that although I never thought of myself as gullible, most of the choices I'd been making all my life—which I'd assumed were the *only* choices—had been defined, if not dictated, by the food and beauty industries. I couldn't understand why virtually all of what I was discovering had been passed over in TV health segments and most government-funded research. Why did I have to go through what I did and nearly forfeit my beauty potential and quality of life (and possibly my life) on things that either didn't work or made matters worse if there were safe therapies that could at least be tried, and at best might be astonishingly transforming—without risk of serious side effects?

THE TRUTH

As I read explanation after explanation, the consensus among doctors was clear: the natural, therapeutic substances that had been at the foundation of my healing and transformation don't fit into the healthcare industry in a profitable (patentable) way and are, therefore, either ignored or subjected to biased scrutiny.

I was stunned to realize that there must be countless therapeutic substances no one was hearing about, but at the same time I was more hopeful for the future—at least my own future—than ever before. In fact, somehow understanding why some of the best information would never be thrust in front of me on billboards or in my favorite magazines made all of my new discoveries that much more valuable to me. But even I never imagined it would take another decade for the public to start hearing about things like fish oil, which is only the tip of the iceberg.

I started to view everything differently: TV ads, billboards, government guidelines, etc. It was as if a filter that had been deadening my senses—and sensibilities—for most of my life was being removed layer by layer. The more I learned, the more I wanted to go out on the street with a megaphone, post notices, and shake people.

I stopped following diet and beauty trends and began to make informed choices based solely on the proven benefit, potency, and purity of my products and regimens. My purchases were no longer dictated by ads and social approval but rather by my *body's* approval. I became keenly aware of the difference between expensive, high-end packaging and the actual *substance* of a product. I was no longer sold on products that merely *contained* good ingredients but came to seek products that were also free of known irritants and toxins. And that was the difference between my own criteria and those of everyone else I knew at that time. Soon I was buying the highest-quality cosmetics and enjoying results I knew even the privileged were not aware of.

NEW PRIORITIES

I soon found myself spending more money on whole foods, supplements, and nonirritating beauty products than on cosmetics and clothes. And if I temporarily reverted to my old habits because access to my new preferences was limited (like when I visited my hometown), then the old cravings and physical agitations returned, reminding me why I'd changed my ways.

By age twenty-six, my beauty began to unfold, and I glimpsed nature's intention in the mirror for the first time. At thirty, I looked about fifteen years younger than I had when I was twenty (a brain-twister, but true!). I saw a different person altogether. One day when I washed off my elaborate makeup job, I suddenly realized that I had an innate beauty that shouldn't be covered up. I soon realized that I had the potential to be one of those women who could get away with wearing little or no makeup. I was stunned. My joy in being a woman began to emerge for the first time.

As for all those models who once seemed like a different species, today I understand who the alien really was. For twelve years I had been an alien to nature's intention for me. When I began writing this book, it was more than nine years since the final breakthrough that changed the physical and emotional course of my life. I haven't weighed myself in many years, but I'm still the same size 4. I don't work out at a gym, but I do like to move, and I do things I had never dreamed I would do, like ski and rollerblade. I dart up the stairs effortlessly now because my body feels good and my cells are well cared for. I don't deny myself any particular food—except fake or blood sugar-spiking ones, which no longer hold any appeal for me. I haven't heard the word "should" in my head regarding food since that night it all finally clicked. Amazingly, what I desire seems to have become one and the same with what makes me feel and look good. It's like "beauty nirvana."

YOU DON'T NEED A CRISIS TO BE TRANSFORMED

The way I once treated myself was not just a result of my eating disorder; it was also a result of our culture and the images and advertising ceaselessly thrust in front of us. For so many years I was in a holding pattern, and each time I started over I dragged along the same stubborn mind-sets about how to live and how to achieve my body and beauty goals while lacking the same crucial information. These deeply ingrained beliefs muffled my instincts, my sensibilities, and my own criteria for what I put on and in my body. It took a crisis for me to challenge them.

As I look around me today, I see a potential in most people that they cannot imagine for themselves. And I know it is within their reach. But by sharing what I learned the hard way, I hope to empower you to avoid the crisis and wasted years on futile, misguided attempts to look and feel better. If someone had shared with me what I will share with you in this book, I might have lived my teens in my teens rather than in my twenties and thirties!

CHAPTER 2

THE PROCESS OF SHEDDING

People ask me: "What did you do differently the day you started losing weight?" But I had begun no diet, no fitness plan, no deprivation, and no drugs. I wasn't transformed by losing weight, and amazingly, I didn't lose weight by setting out to become thin. I had no beauty or weight goals or plans when the pounds started coming off. In fact, my transformation didn't start or end with weight loss. My real beauty story started when I let go of all my beauty goals and began to shed the stubborn mind-sets and the health burdens that had denatured my life and kept my beauty from emerging. The truth is, beauty and comfort in our own skin and bodies is a *natural, effortless state* that is too often thrown off balance by modern assaults, conveniences, and toxins to which our bodies are unable to adapt.

SOMETIMES IT'S WHAT YOU *DON'T* DO THAT MAKES YOU BEAUTIFUL

Beauty is not about buying, applying, and doing all the "right" things. It is what remains in each of us after we lift away the burdens and stop the self-sabotage that prevents it from thriving. I used to spend hours in front of the mirror without taking in the true state of my beauty. For all those years, it had been obscured, not only by layers of makeup, wardrobe "noise," and products but also by a lifetime of built-up, compensatory, and distractive measures and layers of false beliefs I'd adopted on how to achieve my physical goals. As I shed these mind-sets and self-sabotaging practices one by one, I was able to

15

reattune to my own true essence, and once again hear the long-muffled messages from my body that had been there all along.

Before we begin to cultivate our true radiance, we must first recover and reconnect with it by removing the barriers that stand in its way. If you've gotten yourself caught up in a merry-go-round of problem-causing self-care strategies, you can't keep accumulating more products and practices and expect to be transformed. You must first recognize the assaults and then stop them, reverse them, and recover from them in order to reclaim your true potential and take off in a new direction.

THE PROCESS OF SHEDDING

This most critical step toward vitality, which I call "the process of shedding," is a cyclical, ongoing journey of undoing, uncovering, and unveiling. In the following chapters, I'll take you through a process of shedding the self-limiting mind-sets, misguided beauty and lifestyle rituals, and toxic choices you may have accumulated over the years. When this process is powered by the critical motivational, informational, and logistical tools outlined in the next chapter, it can systematically lift away your beauty barriers one by one, until nature's glowing intention for you is uncovered and freed.

SHED THE THREE TYPES OF BEAUTY SELF-SABOTAGE

There are three types of self-sabotage that are important to target in your process of shedding:

- **Unwitting self-sabotage.** These are product choices we haven't scrutinized or have adopted based on incomplete information. These products can easily be weeded out with good information and simple upgrades.
- **Assisted self-sabotage.** This is when we let ourselves be led by fads, dubious diet and beauty trends, industry agendas, or convenience issues at our own expense. Good information and products, the proper motivation, and some practical logistical strategies should nip this kind of self-sabotage in the bud.
- **Compulsive self-sabotage.** These are addictive vices such as smoking, overeating, or drinking. Compulsive self-sabotage is tougher to kick because you have the issues associated with the other types of self-

sabotage as well as the emotional and chemical issues on top of them, all feeding and perpetuating each other. If you have a vice you want to correct, there's nothing wrong with setting a quitting date, but understand that the more contributing factors you shed in the meantime, the greater your odds of quitting, the less your struggle, and the more real your success will be.

SHEDDING BRINGS DEEPER ISSUES TO THE SURFACE

As more and more layers of outer sensory irritation, distraction, and blinders are stripped away, deeper chemical and emotional issues that have been thriving on and driving your most stubborn habits and vices may begin to emerge at the surface with new transparency. By continuing the process of shedding, you can literally starve these emotional and chemical roots of the unhealthy acts and substances that keep them alive, and loosen their grip. Shedding is the best way to break free of the downward cycle of self-sabotage.

As each cycle of upgrades and recovery leads to the next, you'll rise far above that old merry-go-round in an upward spiral toward a thriving state that glows of nature's intention.

APPLY THE PROCESS TO YOUR DAWN-TO-DUSK ROUTINES

Transformation is in the details. The things we do with the most frequency and regularity—day in and day out—are the actions that have the greatest impact on our quality of life and our physical reflections. Too often our routines are on autopilot or by someone else's design. Shedding the unwitting, autopilot, low-grade assaults hidden in your dawn-to-dusk routines is one of the most powerful yet painless ways to jump-start your transformation. For example, you may drink a certain beverage every day. What if you found you liked a new beverage equally well, which saved you the unhealthy effects the other had been causing and offered both immediate and cumulative beauty and health rewards? By switching to the new drink, you would shed one of many assaults your body has to recover from every day; at the same time, you would support yourself in a new way every time you drank it. In fact, the more you drank the old, beauty-sapping beverage in the past, the more dramatic and immediate the rewards of the upgrade. Another example, which I'll cover in chapter 11, is your daily shower. By taking a simple measure, you can painlessly "tweak" that experience so that instead of irritating your skin, dulling your hair, and aggravating your allergies, you could—on autopilot—be enjoying a far healthier bathing experience that allows your skin to recover its protective barrier and become calmer with each day.

Each of the autopilot self-care habits below plays a deceptively powerful daily role in determining the future of your beauty:

- Personal hygiene
- Beverage choices
- Skin, hair, and cosmetic regimens
- Bathroom cabinet staples
- Food choices
- Pick-me-ups

Each negative autopilot choice you shed can be upgraded with a new, rejuvenating one. Because my solutions in the chapters ahead will hold far more appeal and rewards than the second-rate substitutions you may have tried to adopt in the past, I call them upgrades. Upgrading your regimens is both joyful and self-motivating. Each assault you spare yourself is beauty in the bank, and each strategic, pro-beauty lifestyle upgrade will yield generous immediate and long-term dividends.

THERE'S BEAUTY IN THE TRUTH: SHED THE MIND-SETS THAT KEEP YOU STUCK

The process of shedding starts inside our heads. By simply reading the previous pages, your process has already begun. But it's easy to underestimate the invisible barriers that can paralyze our progress or blind our sensibilities to real solutions, even when we think our minds are open. None of us likes to believe it, but much of how we treat ourselves and what we become has been determined by our acceptance of the information, images, and choices we are bombarded with every day. By challenging the myths that kept me in a holding pattern, I hope to clear the way for your greatest transformation.

DON'T FORCE YOUR BEAUTY—SUPPORT IT

We are far too harsh with ourselves. We hire face-sanders and commando fitness trainers; we exercise epic willpower to skip meals; we fight to show our

MYTH: *Beauty requires willpower and self-discipline.*

TRUTH: *Willpower and self-discipline are dead-end roads.*

Willpower and self-discipline require us to disconnect from ourselves and treat ourselves impersonally and unnaturally. They are damage-control measures that stand in for real solutions to unexplored issues. They can be applied to any kind of regimen with the same disconnecting result. From the way you approach a zit—search and destroy!—to the way you approach your weight issue, the drill sergeant's attitude is the kind we often commit to at the dermatologist's office or on New Year's Day. Willpower can even be applied with disastrous results, as demonstrated by the will to skip meals and destroy your own metabolism in the process. While exciting in its extremity and even effective at first, it almost certainly leads to disappointment and compounded problems. The greatest risk in the outside-in, bulldozer, show-your-body-who's-boss approach—which I also call the "do-something" impulse—is that it lures us with shortsighted rewards, as it keeps us from identifying the real problems and solutions that should never require us to drive or deprive ourselves.

Quitting cold turkey, adding more reps, eating rice cakes, or exfoliating our poor skin 24/7 are often the damage control measures we must depend on until we resolve the real emotional, chemical, and logistical issues that feed our problems. Strict regimens and inflexible tactics will never make us beautiful in the long run, and they are dangerous substitutes for authentic needs. They may take pounds off or temporarily smooth our complexion, but they will leave us off-kilter and unhealthy and distract us from other lingering issues that need attention.

hair, our sweat glands, and any other natural part of us who's boss, while underestimating our body's own healing and regulating mechanisms and ignoring our own emotional issues and body chemistry. On top of all that, we pass ceaseless judgment on our reflections in the mirror.

The process of shedding is a gentle, kind one. It is never forced, and it compels itself with joyful, harmonious momentum at each stage. After leaving behind the old harsh approaches, you'll all but forget the discomforts and confusion you left behind—that is, until you try living like you used to for a day. You won't believe what you've been putting yourself through!

Here are a few of the more controversial ideas you will become familiar with as you continue:

- Forcing yourself to exercise when you really hate it may only be a crutch you must rely on until you face the real issues that weigh you down. By correcting your mood, food, and hormonal issues, you'll find that your body will *want* to move.
- Harsh skin regimens won't give you the most beautiful skin in the long run. To regain your most glowing skin, you must help it recover its own pro-beauty and antiaging functions.
- Fighting or denying your sweet tooth is no longer necessary for a beautiful body. Handling your cravings with the new sweet alternatives that don't assault your body will allow you to feel satisfied, get healthier, and change your shape at the same time.
- You needn't beat yourself up because quitting a bad habit cold turkey didn't stick. Attacking your vice, which is merely a symptom, won't help. Starving it of its chemical, ideological, and logistical support system through shedding is the road map to real and permanent freedom.

The painless way is often the healthiest and smartest way, and will cause no setbacks, guilt trips, or new problems. Real solutions require nothing more than the transformational tools I will share with you in the next chapter and then help you apply in the chapters that follow. Best of all, they will make the rest of you more beautiful, too.

RECONNECT WITH THE MESSENGER IN THE MIRROR

Today it is easier than ever to disconnect from our true physical state because technologies have allowed us to cosmetically, chemically, and surgically alter ourselves. With today's sophisticated texture of makeup, skin-resurfacing techniques, and botox, we can look dewy, vibrant, and even emotionally unburdened. We often consider only the "sandability" or "zap-ability" of the

MYTH: *Beauty is a frivolous pursuit.*

TRUTH: *Beauty reflects your quality of life.*

Some of us may be genetically predisposed to hearty physical and even mental constitutions, but none of us are invulnerable to the ravages of time, or worse, the toxic hazards on planet Earth. Even lucky folks need to deftly navigate today's harsh new landscape if lifelong radiance is the goal. Such a goal is neither shallow nor trivial since beauty and vitality are inextricably connected to health and quality of life. To achieve them requires awareness and a strong connection with one's inner voice and purpose.

Beauty is not a frivolous issue, nor is it a vanity issue. It is a quality-of-life issue and a birthright we tend to forfeit far too easily by turning opportunities to *create* ourselves into mundane regimens by which we merely maintain ourselves—or worse yet, let others maintain us.

We attempt to fix or improve ourselves by becoming customers of industry-prompted regimens that cause new problems. We've lapsed in our discernment of the raw materials we use to care for ourselves. With all of our comforts and gadgetry, too many of us are deprived of the joys in the simpler things: the joy in body and spirit that can make living by modest means more rewarding than living with every material advantage money can buy; the joy of connection with our own glowing essence; the joy of priceless vitality. Vitality *is* the universal beauty aesthetic.

flaw rather than what such signs as bloating, blemish patterns, poor circulation, or broken capillaries might tell us about our health and our choices. By failing to link our looks with our lifestyle, we miss out on the opportunity to truly heal our beauty from the inside.

Though they can and should help you sleuth out your health issues, doctors are less and less likely to give consideration to aesthetic cues other than your weight, perhaps because we've become so good at altering those cues superficially. How often will doctors tell you that your under-eye circles, your brittle hair and nails, your varicose veins, or your age spots are revealing something about your health? But any approach to health, wellness, and wholeness must be aesthetically sensitive, if not aesthetically guided. If we continue to obliterate our external "flaws" without first considering the precious clues and responsive guidance they can potentially provide, we deny ourselves the rich opportunity to connect with our bodies and mirrors in a far more nurturing way.

In order to attune ourselves to the revealing dialogue between our choices and our reflections we need to quiet down—and even pare down—to hear it. This sacred communication from our bodies is all too often muffled by sensory bombardment, chemicals, overstimulating foods, and products that short-circuit our body's signals.

But as you detoxify toward a state of healing and thriving, you may notice your body becoming more sensitive to the old toxic choices. It's not that your body is less tolerant; rather, it is improving its communication. As a result, you'll begin to preserve your precious vitality by uncovering crises before they happen, and by learning to follow your body's lead again. Your naked face becomes calmer, yet more responsive if you stray back to a toxic choice, and those occasional skin blemishes lose their ability to cause panic as your faith in your body's ability to resolve them on its own is restored. The best part of this resensitization is that you will taste, smell, and feel like never before.

ESTABLISH A NEW RELATIONSHIP WITH YOUR REFLECTION

There's more to gain from looking in the mirror than assurance that your makeup is right, your teeth are clear of spinach, or your concealer is doing its job. Each morning, really look at your face and take in what it has to say. You'll begin to see marked—even startling—day-to-day fluctuations in your facial shape and features and even in your skin's tone. "Virgin" skin—before all of the acids, peels, and irritants throw it off-kilter—is the ultimate messenger. Facial bumps, circles, and blotches aren't there to embarrass you; they should alert, inspire, and guide you to take steps to correct an imbalance that is likely causing problems throughout your body.

For example, your face can de-puff noticeably within as little as one day after weaning off blood sugar-spiking foods. As we become increasingly adept at tracing little changes in our faces to the offending—or healing—acts, we

SHEDDING THE BODY IMAGE BURDEN

Most of us have something different going on in our heads when we look into the mirror besides concern for our health. We focus on doing what we deem necessary to make ourselves look "presentable." It's the millions of little thoughts that come in and out of our heads during this ritual that make up our body image, which we carry in our subconscious all day, through every situation, long after we've stepped away from the mirror.

Each of us—via commercials, magazines, television shows, billboards, and even well-meaning adult role models—has been instilled with an ever-present "meter" of consciousness by which we evaluate where we fit in or fall short of our culture's ideals for physical beauty. We may be happy with our eyes or our hair, but covet someone else's shape or cheekbones or fashion sense. Ideally, as we mature, we evolve to accept or even love our out-of-the-ordinary features. The curly hair or freckles we may have disliked as a teen becomes our trademark in our thirties or forties.

Whatever your thoughts are when you look in the mirror, the most important assurances that they won't become self-destructive are 1) a foundation of self-love and sense of self that overrides anything physical that may be going on with you, 2) a support system of mutual respect and appreciation for—and from—those around you that is not based on looks, and 3) an emphasis on health when it comes to physical concerns.

This is why it is dangerous to cultivate a social sphere or enter into a career in which success is contingent on looks. If achieving the physical standard is anything but courtesy of incredible genes, then you've got a recipe for emotional and physical problems if you set out to get there by someone else's standards or time frames. Immediately, you're sidetracked from focusing on your own vitality, which is, ironically, the only true way to look your best. Focusing on aesthetic or external physical goals to be admired by (or to judge) others invariably leaves holes and leaks in both our souls and our commitments to our selves.

An extreme example of this is the frustration and danger I've seen models I've worked with subjected to. Often, they don't even have the luxury of putting their own

(continued on next page)

health before the constant pressure to be the size that is printed on their promo cards. In the name of beauty, they purge and starve themselves, subsist on empty, fat-free foods, smoke, or undergo surgery. Some are sent by their agencies to "A-list doctors" who've become sought after in the industry because they will break medical protocols and prescribe dangerous weight loss drugs (meant only for dangerously overweight people) to slim young women.

In the case of plus-size models, I've observed that the ones who take care of themselves have the healthiest self-image. Women who are large because they're abusing their health rarely feel good about themselves, no matter how many well-meaning organizations tell them that being large is just fine. Yes, we must love ourselves, no matter how we look, but maybe that's a reason to listen to what our looks tell us.

The following are ways in which both adults and teens can build (and encourage in others) a foundation on which body image issues are far less likely to thrive:

- Devote time to nurturing your unique talents and interests, be they art, literature, music, sports, or other pursuits that are unrelated to your physical attributes.
- Choose relationships that engage your personality and common interests, not your opinions on fashion and the appearances of others.
- Watch what you say and how you judge people around you. With any comment or thought, you unconsciously subject yourself to that same scrutiny. Choose to comment on others' deeds and character rather than their looks or weight.
- Never skip meals. Not only does this lead to eating disorders, but studies show it will have the exact opposite effect you're looking for (weight gain).
- Seeking health will give you a healthier body image as well as healthier self-esteem. It will also help you look your best, the real way.

The next time you look in the mirror, forget comparing yourself to others. Look more closely at yourself, and see yourself in a different way. Take in the *state* of your health and beauty. Beyond our weight or size or how good our makeup, hair, and wardrobe look, we can learn so much more from the mirror by listening to our bodies.

begin to see flaws as more than nuisances. Each becomes an opportunity to transform our beauty authentically from the inside out. In this way, beauty becomes a motivator that finally serves us. The so-called vanity table becomes the setting for a sacred daily ritual.

The brief, contemplative minutes in front of my own mirror constitute a grounding daily check-in—a "state-of-my-beauty" address that I read from my face. I use this time to take in the astounding rewards of prior adjustments that are still paying off years later, as well as the responses to recent lifestyle shifts. For example, the under-eye circles that occasionally appear in my mirror are usually from lack of sleep, the sulfites in conventional wine, or sweets. But under-eye circles can have dozens of other causes. Starting tomorrow morning, listen carefully to what your face is telling you about your choices and your life.

THE NAKED EXPERIMENT: DECONSTRUCT YOUR BEAUTY AT THE SURFACE

Consider breaking unfounded beauty habits you may have started without thinking and continued for the sake of ritual or fear of stopping: the permanent wave, overzealous brow plucking, or the trademark lipstick you just can't seem to throw out. Start from scratch (obviously if you're a man, this won't be as much of an issue!). If you wear makeup or perfectly coiffed hair, try taking a break from it on weekends—as much as feels comfortable—until what feels naked at first starts to feel okay. Take note of your subtle and unique assets that may have been obscured by constructed makeup and hairstyles, and allow yourself to reevaluate the effects you typically try to achieve. You may notice if you go without powder, for example, that the oily condition you had been trying to control is really natural, healthy skin lubrication. You may notice the natural blush you get after you exercise and favor it over the effect you had created with makeup. Use these discoveries as inspiration for using makeup to subtly augment and even help you visualize your emerging radiance as you progress along your path to true vitality. During this period of paring down and coming to terms with the real you, use only neutral or sheer makeup colors to play up subtle contours without distracting from you.

Most of all, free yourself of any restrictive visual persona that may have confined you in the past. If you'd always felt you *had* to wear makeup, you might want to take a break from it altogether. Then you can be sure that when you do wear it again, it really is your choice to do so. The nature of the reactions this may cause among friends and significant others will certainly reveal the rigidity and extent of the beauty prison you are escaping, as well as the ability of others to focus on who you really are. Continue this external shedding by questioning every augmentation: shoulder pads, pins, scarves, loud makeup, and overly structured hair.

To share an example of one man's process that I helped him through: A friend's son who was still in college was prematurely balding. His reliance on a remaining sprout of hair that he used to cover his bald spot for more than a year was somewhat obvious. I talked him into simply letting me cut it off and nicely shape the hair he had remaining on the sides of his head. Even I did not expect his reaction to the result. For days and weeks following this "letting go" of that crutch, he thanked me profusely, and literally said that getting rid of it had changed his life. I have to admit that my own perception of him was transformed as well. Those little crutches do more than speak to our own insecurities. They communicate them to others as well.

Can you get out the door on short notice without feeling like a disaster? If not, you're not really free. But you will be. As your inner vitality unfolds, your old makeup, hair, and even wardrobe crutches will be shed naturally.

EACH CYCLE OF SHEDDING IS GREATER THAN THE SUM OF ITS PARTS

As you apply the principles of shedding to one area, you'll find that it is only a matter of time before it migrates to others. As your knowledge, self-respect, and ability to think independently increase, your outer beauty practices will simplify. Some will be shed entirely.

The spiritual rewards of shedding are as profound and exciting as the physical ones. Giving up the numbing, false comforts of conventional beauty routines and embracing powerful new choices that resonate with your long-neglected, better instincts restore not only your well-being but also your soul. With each cycle of beauty recovery, and each layer of beauty baggage you shed, you'll feel a new burden lift away, and will soon come to realize just how weighed down and denatured the old you had become. Your perspective will evolve until you look back in amazement at the way you used to care for yourself. You will rejoice to be free of your misconceptions as a whole new world of possibilities and a whole new level of connection with your intended radiance and your self open up.

As you explore each phase of shedding and upgrading ahead, jot down the first round of upgrades and strategies you'd like to try in a notebook or journal. If you focus on your most frequent autopilot routines, your first cycle of shedding will give you enough exciting short- and long-term rewards to inspire and propel you into your next cycle. In honor of the skeptical woman I was, I've carefully sequenced the upgrades ahead to maximize your up-front rewards and build on one another, so the need for blind faith and wondering if this will work for you will be minimized!

From this healing foundation, you will be fully primed to reap the maximum rewards of feeding, cultivating, and rebuilding your beauty in a whole new way with the amazing tools ahead.

CHAPTER 3

THE REAL TOOLS FOR TRANSFORMATION

T he real tools for transformation transcend trends and technology to help us achieve the vitality that the most sophisticated hair and makeup techniques can only mimic. These tools—which took me more than a decade to stumble on—will save you untold struggle, so you can begin your own *real* transformation today. They can free you from the assault-recovery merry-go-round and break through all your beauty glass ceilings. If any of the following tools are missing from any beauty or body approach, success will eventually crumble. By applying these tools throughout the journey ahead, you'll have unprecedented inspiration and support for what might otherwise require a blind leap of faith—which is exactly what I want to discourage—and needless inconvenience.

TOOL #1: THE MAGIC MOTIVATION

Think Health and Beauty Will Follow

I learned the hard way that profound transformation doesn't happen unless the right motivation is in place. To be sexually appealing, look good for the lingerie shoot, win the role, and be lean and mean for the corporate machine are all motivations that keep us at war with ourselves, no matter how "successfully" we change our exterior, because they do not address our essential needs. Superficial goals lead to superficial measures and superficial results that must be maintained through ongoing struggles with willpower and self-discipline. Motivations of self-love and health, on the other hand, work with and never undermine our sense of self-worth, and they engage our self-preservation instinct, whereas other motivations trample it.

The most profound journey to radiance begins when we give up beauty goals and focus instead on health. The vanity motive dies hard, but what die with it are the self-destructive, drastic measures we had mistakenly thought would bring us the greatest and quickest rewards.

Beauty and Self-Preservation

The survival instinct is a primitive one we can sometimes allow to atrophy in our cushy, civilized world. My self-preservation instinct was the final motivator within me as I reached my health crisis, and once it kicked in its power took me by surprise. Self-preservation fully engages both instinct and intellect. It inspires a material vigilance that can guide countless superior choices and bear untold fruit if we let it lead the way, even if we haven't reached a crisis. Survival is as much an issue today as it was in the time when we faced saber-toothed tigers, only the threats today are far less obvious.

Our society accepts sports and car fanatics. We prize the successful pursuit of the perfect bikini wax. But those who carefully evaluate what they put on and in their bodies are often met with attitude or harassment in some circles. Caring about our health doesn't make us fanatics. It makes us rational and conscious. To be passive about health is to be lacking in self-respect and taking for granted our own capacity for beauty and happiness. Your health is the most rational passion there is.

Aim Higher Than the Mirror and the Scale

Most people see a nutritionist, trainer, or doctor for matters of appearance or relief of a symptom. But suppose you went to these specialists to improve your health. For example, you might really throw off your dermatologist if you use him as part of your plan to get or stay healthy. Imagine going in only for a comprehensive diagnosis to get to the cause. Imagine making your doctor aware of your other symptoms and your history, asking him to consider the possible side effects your habits or prescription drugs may be causing, and swatting his hands each time he reaches for the prescription pad or a free sample of steroid cream.

MYTH: *A hard body is the healthiest body.*

TRUTH: *Cellular health is what counts.*

A heavy person can be healthier and more radiant than a hard body (though the healthier you are, the harder it is to stay heavy or sedentary). How healthy you are on a *cellular* level determines your vitality and how much you feel like moving. It also shows in your face, your hair texture, and your sense of well-being, not to mention your doctor's blood tests.

It is possible to be a "healthy weight" and be far less healthy than someone whose weight is considered too high. A mother may keep more weight off in the long run with less struggle and healthier results by chasing her two-year-old around than by joining an aerobics class. But being guilted into thinking that she should add a workout to her already physically demanding day keeps her from facing the emotional, biochemical, and hormonal issues that affect her weight. Give up the mind-set that health is about sweat or that a cut body is always the healthiest body. While regular activity is important and will help make you beautiful, your shape and even your desire to move are largely affected by your nutrient and hormone balance and the vitality of your cells. The beauty you exude glows from your cells, not from your muscles.

Sometimes even your doctor isn't operating on the best information or motivations. For example, it's one thing to restrict calories or take a potentially dangerous drug to achieve a "healthy weight"; it's quite another to focus on getting healthy and drop the excess weight in the process. I have never heard of this approach being advocated by a conventional doctor, but it's the healthiest, most successful, and most painless approach of all, and the best approach to skin problems as well.

Similarly, the most effective motivations to exercise go beyond weight loss. If you focus instead on its antidepressant, stress-busting, and bone-strengthening effects, then the attitude you'll adopt toward exercise will be more likely to uplift you than make you feel self-judgmental. There's nothing negative about 100 percent healthy motivation!

Aim higher for yourself. And make sure that the professionals who advise your choices are aiming high enough for you, too.

In the name of beauty, focus on your health. Change your New Year's resolutions from weight to targeted health goals, like "stabilize my blood sugar," "look into my hormones," "balance my moods and chemistry," or "close my nutrition deficits." Beauty payoffs will follow once these health goals are set and nutritionally informed.

Summary

- Think *health* and beauty will follow.
- Superficial goals lead to superficial means and superficial results.
- Trade in the thin and sexy goals. Focus on the magic motive: health.
- Celebrate your beauty as it emerges, but be motivated by health.

TOOL #2: COMPLETE INFORMATION

The More You Know, the Better You Live and Look

As powerful as it is, the health motive can only take you so far if you are limited by incomplete information. If you rely on TV health reports and other sources currently sponsored by food, body care, and drug companies, you're not getting the whole story. And believe me, we all need the unsponsored information we haven't been getting.

Even if we apply our best instincts to our choices, there's a need for a heightened awareness in today's world. And we can only protect ourselves from the beauty wild cards—environmental toxins, agricultural, food and drug experiments, and untested chemical combinations—if we are aware of them.

New World, New Tools: Why Instinct Is Not Enough Today

A hundred years ago, when unprocessed foods, clean water, and truly fresh air were commonplace, becoming informed might have been more of a luxury than a necessity. You could pretty much learn what was good for you by listening to your grandma. But our mothers' generation may have been the last for which basic beauty advice could suffice. "Eat right, drink enough water, exercise, get your beauty sleep, and get plenty of sunshine" may have been enough back then, but life has become more dangerous in less obvious ways. Conventional beauty wisdom is no match for our modern beauty challenges. In order to thrive—not merely survive—in today's world, we must re-inform our beauty instincts to navigate the changing landscape. And though unglamorous truths can be disturbing at first, acting on them can knock down the biggest barriers that keep us from our true, vital potential.

Good Information Replaces Hard Work

It doesn't take hard work or deprivation to end dry skin or cravings; it just takes information. For example, it isn't painful to install a water filter in your shower that will spare your skin—and the rest of your body—a fair amount of premature aging while making your hair silkier and your body ecology healthier. It's not work to take supplements that reduce varicose veins or cravings, or to upgrade a harmful product to a proven alternative. Complete information can lay to rest the myths and rationalizations that have kept you from thriving. It spares you all kinds of "rides" and puts you on firmer ground so your beauty can really take off. Favoring beauty-sparing, nontoxic choices is the result of getting informed.

Are You an Obedient Consumer?

Whether we think we are gullible or not, as naturally trusting beings we let marketing deceptions have an impact on our lives. By accepting as truth what we hear most often, what comes in the most appealing package, or what is endorsed by most medical spokespeople, we too often reward the companies that spend their millions on everything but the actual product. Appealing poetry, packaging, and synthetic smells and tastes distract us from the actual substances we're being sold. And to keep us off the trail to any truths we're not meant to discover, every effort is made to keep consumers from demanding the details: "Trust us. We're the professionals." "You don't understand the science." "It's more complicated than that." "You don't have the facts." "It's best to go ahead with the conventional approach." "Take control and take this . . ." "It's the number-one recommended choice." Don't let anyone shame or distract you from demanding details, reading the small print, and becoming the only expert you need to trust. Remember: Science is there for everyone. Don't be a "good" customer; become a discerning connoisseur.

Becoming Your Own Best Expert Is Easier Than You Think

Some people put off getting informed, and I can't blame them. Unless you have easy access to sources of unfiltered information, it can be a chore to dig it up. My goal is to spare you the searching and give you a healthy infusion of the facts, strategies, and resources you haven't been getting, so you can become an expert on what's best for you in a very short time.

For example, after familiarizing yourself with the proven nutritional options for improving your specific skin condition, you may, after one sitting, know more about cultivating good skin than you might ever learn from your dermatologist. Western medicine is still almost exclusively about alleviating symptoms, not about health-supporting solutions or achieving vitality. However, if you set about to learn what is best for you, the results will not only be liberating clarity and simplicity, but a far more radiant future. It is within all of us to become our own best expert and advocate. If we don't, no one else will.

Get the Straight Science: Beauty Shouldn't Require Blind Faith

Most people would like to *think* they could get beautiful without harsh skin regimens, drugs, or epic willpower, but they don't believe it. I know what it means to be resistant and skeptical. Despite my belief in the solutions I've uncovered, I encourage skepticism and discourage blind faith. Science is there for the people, but it is not always reported. Science shouldn't be left to industry interpretation or "professional use only." The body of science that validates the natural solutions that big industries tend to omit or disparage in their media press releases is growing by leaps and bounds. And since they are suppressed for lack of profitablity, the only way to learn of these transforming findings is to get hooked up to the stream of unfiltered information that can complete the whole—not just the familiar—picture of your options.

Patents Equal Profits: The Catch-22 That's Been Keeping You in the Dark

Unadulterated forms of natural substances cannot be patented, and therefore they don't make companies the kind of profits patented drugs and beauty products can. Many supplements and herbal remedies have been shown to have healing or protective effects at much lower cost and with fewer side effects than the corresponding drugs. Yet without the quantifiable financial

MYTH: *The media will keep me informed.*

TRUTH: *The media is not a source of balanced information.*

The published science that verifies natural approaches is often overlooked by the media due to the financial support that patented, money-making drugs get but natural alternatives don't. Loosening of media regulation in the 1990s led to the rapid consolidation of media control into the hands of the few mighty corporations that now handle the nation's entire broadcast media industry. Talk show health segments are often sponsored by pharmaceutical companies. We are living in a new era of industry-owned information flow and even industry-influenced scientific reporting.

Even though some important stories regarding your health and beauty do make it to prime time, they are often quickly upstaged if the moneymaking potential is not there. Stories like those on the benefits of supplements or the dangers of antibacterial soaps get lost due to lack of industry sponsorship. Consequently, not only do we not hear about lots of products that work, but perhaps of even greater concern, we also don't always hear about some of the dangers in what we currently eat, take, and apply.

For the same reason, research discrediting nondrug treatments often garners wide attention, even when it might only be one negative—and perhaps poorly designed—study out of dozens of underreported positive ones. Though not a beauty product, one clear example of this skewed media coverage is the attack leveled at the herb St. John's wort, a natural (read: unpatentable) substance shown in at least twenty-five double-blind clinical studies to effectively treat mild to moderate depression. But what most of the public heard about was one study that found it failed to alleviate severe depression, a condition for which it was never historically used or intended. This study was funded by Pfizer, a pharmaceutical company whose own drugs, according to the Merck Manual guidelines, are not considered effective against severe depression when used alone.

payoff that patent protection affords—which pays for slick ad campaigns, TV health segments, and celebrity endorsements—there is little corporate interest in funding expensive clinical trials for FDA approval of natural substances. The multimillion-dollar price tag of FDA approval is far out of the range of most sellers of natural products, which—because they can't patent them—could never recoup such an investment. Keep this in mind as you view impressive billboards, advertisements, and TV health segments, and as you peruse the decidedly unslick aisles of a natural products store. Don't be deceived...

It is also worth noting that pharmaceutical and chemical industries are in the habit of developing synthetic—and therefore patentable—versions of existing natural substances and then marketing them to the public as the best or only effective treatment. For example, scientists are now working to create an anti-breast cancer drug synthesized from the natural substance sulforaphane, a component of broccoli. The patented synthetic version (likely with side effects) may be available soon, but sulforaphane has been available as a supplement for years. A related substance from broccoli called I3C—also currently available as a supplement—has been shown to inhibit the growth of certain human breast cancer cells better than the drug tamoxifen under laboratory conditions, without the side effects that have made tamoxifen so controversial. While you probably haven't heard about I3C, much pharmaceutical-grade advertisement, media fanfare, and inflated costs will likely come with the announcement of its synthetic counterparts.

Similarly, the manufacture of progestin was the product of the goal to synthesize a patentable (profitable) form of progesterone from foods like wild yam and soy, which have often been publicly ridiculed and dismissed by the very industry that scrambled to synthesize them. Incidentally, the synthetic hormone showed immediate evidence of serious side effects, while the natural, bio-identical hormone produced none when properly dosed.

The Ultimate Beauty Secret: A Healthy Dose of Disenchantment

Unfortunately, the search for complete information inevitably leads to the shocking revelation that some companies we all grew up trusting are, in fact, led by quite a different set of motives. I encourage you to think critically and never assume that a treatment, product, or food is safe or good for you just because your grandmother did.

MYTH: *My doctor will keep me informed.*

TRUTH: *Your doctor may not know about or consider natural treatment options.*

Many doctors are too busy and—believe it or not—not required to look at independent research in medical journals for new treatment options even if they are found more effective than drugs. Some doctors depend entirely on pharmaceutical sales reps for ongoing treatment information. Pharmaceutical companies have historically spent upwards of $13,000 per doctor per year to court physicians with ceaseless perks and incentives—like frequent flyer miles, Broadway shows, exotic trips, and free gas fill-ups—to sell drugs. Wooing doctors and the media is expensive business, and unpatentable natural product manufacturers could not begin to compete, even if the establishment were in their favor.

Even *science* is no longer sacred. Scientists are currently allowed to accept money or stock from a company while conducting research on its products.

A review of literature and interviews conducted by Dr. Thomas S. Bodenheimer of the University of California, San Francisco, concluded that when drug companies paid for a trial of a new drug, "biases can be, and have been, intentionally introduced that favor the company funding the study." One FDA official was quoted as saying that the consequences of these conflicts had gotten "completely out of control."

When the government attempted to impose restrictions on these conflicts of interest, the industry lobby prevailed. Until these conflicts are effectively prohibited, wouldn't it then be prudent to assume that any drug may carry far more risk than we are hearing about? Protecting your vitality means doing your own research before taking such risks, and seeking nontoxic solutions.

Corporations that damage the environment and harm us can still run the most heartwarming ads and employ good, upstanding—though perhaps misled—people. Doctors, scientists, and farmers of conscience can still serve as unwitting pawns of unscrupulous companies or industries. When the hands-on

DID YOU BUY THESE EXPERIMENTS?

These controversial diet and personal care products have been hotly debated because of their possible negative effects on the body. If you bought these products, it's probably because you were told they were safe. But did you get to hear both sides of the debate? Here are some widespread medical views that were mostly lost in the media due to lack of corporate sponsorship.

- **Wow potato chips and other Olestra-containing products:** Several countries, including Canada, denied approval of Olestra as a food ingredient because it blocks the absorption of crucial fat-soluble vitamins.
- **Antibacterial soaps:** Like antibiotics, these soaps have been found to give rise to microbes that are resistant to these products. Though doctors agree that they're harmful, there's no profit in removing them from the market.
- **NutraSweet/aspartame:** Routine consumption of aspartame-containing products may create a buildup of methanol in the body, leading to neurological and other problems.
- **Fat-free foods:** The well-known consequence of high-glycemic foods—as fat-free foods tend to be—is that they raise triglycerides and can lead to insulin problems, unhealthy blood sugar metabolism, weight gain, and even diabetes.

GOVERNMENT REGULATIONS: TOO LITTLE TOO LATE

Because of ongoing conflicts of interest in our regulatory bodies, we face a modern-day minefield of potential threats to our vitality. Today, it's easy to dramatically reduce these dangers by overhauling not only your choices, but your sensibilities. Hindsight is 20/20.

- For years, fat-free recommendations from government scientists were based largely on profit-driven speculation, and conflicted with common medical knowledge about the actions of insulin.

- As early as 1979, reports indicated the dangers of phenylpropanolamine, an ingredient in diet pills and cold remedies. But it wasn't pulled from the shelves until 2000 and not before it caused needless strokes in hundreds of healthy people.
- Fenfluramine-phentermine (Fen-Phen) was an ingredient of anti-obesity drugs such as Redux and Pondimin. According to a Mayo Clinic study, as many as one-third of users studied showed heart abnormalities by the time the drug was recalled in 1997.
- Putting a cosmetic on the market does not require safety data on ingredients or any pre-market review, and manufacturers do not have to report consumer complaints about their cosmetics. Of all cosmetic chemicals used, only a small percentage have been adequately studied, and nearly nine hundred are toxic, according to the National Institute of Occupational Safety and Health.
- The Environmental Protection Agency (EPA) has found traces of shampoos, antibiotics, hormones, and chemicals from synthetic drug and personal care products in rivers and waterways all over the United States, yet it has made no long-term plans for cleanup or restrictions as other countries have begun to do.

people we're taught to trust, from pest control technicians to doctors, aren't held accountable for—or even fully informed about—their own products or services, it's easier for disconnected decision makers to do what would ordinarily seem unconscionable: put profits before human lives. From the use of mercury or fluoride in dentristry to the use of toxic products by your manicurist, we are talking about people who are actually unfamiliar with large bodies of compelling research.

Moral of the story? The more you know, the less you have to take anyone's word for it and the more power you have to preserve and transform your own health and appearance.

Do your body and your beauty a serious favor: don't put your unquestioning trust in professions and industries, brand names, number-one recommended products, lab coats, or government guidelines, no matter how respectable they seem. The only people you ever needed to trust entirely were your parents, and just as every parent has very human weaknesses and personal agendas, so does every regulatory agency and authority figure that influences your lifestyle choices. The sooner you let go of any remaining blind faith you have in anyone else's ability or incentive to protect you, the sooner you can put that faith and the role of protector where it belongs: with *you.*

Informed Choices Depend on Full Disclosure

If you're informed, you can make wise choices. But some industries have been quite successful in their efforts to keep certain information from public knowledge. For example, in the United States, the majority of people eat

MYTH: *If it really worked, I would have heard about it.*

TRUTH: *Results of important research are not always made public.*

For example, it was long suspected but finally proven in 1999 in a stunning court ruling that the FDA had unjustifiably censored health claims backed by good science from appearing on nutritional supplement labels, in the name of "protecting the public." The federal appellate court found that claims about the important reproductive health and birth-defect-preventing benefits of folic acid had been unconstitutionally suppressed by the FDA. For years, tens of thousands of women weren't hearing about a substance that was crucial to the health of their babies. Countless similar obstructions to well-researched health claims exist today.

In a TV interview in July 2000 Dr. Bill Fair, former chairman of urology at the prestigious Memorial Sloan-Kettering Cancer Center, was asked by NBC 4's Dr. Max Gomez, "Has the conventional medical world been arrogant in its rejection of Eastern medicine?" Fair hesitated and then replied, "Yes, I would have to say that. I would like to think that this movement back toward more primal systems was something that originated within medicine, but it hasn't. It's the patients doing the originating. They're leading it."

genetically modified foods (also known as genetically modified organisms, or GMOs) without even knowing it, much less knowing what they are. GMOs are foods that have not been subjected to long-term studies (and several studies have revealed problems), and are considered unpredictable and dangerous by many prominent scientists. Though such foods are either labeled or not allowed in many other countries due to safety concerns, in the United States they are sold without a label. Unless a product is 100 percent organic, there is no way for consumers to avoid GMOs. Industry lobbying and pressure against laws that would require labeling and allow consumers to make informed choices is intense. With regard to milk, for example, the manufacturers of the genetically modified bovine growth hormone known as rBGH have even tried to prevent dairy producers who don't use it from stating so explicitly on their labels. Without full disclosure, the concept of choice is merely an illusion. If we reward the actions of such shrouded industry with our uninformed patronage, we give ourselves up as guinea pigs.

Declare Your Independence

Mainstream guidelines, mass production, and standard care have created the alarming statistics and compromise in quality of life we hear about and experience every day. But where society has headed doesn't have to be where you're headed. Don't be another beauty statistic. Learn for yourself. Think for yourself. Don't be duped into thinking of alternatives as unproven or unpatriotic. Look beyond headlines (they are very often incorrect). Vote with your dollars. Declare your independence from standard self-care strategies and start opening your eyes to the new world of safer, science-backed, and self-affirming solutions.

Summary

- The more you know, the better you look and live.
- Incomplete information keeps us stuck. Complete information sets us free.
- Feed your self-respect with informed acts.
- Trust solid science, your instincts, and the individuals you choose—not lab coats, professions, and industries.
- Look beyond mainstream media for unpatented, natural solutions.

- Distinguish raw science from industry interpretation and bias.
- Demand full disclosure about everything that goes in and on your body.
- Become your own best expert. It's easier than you think.

TOOL #3: ACCESS TO THE BEST PRODUCTS AND RESOURCES

Convenience Spells the Difference Between Intentions and Results

All the motivation and information in the world won't help you if there's no easy way to follow through. It's important to have practical, appealing solutions in order to gain the courage to leave old mind-sets and habits behind. By experimenting with the superior pro-beauty products and lifestyle options presented throughout this book and in the Resources section at the end, you can reset your own informed criteria for what goes on and in your body.

Each time we simply accept the choices we feel we are stuck with, we resign ourselves to a physical destiny nature never intended for us. There is no longer any reason for this kind of compromise. With Internet and mail-order retailers of better products and services popping up all over the country, you can now access the good life wherever you are. Living a pro-beauty lifestyle is not only practical for the first time but also far more uplifting than the standard choices we've come to accept at our own expense. As you evolve your purchases to align with your expanding tastes and knowledge, your definition of decadence will change completely, and your quality of life will soar.

Our Social Connection with Name Brands

Name brands are part of our social fabric. As it is with many adults, brand identity is important to kids, who are harshly judged by the labels they wear and the foods they trade with friends from their lunch boxes. But making inferior choices for yourself or your family based on unearned brand loyalty comes at a price you will only fully understand once you've made the switch to brands of true substance.

If you look at the ingredients lists on two bottles of shampoo—one from a well-known beauty product manufacturer and one from a health-conscious company—you'll realize that one company has spent all its money on packaging and

SHELF LIFE VS. QUALITY OF LIFE: WHY THE BEST-KNOWN BRANDS AREN'T ALWAYS BEST

It often appears that the most familiar, trusted brands are the best. But this is rarely the case and is, in fact, quite ironic if you look beyond the packaging to the actual substance you're buying—the part that has real impact on you and the quality of your life.

Indefinite shelf life and third-party warehousing are the backbone of mass-marketed food and body care manufacturing. Removing vital oils and biologically active components from mass-produced foods and cosmetics, and substituting cheap refined oils and fillers, ensure not only the longest shelf life but also the best returns on a manufacturer's investment in raw materials. By using refined and denatured raw materials that have literally had the life sucked out of them, manufacturers not only save big on the cost of materials but can also store products indefinitely, give quantity discounts, and still rake in the kind of profits it takes to run the most endearing ad campaigns. But this win-win situation for the manufacturer is a serious loss for your beauty and quality of life.

The common thread between our souls and our physical bodies is the interconnection between ourselves and nature. Biologically harmonious products and fresh whole food are crucial to achieving radiance in today's denatured world.

Let's compare the ingredients of two brands of cream of mushroom soup. One is a brand your grandmother may have trusted; the other, less familiar.

"Famous Brand" Cream of Mushroom
Ingredients: Maltodextrin, whey, partially hydrogenated soybean oil, cornstarch, salt, guar gum, mushrooms, yeast extract, lactic acid, sodium caseinate, sugar, natural flavors, onion powder, garlic powder, artificial flavor, caramel color, lactose, disodium guanylate, disodium inosinate

"Healthy Brand" Creamy Portobello Mushroom Soup
Ingredients: Filtered water, portobello mushrooms, organic onions, organic soy milk (filtered water, organic soybeans), mushrooms, organic celery, organic rice flour, organic expeller-pressed safflower oil, sea salt, organic spices

Which of these do you think your body recognizes as food?
The famous soup, hair-color, cosmetic, wholesome-snack, instant-bake-mix, soap, and diet-shake names ring in our heads, not because these products are exceptional but because of the priority placed on marketing them.

MYTH: *Synthetic products have surpassed natural ones.*

TRUTH: *Nature's sophistication is inimitable.*

We think of man-made technology as being more sophisticated, but in reality it is nature that is inimitable. Technology may help isolate, stabilize, or deliver the power of nature, but it cannot replace it. Nature works by countless mechanisms and synergies. Synthetics work by only a few, and invariably fail to take the place of natural substances in and on our bodies without creating new problems.

Many plant substances, because they are bio-identical to those in the body, have the amazing ability to balance our chemistry, whether we are deficient in—or suffer an excess of—those substances. No synthetics can do this. For example, plant estrogens can successfully mimic and displace harmful estrogens in our bodies with weaker, beneficial estrogens, and at the same time alleviate certain symptoms of estrogen deficiency.

Similarly, plant sterols can calm overreactive immune responses while increasing inadequate immune response. They can even normalize cholesterol levels by successfully mimicking and displacing harmful cholesterol in the body without creating the imbalances or side effects associated with widely prescribed cholesterol-lowering drugs.

Many natural antimicrobials such as tea tree or oregano oil have been shown to work as well or better than synthetic ones without creating resistant bacteria as synthetics like trichlosan can. Some scientists believe that natural antimicrobials are too complex for bacteria to develop resistance to.

Most amazingly, in recent years several natural substances such as pterostilbene from blueberries have demonstrated a wide range of positive effects on gene expression, up-regulating many disease-protective, antiaging genetic functions.

Negative side effects rarely occur from natural substances, and are generally resolved upon adjusted dose or discontinued use. But because of their complexity and multipurpose nature, when they help you with one problem they are also likely to have numerous good side effects.

MYTH: *If it's derived from nature, it's natural.*

TRUTH: *It's not where it comes from but what's been done with it that counts.*

I recently attended a beauty technology trade conference here in New York. It was exciting to see the emergence of natural substances as the undisputed superstars of cosmetic formulations. However, some company representatives appeared confused in their eagerness to capitalize on the natural craze without changing their ingredients, claiming "our ingredients are *derived* from nature, so they're natural." Nice try. Many substances "derived from" nature are anything but. Super-cheap mineral oil and petroleum jelly may be derived from natural petroleum, for example, but they are so highly processed (exposed to heat and pressure) that they no longer readily break down in the environment or on the skin. They displace natural skin lubrication (sebum), disrupting the skin's ability to regulate and receive real moisture, according to cosmetic and plant chemist Aubrey Hampton, PhD. Similarly, hydrogenated trans fats, such as margarine, displace healthy fats in our cells, confusing and disrupting anti-inflammatory, immune, and hormonal processes in the body. Even nutritional supplements generally work better if they're in the natural—as opposed to the petro-derived, synthetic form—as is seen in the case of vitamins E and D. Perhaps our bodies are the best judge of when the line between natural and refined has been crossed.

The irony is that extreme cheapness and indefinite shelf life are what afford synthetic cosmetic, food, and drug manufacturers the million-dollar marketing campaigns that get us to think that synthetics have come to improve on nature. Don't buy it.

marketing while the other has actually put real, perishable bioactive (expensive) ingredients inside the bottle.

Even if the smell and the packaging have won you over, the body knows the difference. Don't be brand loyal—be ingredient loyal. Go for substance over packaging. Get past the smell, the bright colors, and the poetry, and get down to the contents. Why reward money spent on the PR and not on the

MYTH: *Beauty is expensive.*

TRUTH: *Keeping up the illusion of beauty is expensive.*

My beauty career has given me continual contact with some of the world's most privileged people—people who can afford just about every beauty advantage they desire: personal trainers, Pilates and yoga gurus, facial peels, massages, and relaxing trips to Baja. But the truth is that the little mundane choices we make day in and day out far outweigh the impact such luxuries can have on our beauty, even if we do achieve the hard body we've just paid big bucks for. If you find yourself worried about the money you'll spend on upgrading your food and personal care products, consider how much you might be willing to part with for another tube of lipstick, a pair of shoes, or a manicure. Then consider how much you would be willing to pay for products that can help make you radiant for the rest of your life, not just this season. Many women would rather spend $100 on one skirt that makes their backside look good than pay for pure, potent body products and supplements that could actually change their skin and shape and make strategic dressing unnecessary. They consider these expenses extravagant. But they are the real beauty splurges. They're actually much less expensive than the additional cosmetics, procedures, quick fixes, compensatory clothes, and temporary cover-ups we resort to in order to maintain the mere *illusion* of beauty.

I once spent a fortune keeping up with my weight fluctuations. I never had anything to wear or enough time for the elaborate makeup job or perfect hair I depended on to compensate for the rest of me, which was falling apart. And the cost of the resulting medical crisis was nothing to sneeze at.

After I experienced my first real physical rewards, I came to consider each purchase as an investment in my future vitality. I learned that health was not only hope but also happiness. Once your beauty shines on its own, you don't need the expensive arsenal of clever cover-ups and distractions.

Remember: beauty isn't expensive. Focusing on surface pursuits while taking the real thing for granted is what will cost you untold beauty and dollars down the line.

ingredients? Why not buy the best of the best, not merely the best of the mass-marketing campaigns?

Warning: For Some, Solutions Aren't Sexy

Some of us become so absorbed in the social and cultural allure of prestige-based food and cosmetics that the transition from novelty to solution may alter the very structure of our lives. The pursuits of beauty, the perfect body, and even social esteem connected with the "right" products displayed on your bathroom counter can actually provide a sense of purpose, accomplishment, and social camaraderie. This never-ending cycle of trend-following leads to ceaseless "research," boastful splurges, short-term fixes, and exploitation of hopes and dollars. But you'll no longer be satisfied with such "play" once you truly inform yourself and taste the rewards of getting serious about your beauty. Getting hooked in to a better world of personal care and lifestyle options will make your new, higher beauty pursuit more rewarding and successful and liberating than any before it.

Summary

- Convenience counts. Easy access to better options fosters change.
- Demand purity, potency, proof, and appeal. You can have it all.
- Go for substance over packaging. Look beyond well-known brands.
- Get and stay hooked into the world of products and resources that support and serve you—materially, not just with heartfelt slogans or "green" images.

YOU'VE CREATED WHAT YOU ARE TODAY; ONLY YOU CAN CREATE WHAT YOU BECOME TOMORROW

As much as I was a victim of the ceaseless suggestions that perpetuated my self-sabotage, only *I* was ultimately responsible for it, and nothing or no one could have made me change until I took charge of healing myself.

Though I regularly refer to the dubious information and negative messages that we are all bombarded with, make no mistake: you have created what you are today, with varying degrees of help from countless influences. Today you will create what you will be tomorrow. There's no point in blaming doctors, irresponsible companies, unresponsive politicians, or the "system" for the problems of the world around us that have invaded our lives and our beauty. Relying on cultural or commercial cues for our choices is what causes us to stray from our better instincts in the first place. If you start sentences with "My doctor has me taking this" or "My trainer has me doing that," stop yourself. Only *you* have *yourself* doing whatever it is you choose to do. Stop following and start setting your own course.

What I never learned in beauty school or from any doctor, weight-loss counselor, or nutritionist was the importance of masterminding my own transformation by getting informed and rejecting self-defeating motivations. Only we can transform ourselves, and we must identify and cultivate our assets and discern our raw materials with the passion of an artist.

USE THE TOOLS TO CREATE YOUR SELF

Beauty comes not of obligatory self-maintenance but of joyful self-creation. You are the only expert on yourself there can ever be. If you forfeit that role, a huge part of your potential and your truest gift to yourself and to others will be lost.

Why be content to merely survive when you can thrive with glowing, vital radiance? Aren't we each worthy of being our own passion-driven project? No one ever called a painter a fanatic for refusing to use second-rate brushes and supplies on his artwork. No one ever called a chef high-maintenance for being a stickler for freshness and quality or for demanding to know the origin of the ingredients that go into his creations. We, too, must become such passionate connoisseurs of ourselves.

Use these tools to customize your lifestyle and cultivate your beauty solely from the inspirations of truth, your connection with yourself, and the awe-inspiring dialogue between your body and nature's intention.

Beauty comes not of obligatory self-maintenance
but of joyful self-creation.

Applying these tools to the process of shedding will enable you to re-attune to long-neglected needs and instincts, and to rebuild each area of your life, from your New Year's resolutions to your beverage choice, skin care, and pick-me-ups, to your bathroom cabinet staples and even your healthcare objectives. These tools will help you to build your own permanent sanctuary from bombardment, disruption, and deception. This sanctuary will be a place in which to nurture your self-creating spirit and cultivate your glowing potential on a new foundation of the healthiest motivations and the wisest, most powerful choices.

PART II
FEEDING AND CULTIVATING BEAUTY

CHAPTER 4

DRINK YOURSELF BEAUTIFUL

It's easy to become mindful of what we eat while tuning out how we quench our thirst. This first priority upgrade to jump-start your transformation may surprise you, but the consistency, frequency, and sheer volume of our drink choices mean that our habitual sips, slurps, and gulps can have more impact on our looks and well-being than just about anything else we do. Virtually every beauty factor—skin, hair, bones, weight, breast health, and overall vitality—is dramatically affected by the beverages we drink every day. Whether that effect is positive or negative is up to us. Fortunately, our drink habits are incredibly easy to tweak for astounding immediate and cumulative beauty rewards. You may already be the proud owner of an evolved palate and enjoy beauty-enhancing beverages like pure water, green tea, herbal concoctions, and even creamy or sweet drinks with minimal sugar and caffeine. If that is the case, this chapter will give you added motivation, an expanded repertoire of exciting new pro-beauty beverage tastes, and increased physical rewards. But if you are a regular drinker of such beauty-stealing beverages as sweetened commercial teas, sodas, fruit drinks, iced-coffee concoctions, or even juice and are apprehensive about giving them up, it is you who stands to reap the most dramatic immediate rewards if you change what you drink. Your face may respond to a well-chosen upgrade with reduced puffiness and under-eye circles as soon as tomorrow morning. If you are currently a slave to your fifteen-dollar-a-week mochalattechococcino habit, you may enjoy clearer, smoother skin in as little as two weeks simply by upgrading to truly hydrating brews in lieu of dehydrators like coffee.

THIS IS NOT ABOUT CALORIES

As kids we learn that sugar rots our teeth. As grown-ups we learn that sugar drives up the *calorie* content of what we eat and drink. Further, we learn that coffee speeds up our metabolism so we can burn more *calories* and that sugar-free drinks won't affect our diets because they contain no *calories*. But the problem is not the calories we tally; it's the unstable chemistry of cravings, energy, and moods that sugary, caffeinated, and diet drinks can perpetuate. As you continue with your series of upgrades, you'll see that it is the healing, balancing, and truly satiating qualities in drinks and foods that matter most to your looks and your life in the long and even the short run.

We make jokes all the time about our sugar and caffeine addictions without really considering the truth behind our words. These addictions have real physiological effects on our bodies. The secret to breaking this cycle is strategic upgrading—not sacrificing.

STRATEGIC UPGRADES AND TASTE-BUD TRAINING

Your initial goal should be to find satisfying and revitalizing upgrades for any beauty-robbing beverages you drink. Doing this will have quick physical payoffs and free you of the chemical pendulum that can cause you needless cravings and energy slumps. Upgrading your beverages also changes how you taste foods, which is why this chapter is the crucial strategic springboard to the series of food upgrades that follow in the next chapter.

Well-chosen upgrades that are right for you won't feel like substitutions at all after the first few days. Finding them sometimes requires a little experimentation, but once you find the right ones, rather than feeling deprived, all you will feel are the old burdens lifting away, the new beauty effects setting in, and new taste sensations pleasing your palate. You'll wonder how you ever did without your new choices.

START WITH PURE WATER: THE LEAST AND THE MOST YOU CAN DO FOR YOUR BEAUTY

At least 70 percent of the skin's blemish- and wrinkle-fighting hydration comes from the water we consume. If I've just motivated you to drink more water—good! Just be sure you're not drinking more *tap* water. If you haven't done so already, switching from chlorinated tap water to reliably purified water will be

ARE BLOOD SUGAR ISSUES SABOTOGING YOUR BODY AND YOUR BEAUTY?

The way we metabolize sugar is one of the biggest problem factors when it comes to our weight, our vitality, our skin, and premature aging. The hormone insulin normalizes blood sugar levels in the body. Insulin resistance, which now affects nearly sixty-five million Americans, is a condition in which a body's cells build up tolerance to insulin, which makes it less effective at doing its job of keeping blood sugar stable. Feeling tired after or before eating and being overweight are common symptoms of insulin resistance. Sometimes called "Syndrome X" or "metabolic syndrome," it can lead to more serious problems such as diabetes and heart disease. Foods and beverages high in refined sugars contribute to insulin resistance by causing a spike in blood sugar levels. The more our blood sugar is spiked over time, the more likely we are to become overweight and challenged with cravings, insulin resistance, and its eventual result if we don't halt it—diabetes. Those of us who grew up drinking sweet drinks and eating starchy foods have a head start toward these issues. Humans are just not built to handle that much sugar, and we don't show any sign of adapting to it. Fortunately, we can prevent, greatly improve, or even reverse this condition by avoiding sugar and other blood sugar-spiking drinks and foods, eating more fiber, being active, and stopping smoking. Luckily, there's a sweet yet healthy upgrade for every drinkable sugar fix you might crave. Find yours now, and begin an amazingly quick reversal of much of what troubles your body and your looks.

perhaps the most important health and beauty lifestyle upgrade you will ever make. If you do not have a water purifier, then I would wager that you are not much of a water drinker. It's hard to make yourself drink a healthy quantity of water if it tastes bad, and it is unhealthy to drink a lot of heavy metals, volatile organic chemicals, and chlorine—which age the body and skin and degrade the body's ecology.

Here are some motivations to upgrade to pure water:

- Clearer, more comfortable skin as body ecology is reestablished

- A reduction of the toxic byproducts and aging associated with chlorine exposure
- A healthier digestive tract and better absorption of nutrients
- Diminished allergies and yeast infections thanks to improved bacterial balance

Pure water will boost the value and appeal of every tea, soup, and beverage you make at home. See the Resources section for some of the best water purifiers and distillers for the money as well as the first pitcher-type and portable purifiers that work well and are affordable. Bottled water is less preferable, as it is not reliably pure and puts a great strain on the environment. Water purifiers are the best beauty bang for the buck!

SWEET DRINKS ARE EVEN WORSE THAN SWEET FOODS

Few autopilot choices offer more of a surefire shortcut to beauty and body self-destruction than sweet beverages. A jolt of sugar, such as your morning juice (and for some people even milk), will give you a slight "buzz" and then start a heavy pendulum of mood swings and cravings that will continue to peak and drop again throughout the rest of the day. Liquid sugar does crazy things to the body. In addition to causing the pancreas to spew too much insulin in order to neutralize the massive sugar rush, it also causes the excess sugar (or carbohydrates) to be stored as fat. In this way, sugar turns our bodies into fat-storing machines, *even if we're not eating any fat*. Because they contain little fiber, fat, or protein, most sweet beverages cause sugar to enter the bloodstream more quickly and are thus more likely than food to cause fat gain, blood sugar swings, and the cravings that always come with them. Let's compare drinking juice to eating the whole fruit. Eating an apple, for example, introduces sugar into the bloodstream more slowly because of the fruit's fiber, but drinking apple juice is more like injecting sugar. It's easy to become addicted to liquid sugar's immediate lift while becoming a victim of its unwanted consequences, but it's avoidable by strategizing some palate-pleasing upgrades.

SUGAR AND SKIN

In his book *The Perricone Prescription* (HarperCollins, 2002), Nicholas Perricone, MD, did a great job pointing out the compelling scientific connections

SMART SWEETENERS

Erythritol

A new arrival on the market, this natural "sugar alcohol" (sugar alcohols contain neither sugar nor alcohol, by the way) is fermented from cornstarch and has 70 percent of the sweetness of sugar. It's safe for teeth, easily digested (doesn't usually produce the laxative effects of some other sugar alcohols), has no calories, and clinical studies have shown it to be safe for diabetics.

Inulin and Oligofructose

These newly celebrated, seriously "functional" sweeteners derived from roots like chicory (or Jerusalem artichokes) are just becoming more widely available and have some of the most impressive health benefits ever documented for a natural sweetener. A quick PubMed search reveals that inulin and oligofructose increase calcium absorption and contribute to bone health. As soluble fibers, they lower insulin, blood sugar levels, and triglycerides, and reduce not only constipation but the incidence of colon cancer. As "prebiotics" they encourage the growth of healthy bacteria, reduce pathogenic bacteria in the digestive tract, and improve immunity. The sweetness of inulin may be 10–50 percent that of sugar, while oligofructose is generally 30–50 percent of the sweetness of sugar, so they are usually used in combination with other natural sweeteners, such as stevia and lo han.

Lo Han

Lo han fruit is the key ingredient in a number of natural, no-calorie, low-glycemic sweeteners. A fruit that comes from the mountains of China and Japan, lo han was found to have antidiabetic effects in one Japanese study.

Maltitol

Maltitol is another sugar alcohol (also called a polyol) that has a long history of use, particularly in candies recommended for diabetics, and is considered to be natural but has a more pronounced laxative effect than the other sugar alcohols. While I would choose it any day over a synthetic sweetener, I much prefer xyliltol, inulin, stevia, erythritol, or lo han-based sweeteners.

(continued on next page)

Stevia
Stevia is an herb three hundred times sweeter than sugar. It has been a staple sweetener in other countries for centuries and, amazingly, has even been shown to help stabilize blood sugar in some studies. But despite its incredible safety, it's been kept off the sweetener shelf by the FDA, which required it be called a "dietary supplement." I use either the vanilla stevia liquid or the powdered, de-bittered type (see Resources), as I find it far more sugarlike than typical stevia, which has a slight aftertaste.

Xylitol
Probably my favorite sweetener, xylitol is very sugarlike, natural, low-glycemic, and has recently been embraced by the American Dental Association for its anticavity benefits. There are numerous other health benefits attributed to xylitol, from inhibiting ear infections to building bone to stimulating collagen synthesis. Use measure for measure like sugar. Has a slight mouth-cooling effect. Not recommended for making sweet drinks, due to its potential laxative effect if consumed in large quantities.

between sugar and everything from inflammation, blemishes and edema-related puffiness, and under-eye circles to wrinkles, sagging, brown spots, and overall accelerated aging. Sugar wreaks havoc on collagen and leads to the cross-linking of the fibers that give elasticity to the skin, thereby causing wrinkles. In addition, another aging process caused by sugar, called glycation, results in an ugly type of protein breakdown occurring in the skin and throughout the body.

If you regularly consume beverages with upwards of 18 grams of sugar per serving—the same as a Hershey bar and less than in a glass of grapefruit juice—you not only have serious motivation to make the substitutions suggested in the following chart, you also have some incredible beauty rewards to look forward to in less time than you might imagine.

Here are some motivations to upgrade your sugar fix beverage:
- A slimmer, sleeker body
- A dramatically refined facial appearance due to diminished puffiness
- Smoother, clearer skin—and fewer wrinkles in your future

- Better skin color with reduced sensitivity and decreased inflammation
- Elimination of a primary cause of premature aging
- Victory over cravings, which—for many people—will mean a trans-formed body

Switching to smartly sweetened or super-low-sugar drinks will naturally help you to painlessly do the same in your food choices. After only a two- or three-day break from the old sugar assaults, your cravings for sugar will diminish, and you will begin to taste the unique flavors in real drinks and foods with much greater appreciation.

GET THE SUPPORT YOU NEED TO WEAN OFF SUGAR

Though the body's call for nourishment is seemingly silenced by a sugar fix, many people don't realize that nutritional deficiencies can actually be caused by sugar. These deficiencies are widespread—even for those who eat a balanced diet. With the support of the beverage and food upgrades to come and the blood sugar-stabilizing supplements you'll read about in chapter 9, your body's needs will be met in a way that satisfies its deepest hunger and thirst, and it will remain satisfied until true hunger—not just rebound craving—strikes.

SYNTHETICALLY SWEETENED DIET DRINKS MAY BE DANGEROUS

Scientific studies have not shown any long-term weight loss or prevention of weight gain from consumption of artificially sweetened diet drinks. In fact, beyond the bone-destructive phosphates in diet sodas, there may be some serious dangers lurking in all aspartame- or sucralose-sweetened diet drinks.

According to nutritional pioneer Dr. Michael B. Schachter, co-author of *Food, Mind and Mood,* 80 to 85 percent of all complaints received by the FDA were attributed to aspartame before its recent decline in use. Between 1984, when the FDA approved aspartame, and 1987, the FDA had received more than six thousand complaints concerning it, including 250 involving epileptic seizures. Dr. Shachter explains: "If an approved drug had as many complaints as aspartame, it probably would have been removed from the market long ago. But, aspartame has been approved as a food additive, not a drug, so the manufacturer doesn't have to track adverse reactions as they would with a drug.

SPRITZERS: THE PERFECT SODA UPGRADE

In recent years, soda has been directly linked with obesity, diabetes, mental problems, and even genetic damage. Smartly sweetened spritzers are the answer and quench thirst on a whole new level. They're so easy to make that you can make a pitcher of them at home, using unsweetened cranberry juice and lime seltzer, or make a modified version of it at your favorite restaurant or bar by ordering plain soda water and adding your own flavored liquid stevia, or stevia-sweetened herbal concentrates (find them in dropper bottles at the health food store and keep one in your pocketbook).

Kat's Favorite Flavored Spritzers

Fill a glass two-thirds full with plain seltzer and some ice. Add an ounce of unsweetened cranberry juice for a beautiful blush and a tart flavor, and several drops of plain or flavored stevia, such as lemon or vanilla (see Resources) for a sweet flavor even your kids will love. You can also use the flavored stevia alone if you don't have cranberry juice. The unsweetened cranberry juice is expensive but very concentrated, so it lasts a lot longer than sweetened cranberry juice (and doesn't carry the consequences). Add a slice of lime or lemon if you like. You can even create a Fresca-like refresher by adding a drop of grapefruit food-grade essential oil (see Resources) to lime flavored seltzer (or plain seltzer with a squeeze of lime), along with a smart sweetener. These spritzers will satisfy any sweet, fizzy soda craving and quench thirst deeply, without hurting you. If you're weaning off caffeine from cola, substitute green tea for half the seltzer for a healthier lift. This is an ideal drink for both you and your kids that could very well reshape your future since each sugary soda you drink per day dramatically increases your chance of becoming obese. Another variation? Use cocoa extract with vanilla stevia, and even add half-and-half to the seltzer to make an "egg cream." Between all of the flavorings, flavored green tea concentrates (many of them decaffeinated), and food-grade essential oils, the taste possibilities are endless (see the Resources section for all ingredients mentioned above). Half the fun is in discovering your own new flavors!

"Aspartame, like MSG, is an 'excitotoxin,'" Dr. Schachter further explains. "Because its effects are cumulative, one may feel fine consuming it at first, then begin to experience problems characteristic of the headache, vision, and other neurological complaints regularly called in. An additional concern about aspartame is that it tends to lower serotonin in the brain. Low brain serotonin levels are associated with depression."

The FDA responds to concerns about aspartame by saying that methanol (a potentially harmful byproduct of aspartame) is commonly found in fruits and vegetables. But several prominent scientists, including Dr. Schachter, board-certified neurosurgeon Dr. Russell L. Blaylock, and Dr. H. J. Roberts, author of *Aspartame (Nutrasweet): Is It Safe?*, note that while natural methanol in fruits is commonly offset by the presence of ethanol, the methanol in aspartame does not have protective ethanol, so it can be absorbed and may cause harm as it accumulates.

Splenda (main ingredient, sucralose) has its own issues. FDA findings regarding the animal tests done with Splenda showed thymus gland shrinkage and kidney swelling when Splenda was administered in high quantities. Splenda should have undergone more independent, long-term investigation, as should any synthetic chemical that has no history of compatibility with the human body. The main concern of some scientists and healthcare professionals is that sucralose's chemical structure closely resembles a class of chemicals that have a history of toxicity in the body.

Acesulfame K and Saccharin

Acesulfame K (Sunette), also listed as acesulfame potassium, has increasingly been used in protein shakes and other beverages since 1988 and, like saccharin, in animal studies has been linked with tumor growth.

Tagatose

This highly processed sweetener derived from lactose has no aftertaste and has captured the interest of food industry giants. You will see it soon in your convenience store soft drinks, certain cereals, and more. Because it goes through a good amount of processing and doesn't show much health benefit, I am not as keen on it personally as I am on beneficial sweeteners such as xylitol or the fiber inulin. Some of the polyols are also processed but are still familiar molecules to the body, and have a long history of use.

Fortunately, you now know about the safer alternatives, so you needn't be part of a lab experiment. Here are some motivations to upgrade your diet drinks:

- Stronger bones if you upgrade from sodas, which contain bone-eating phosphates
- Peace of mind and freedom from the unknown consequences of synthetic or poorly tested sweeteners

Diet Soda Upgrade

Steaz Diet Black Cherry Soda is the very first American diet soda sweetened without synthetic sweeteners. Technically sweetened with a few grams of sugar, it gets most of its sweetness from the sweet-tasting stevia herb and black cherry flavor. It is green tea-based and is the soda I serve on my programs. It even tastes great diluted by half with plain water or seltzer once you've resensitized your palate to require less sweetness (though kids will love it straight). Though other companies are poised to follow suit, Steaz has led this innovation by several years. Here's to the pioneers!

Consider the aforementioned spritzers or the upgrades I suggest in the "Beverage Makeovers" chart (pages 79–81) as your new diet drinks. Use only smart sweeteners from the sidebars on page 57–58 for your teas, coffee or herbal coffee, spritzers, and lemonade—and of course, in all your sweetened foods.

CAFFEINE, CRAVINGS, AND FATIGUE

Dr. Schachter explained the caffeine-fatigue connection to me: "Coffee and other caffeine sources cause the release of stress ('fight or flight') hormones, which has at least two negative effects. The first is a blood sugar drop, followed by increased sugar cravings; the second is increased fatigue over time that is caused by the exhaustion of the adrenal glands, which inevitably occurs in those who consume caffeine throughout the day over extended periods. The result is burnout and fatigue."

Caffeine can also cause insulin resistance. Furthermore, caffeine can contribute to elevated cortisol, a stress hormone, according to Stephen Cherniske, MS, author of *Caffeine Blues*. In his book, he describes how this condition affects sleep and causes immunity problems, accelerated aging, and mood changes. Cortisol has also been linked to accumulation of abdominal fat. As cortisol rises, the body's level of DHEA—the "youth hormone"—decreases. As you'll learn in the coming chapter on supplements, decreased

DHEA is bad news for your weight and your quality of life. I am very happy that my body started to reject coffee naturally after I fixed my liver and blood sugar issues. I finally realized that this so-called diet-friendly drink was a huge barrier to normalizing my cravings and my weight.

Here are some motivations to upgrade your caffeine fix:

- Freedom from cravings caused by coffee's blood sugar connection
- Clearer, healthier skin due to increased hydration and alkalinity
- Less taxing of adrenal glands, which leads to more energy and less-reactive skin
- Diminished under-eye puffiness as cortisol- and adrenal-related water retention is reduced
- Stronger bones due to improved mineral absorption and digestion
- Deeper sleep, and thus more beautifying human growth hormone (hGH) secretion during sleep
- Easier weight loss, a flatter abdomen, and slower aging from raised DHEA and lowered cortisol levels

WEANING OFF SUGAR AND CAFFEINE

All sugar and caffeine fixes are related to—and affected by—each other. If you focus only on omitting your afternoon cola fix and continue your morning juice habit, for example, you are overlooking a huge contributor to your day-long energy swings and cravings and thwarting your own progress toward freedom from them. It is much easier to gradually upgrade by consistently reducing caffeine and sugar content in all beverages throughout the day. For example, if you normally drink a sweet beverage in the morning and another in the afternoon and each contains more than 20 grams of sugar, try upgrading both to beverages with only 5 to 10 grams of sugar each. You can always easily do this by diluting your beverage by half using water or seltzer, or in the case of coffee, an herbal coffee (see sidebar). This is a terrific trick to save your kids' health, too. On the occasions when they insist on having soda, buy one soda and one seltzer water and mix the two. After they get used to that, increase the proportion of plain soda water. It's always amazing how sweet even the watered-down combination is! I used to order soda water with a splash of lemon-lime soda at the movie theater. Today even that is too sweet for me and not as refreshing as real, unsweetened lemon or lime seltzer.

STELLAR COFFEE UPGRADE: TASTING IS BELIEVING

Teeccino is an herbal beverage that tastes, smells, and brews almost exactly like coffee in your machine, drip cone, or French press. Even die-hard coffee drinkers will be impressed. It actually restores energy (via potassium), alkaline balance (more on that ahead), hydration, and mineral reserves rather than draining them like coffee does.

I like it with lots of organic half-and-half. It is also great iced. Sweeten, if you'd like, with a smart sweetener.

Unfortunately, most movie theaters and convenience stores don't even offer plain seltzer water (or especially the lime and cherry ones that really scratch the soda itch), which is why it's wise to tote your own. These actually quench thirst, without perpetuating the need for more "fixes."

Like any other vice, the allure of addictive beverages is connected to the sensory experience, chemical effects, ritual, and situation. Don't ignore your very real needs by attempting to become your own stoic drill sergeant. Deciding to quit coffee today without considering those needs will only limit your success. Instead of focusing on self-denial, focus on satisfying each area of need your coffee fulfills with something equally satisfying but more healthful.

THREE COFFEE-WEANING TECHNIQUES

1. More milk, less coffee. To start? Latte over cappuccino. Ask for only one espresso shot when you order the large size. Better yet, order regular coffee but ask them to fill it only halfway and top it off with milk or, as a treat, steamed milk. Over time, increase the milk to three-quarters. (Stop worrying about fat calories—just skip the sugar!) Use low-fat milk if it makes you feel better, but letting go of the fat phobia will give you a more satisfying beverage.

2. Mix brews. Start mixing Teeccino in with the coffee grounds you brew at home or the office. Gradually increase the portion of Teechino until you are drinking little to no coffee.

3. Half-caf. Drink coffee that's a combination of regular and decaffeinated coffee. Keep in mind that even with decaf, you are still left with several issues that work against beauty, such as acidosis and malabsorption. Use this technique as a last resort and choose Swiss water process decaf whenever possible, since other decafs generally contain toxic solvent residues like hexane.

GREEN AND WHITE TEAS: THE ALL-STAR BEAUTY BEVERAGE

A great place to start—and maybe even end—your search for the perfect beauty drink is green or white tea. Green tea has proven anti-inflammatory benefits to the skin, strengthens the teeth, decreases insulin resistance, inhibits breast cancer, burns fat, and is good for the heart. The list goes on and on. Studies have shown decreased breast cancer risk in Japanese women who drank upwards of six small cups per day. *Camellia sinensis*, the only plant leaf properly called "tea," gives us black, green, oolong, and white teas. Because white tea is the least processed, it is believed to possess even more benefits than green. Hot or iced, smartly sweetened or not (I prefer to experience them without sugar), they are a powerful upgrade to your autopilot beverage routine. Note that adding milk or cream to true teas has been shown in at least one study to reduce some of their health benefits. If you are very sensitive to caffeine, you might not have a problem with green or white teas, as they have substantially less caffeine than coffee, and they contain a relaxing amino acid called L-theanine, which has been found to counter the effects of the caffeine in teas. For very sensitive people, decaffeinated teas are the best option.

Most organic decaffeinated versions use the CO_2 method of decaffeination, which preserves the health benefits of the tea while sparing you the solvent residues left behind in cheaper decaffeinated teas. Another way to cut caffeine is to drink mostly white tea, which contains a third or less of the caffeine of green teas, and is available in Earl Grey, jasmine, chai, and countless other flavors at health food and gourmet stores.

Exotic Green Teas: A Connoisseur's Beauty Splurge

Creamy Taiwanese oolong, Earl Grey green, heavenly jasmine tea: these are all green teas, but they taste very different from basic green tea. (Taiwanese oolong is actually buttery, and drinking jasmine tea is like drinking flowers.) It is hard to believe that something so delicious can be so powerfully healthy.

BETTER BOTTLED DRINKS AND TEAS

If you're in the habit of drinking bottled beverages containing 30 or more radiance-robbing grams of sugar, you might either stop the sugar cold turkey (which is really not painful if you sweeten the drinks smartly) or progress gently down the sugar gram scale as your taste buds evolve. Once you're down to less than 3 grams of sugar in a beverage, you'll start to shake any remaining cravings altogether and feel a real change in energy, inflammation, and weight issues. Any more sugar than that—unless you're naturally slim or a dedicated athlete—will, unfortunately, thwart your progress toward achieving the kind of vitality, fat burning, and freedom from cravings I want you to experience. Athletes should immediately upgrade their sports drinks to unsweetened coconut water, the world's most perfect sports drink, which offers at least ten times the electrolytes without all the sugar and artificial stuff. Here are a few widely available low- and no-sugar natural bottled beverages:

Sugar content in grams:
- Ito En Teas: 0 g
- Steaz Diet Black Cherry Soda: 5 g
- Honest Teas: 0–9 g
- Tazo Enlightened Lemon: 8 g
- V-8 juice: 11 g
- Zico coconut water: 14 g (recommended for athletes or slim folks only)

Just a liter of oolong tea daily helped reduce allergy-related dermatitis lesions in test subjects over a few weeks. Once you find a green you love, you've settled on one of the ultimate pro-beauty upgrades. Mail-order sources for these and some other high-end teas and herbal infusions are listed in the Resources. Quality is important, as cheaper teas can be grown in polluted soil and have even been found to harbor high amounts of fluoride, which can inhibit thyroid function.

For those who are not yet lovers of classic teas, but want to experiment with a variety of scented teas and herbal infusions, I have found the following varieties to appeal to a wide range of tastes.

Chai (Minus the Sugar)

Everything in unsweetened chai is great for you. The black tea, turmeric, and clove all have rejuvenating effects. The problem lies in the sugar that manufacturers and coffeehouses add so you will stay addicted to it. At the coffeehouse, if you crave a creamy treat but don't want the bodily devastation caused by the loads of sugar in most coffeehouse concoctions, ask them to use a chai tea bag instead of their prepared chai, and just have them put the bag into a tall organic "steamer" (steamed organic whole milk). A sprinkle of nutmeg really puts this over the top. The sweetness from the whole milk alone is surprising (whole milk has around 11 grams of natural sugar, but its fat content slows its effect on the bloodstream, as does the fact that you sip this drink, rather than chug it). If you need it sweeter, use a smart sweetener from packets you've tucked in your pocketbook (note to self to remember to do that!).

Black Tea

An easy full- or part-time substitute for hot or iced coffee with antioxidant benefits similar to—though less powerful than—those of green or white tea is black tea. It contains about half the caffeine of coffee. To the evolved palate, unsweetened iced tea is divine! Don't drink too much, as it can dehydrate you.

Earl Grey Tea and Earl Grey Green Tea

The bergamot oil that gives Earl Grey its distinctive taste is heaven. It's fantastic with a little organic half-and-half and incredible iced.

Cocoa Spice Tea

Cocoa Spice Tea, from Yogi Tea, is made from cocoa beans and spices and, with a little milk, fills the cozy, creamy, and chocolate need. It's a viable substitute for hot cocoa—which is essentially chocolate-flavored sugar-water, unless you make your own the healthy way, with real unsweetened cocoa, organic whole milk, and a smart sweetener. More on the benefits of cocoa in a moment...

Tulsi Teas

While not a true tea, tulsi, or Holy basil, is one of the most prized ayurvedic herbs, traditionally used to relieve stress and boost stamina. Holy basil has also been found to lower cortisol levels. The flavor is slightly lemony-minty, and there are a variety of blends made with this amazing herb. I find it to be another energizing coffee alternative.

MY GLASS-JAR TRICK

Today I brew green teas and herbal infusions almost every day. I fill a half-gallon, heatproof Mason jar with not-quite-boiling purified water (or cold water, if I brew overnight, which requires no boiling and you can leave the leaves in all night), fill with loose leaves or bags, and brew as directed. I love to watch loose jasmine pearl leaves unfurl gracefully through the glass. I choose my brew based on the kind of support my body needs that day or that week.

To familiarize yourself with the beauty and body benefits of various herbal teas, see the "Drinkable Herbs" chart on page 69.

TARGET SPECIFIC BEAUTY REWARDS WITH DRINKABLE HERBS

Your initial upgrades for coffee and sugary drinks, and temporary break from alcohol, may collectively have the most significant immediate effects on your looks and well-being of any lifestyle upgrades you could make. But once you've stopped all the worst assaults and adjusted biochemically to life without them, why stop there? With a more refined, resensitized palate and a growing appreciation for a wider range of tastes, you are ready to go beyond mere damage control to pro-beauty beverages with the specific effects you want. By targeting your particular concerns, you can quench an even deeper bodily need while addressing issues such as rashes, fever blisters, bones, hair, nails, teeth, breast health, varicose veins, and even your libido. To gain a therapeutic effect from herbal infusions and teas, you generally need to drink several cups throughout the day, so it's important to experiment with several to identify tastes you truly enjoy.

TARGET YOUR BEAUTY ISSUES WITH DRINKABLE HERBS

	Burdock	Nettle	Green Tea	Horsetail	Ginseng	Red Clover	Chamomile	Ginger	Tulsi
Acne	✓	✓	✓	✓	✓	✓	✓	✓	✓
Beauty Sleep							✓		
Bones		✓	✓	✓					
Breasts	✓		✓			✓			
Circulation								✓	
Detox	✓	✓	✓			✓		✓	
Energy			✓		✓				
Hair				✓					
Rashes and Inflammation	✓	✓	✓		✓	✓	✓	✓	✓
Nails				✓					
Stress			✓		✓		✓		✓
Weight			✓		✓				✓
Wrinkles			✓						✓

MAKE A BETTER DETOX ELIXIR

If you want to add a real detoxifying boost that perks up both body and skin, be sure to get a regular dose of beautifying dark green vegetable juices. They can taste a whole lot better than you'd think. Green drinks are super-alkalizing and rich in healing enzymes and chlorophyll, which has been shown in studies to carry heavy-metal pollutants out of the body. Unlike fruit juices, green vegetable juices are less likely to throw off your blood sugar (though a shot of wheatgrass can still spike some people) and are, therefore, a truly energizing way to infuse yourself with cleansing nutrients. I prefer to make so-called "whole" juice over conventionally extracted juices (see sidebar "Kat's Beauty Detox Elixer" on the next page to learn more about whole juice). If juicing is impractical, you might find a juice bar or health food store that will make you a primarily green juice or my tastier Beauty Detox Elixir.

If you can't find time for these things at all, it is all the more important to get enough dark green vegetables into your lunch and dinner (more on that ahead) and use powdered "green drinks" (see Resources) that you can mix with water or make into smoothies a couple of times a week. We all need green! Finally, speaking of detox, I do not believe in juice fasts for overweight or metabolically challenged people, as it is well known that fasting can aggravate tenuous blood sugar issues and even lead to subsequent weight gain and bingeing. This book will show you how to detox every day, through everything you eat, drink, apply, and even think.

CHOOSE YOUR BEST MILKS

Though I've long been aware of the controversies surrounding processed soy, which I mentioned in the first edition of this book, more recent findings have led me to stop recommending soy milk, even for those who can't digest milk. A 2007 study on ultra-heat-treated (UHT) soy products (most soy milks are UHT), suggested that UHT soy destroys much of the benefits soy is known for. I weighed this along with the fact that soy is widely believed to be a thyroid hormone inhibitor (goitrogen), which most people don't need. This is not to say that minimally processed soy foods, such as tofu, aren't healthy foods. But soy milk is off my list.

Because rice milks are highly sweetened, I recommend unsweetened nut milks or the amazing new hemp milk as a frequent choice. Always consider

KAT'S BEAUTY DETOX ELIXIR

The benefits of this tasty (really!) drink are out of this world: Dark greens (the main ingredient) are the ultimate detoxifiers and bone builders. Cabbage is healing to the stomach lining. Beet is a terrific blood cleanser and wonderful for the skin. Carrots are loaded with skin-, vision-, and body-healing carotenoids. Lemon alkalizes the body, and the peel is loaded with bioflavonoids, which strengthen the vascular system throughout the body and are anti-inflammatory (again, great for the skin!). Ginger improves circulation and digestion.

I've modified this recipe in recent years to make a lower-sugar, more fibrous "whole" juice elixir with a Vita-Mix, which also uses only about one-tenth the produce and one-tenth the time and effort of extracted juice. This method also liberates many more nutrients from the cell walls and seeds of the produce and preserves all the minerals from the fiber, making a more alkalizing drink (more on that to come).

If you do use a conventional juicer, dilute the final drink by half to keep the blood sugar impact as minimal as possible. If you're having this prepared for you at a juice bar, it may help to give this list of ingredients to the person doing the juicing for easier ordering. Using a smart sweetener is the secret to a much smoother taste than other green drinks. Feel free to adjust the produce and herbs listed to use what's in season or available to you. Just keep it primarily green!

Ingredients (for conventional juicer, multiply produce by five):
  1 cup cold water or aloe juice (great for digestion)
  1/3 cup of fresh parsley (heavy metal detoxifier)
  1 3/4" wedge red cabbage (stomach healer, contains skin-protective pigments)
  1/2 cup of fresh dark, bitter greens (detoxifying and stimulating to the liver)
  1" piece of ginger, peeled (circulation stimulator, anti-inflammatory)
  1/2 lemon, scrubbed but not peeled (body alkalizer, bioflavonoid-rich)
  1/2 small beet (blood cleanser)
  Pinch of cayenne or 1/4" slice of small jalapeño pepper (peppers reduce pain)

(continued on next page)

Smart sweetener (smoothes out the taste, and adds health benefits)
1 cup ice
Bonus: a sprig of fresh herbs, such as thyme, tarragon, or basil

Procedure:
Put all washed produce into a Vita-Mix. Add liquid to only half the level of the produce. Run the machine on high for 15 seconds. Taste and make any sweetener adjustments, then add the rest of the water, plus any more needed to make an extremely thin drink (it will thicken quickly due to the soluble fiber). Makes two 10-ounce servings. If you have any left over, you can use it up to half an hour later by refreshing it with cold ice and more water.

the sugar content. No matter what the health benefits of a milk are, a blood sugar spike will always thwart your progress on the path to health, as well as freedom from cravings and excess fat storage. I don't serve any sweetened milks (except smartly sweetened) on my programs because sugar prevents all of the beauty and body benefits I want to facilitate. Hemp milk, which hit health food store shelves in late 2006, introduces amazing new properties that no other milk has: a balance of omega-3, -6, and -9 fats, including GLA, and

MAKE YOUR OWN NUT MILK

Soak any nut for several hours (soak almonds overnight). Blanch nuts that have skins in boiling water and then under cool water. After this is done, you can peel off the brown skin (an optional step that makes the milk smoother). Then just throw the nuts in a blender, covering halfway with water to start, and process until thick and creamy. Add water until the resulting milk is the consistency you want. Filter the milk through a cheesecloth or a gold coffee filter to remove grit (an optional step). To taste, you can sweeten smartly and add unsweetened almond, vanilla, or maple flavor.

an anti-inflammatory omega-6 fat. Look for only the newer, unsweetened hemp milk, and be sure to read the labels to confirm that there's been no sugar or other high-glycemic sweetener added.

You might also choose to buy or make your own nut or hemp milk. Brazil nut milk is particularly wonderful and one of the best sources of skin-loving, cancer-preventing selenium you could consume.

How Cow's Milk Fell from Favor

The decline in cow's milk's true nutritional value has come from a variety of technological interventions with hormones, pesticides, and the use of heat pasteurization, which destroys the enzymes that once made milk easy to digest. Milk can also spike the blood sugar of metabolically-challenged people. Unfortunately, even organic milk is pasteurized and a challenge to digest for many people.

It's important to note that because dairy milk contains natural sugar, the fattier a dairy product is (and the slower you drink it), the less likely it will be to spike your blood sugar. Chugging a glass of whole milk, for example, will spike blood sugar. But half-and-half, cream, sour cream, cottage cheese, and luscious Greek yogurt will probably not. If I use milk in a smoothie, I use half water, then add coconut oil, fiber, berries, and protein for the lowest-impact smoothie possible. Low-fat and fat-free dairy products are not only more likely to spike blood sugar, but are also not good sources of calcium, since fat is required for its absorption. More often, I use half-and-half or cream and water in smoothies (and half-and-half in cocoa), which have a lower glycemic impact. This also makes either drink more like a meal or a filling snack. While I don't drink a lot of milk, I have evolved to eating a lot of full-fat organic and grass-fed dairy products. I once had a problem with dairy, but once I cut out sugar and grains and got my digestion and autoimmune systems in order, I became a fine digester of dairy. One study found full-fat dairy products caused weight loss compared to a calorie-equivalent diet without them. One of the most nutritious milks, though one that can still spike blood sugar if gulped down, is raw milk. People are rarely allergic to it because of its natural, self-digesting enzymes, which are unfortunately destroyed in the pasteurization process. I do not buy in to the idea that we weren't meant to eat dairy or that milk is inherently bad or allergenic. Raw

RESTORE YOUR PRO-BEAUTY ALKALINE BALANCE

One of the surest steps to better skin and vitality is to alkalize your body pH. According to Dr. Susan Lark, the editor of *The Lark Letter* and co-author of *The Chemistry of Success*, "Most of the chemical processes within the body work optimally in an alkaline pH of 7.3 to 7.4." Lark recommends a mineral rich diet to achieve this.

Upgrading acidifying coffee to re-mineralizing Teeccino, as well as the addition of alkalizing green drinks (and foods) such as my Beauty Detox Elixir, or homemade nut milks, kefir, and smartly sweetened smoothies with quality raw milk whey or hemp proteins, and avoidance of alcohol, in addition to the food upgrades to come, will go a long way toward alkalizing the body. I use a water purifier with an alkalizing attachment (see Resources). Adding lemon to water is another alkalizing trick. Testing your own alkalinity with pH paper from the health food store is a fun way to track your progress.

milk had a very healthy history before man decided to "improve" it with heat, hormones, and chemical intervention. It is not always available or legal in all states. See if you can find a local organic dairy farmer who sells it through www.realmilk.com.

Finally, cultured dairy products like buttermilk and kefir (a yogurt drink) may be the healthiest dairy products of all. Sour cream, cottage cheese, yogurt, and my favorite, Greek (strained) yogurt, are all cultured, and, therefore, easier to digest than milk. The active, beneficial bacteria cultures these foods contain actually digest their own lactose and help your gut build up its own defensive "army" of good bugs. These good bugs are called probiotics. Probiotics have been found to reduce some types of inflammatory skin problems. The skin benefit is a predictable side benefit of healthier digestion and immunity, as I discovered from my own skin dramas.

BUILD A PERFECT SMOOTHIE

The terms "protein shake" and "smoothie" always sound like a healthy snack or breakfast choice, and when made right, they can give you the perfect stable energy and nutrients and good fats you need. But they can also invite a lot of rationalization when it comes to the blood sugar–spiking concoctions some people harm themselves with each morning. The best way to upgrade your smoothie is to:

- **Start with a better base.** Whole organic yogurt, goat milk, unsweetened hemp milk or almond milk, raw nuts, avocado, whole organic (raw, if you can get it) milk, or kefir are all great.

- **Use an unsweetened (or smartly sweetened) whey or hemp protein.** I avoid soy protein isolates (which might be genetically modified) and high-glycemic or artificially sweetened protein powders. Whey protein—either cross-filtered, ion-exchange, or even better, raw milk or goat milk whey—raises glutathione (a detoxifying compound in the body) and also boosts serotonin levels and mood, while giving you steady energy. Another good one is the newer hemp protein, which offers unprecedented fiber and chlorophyll in a protein, and is also highly digestible. A green powder can also be added. See the Resources section for raw milk whey, hemp protein, and green powders.

- **Upgrade sweet ingredients** like sugar, juice, or banana (all will spike your blood sugar) to a smart sweetener and fruits such as berries or unsweetened Amazonian acai fruit, available in a frozen purée. Goji berries are also a terrific smoothie ingredient and are incredibly rich in skin-loving carotenoids. They give a fantastic color as well! Unless you use a Vita-Mix, you might need to soak them in water overnight to increase their blendability into a smoothie.

- **Add a couple of tablespoons of good oil,** such as virgin coconut (energizing, slimming, and antifungal) or hemp seed oil (full of the fatty acid GLA, which is anti-inflammatory and great for the skin). Adding these oils will increase the energy-stabilizing, satiating, and—believe it or not—weight loss effects of your smoothie, once you've cut out blood sugar–spiking drinks and foods altogether. I'll explain more about this in the next chapter. A couple of tablespoons will do.

- **Add additional fiber** if you're not using hemp protein. My favorite is the newly available coconut fiber (see Resources), which, for the first time, enables you to get more fiber than psyllium (the fiber used in typical fiber drink powders) in a form that actually tastes good. Add at least a rounded tablespoonful. Freshly ground flaxseed also works (grind seeds in a coffee mill; use the same day).

THE TRUTH ABOUT ALCOHOL

I used to drink heartily while I had my eating disorder. But as my body detoxified, my desire for alcohol diminished each year. Now a very little goes a long way. That sensitivity is a good thing, as it means I can finally feel the impact that things like sugar and alcohol were having on me all along. I do not forbid myself to drink. I just don't think twice about ordering only

FLAVONOIDS, COCOA, AND THE SKIN

In a 2006 German study, flavonoids—which are found in almost all healthy drinks I've covered, from green tea to cocoa, from unsweetened cranberry to my Beauty Detox Elixir—showed some amazing skin benefits when ingested by drinking high-flavonoid cocoa. Twenty-four women drank high- or low-flavonol cocoa powder mixed in water for twelve weeks. The high flavonol cocoa contained roughly the amount of epicatechin and catechin found in 100 grams, or a large bar, of very dark chocolate. The low-flavonoid group got less than a tenth of that amount of flavonols in their cocoa powder. At the end of the study, there was no change detected in the skin of the low-flavonol group. However, the change in the high-flavonol group was significant: their skin had thickened, water loss was decreased, skin surface roughness and scaling had decreased, and blood flow, hydration, and skin density had increased. Additionally, they had a 25 percent decrease in skin reddening (erythema) from UV exposure. In other words, the high concentration of flavonoids gave them internal sun protection. Pretty impressive! But does this mean we have to eat a ton of dark chocolate every day? I doubt it. Getting a comparable amount of similar flavonols is easy if you have them coming from a variety of delicious sources. I do recommend that you indulge regularly in quality, smartly sweetened real cocoa made with whole organic or raw milk and dark chocolate. See the Resources for brands with little or no sugar.

sparkling water with lime along with an Italian meal. Or, if I'm having Asian food, just ordering a fragrant pot of tea. Or a virgin Bloody Mary at brunch. I'll have a really good glass of wine with the occasional, celebratory meal, but for people like I was—food-addicted and pre-diabetic—once you have completely freed yourself from cravings, and you do have a drink or something sweet, you actually feel a "yuckiness" in your body that reminds you of that merry-go-round you left behind. Because I take supplements that help keep my blood sugar stable (more on that to come), I am able to have a drink here or there without even starting the sugar pendulum swinging, but certainly for those of you who would like to experience the maximum potential of my approach, it is best to get off alcohol completely at least for the first couple of weeks. Those who are most uncomfortable with this idea are those who will surely benefit from it the most. I can tell you firsthand that not only is it possible to biochemically snuff out typical sugar and mild alcohol cravings in under a week using only nutrition, but the rewards are stunning. If you regularly drink alcohol, here are some immediate rewards you may see and feel the first week of abstaining:

- Dramatically reduced head-to-toe puffiness, if you were drinking often
- Sharper vision, if you are insulin resistant
- Clearer thinking and greater productivity
- Much more energy
- Greatly reduced under-eye circles, due to decreased inflammation

According to one of the largest studies on alcohol and breast cancer, published in February 1998 in the *Journal of the American Medical Association (JAMA)*, the alcohol equivalent of two to four shots of hard liquor per day increased breast cancer risk by 41 percent. Similarly, a more recent analysis of fifty-three epidemiological studies found that a woman's risk of breast cancer increased by 7 percent for each alcoholic drink consumed per day. Alcohol also interferes with deep-wave sleep, the type of sleep during which human growth hormone, or hGH—which heals and rejuvenates the body and skin— is released. The preservatives in wine and beer, which include sulfites, can also give many people that puffy "hangover" face, under-eye circles, and headaches.

Even though drinking moderate amounts of red wine was shown to protect against heart disease, don't delude yourself into thinking that it is better to drink than not to drink. A review of population studies linking moderate drinking with longer life found that the majority of the studies suggesting benefits could have been influenced by people's choice not to drink because they did not feel healthy (and thus the higher mortality in the abstaining group!). Just as with caffeine sensitivity, the slightest genetic predisposition (and they are extremely common) can make alcohol an immediately negative choice for many people. Resveratrol, the well-known antiaging (at least in rodents) flavonoid from red grape skin believed to be responsible for wine's supposed heart benefits, has been available in supplement form since the mid-nineties. I prefer to leave the blood sugar spikes and under-eye circles I get from wine for special occasions.

Finally, if you are battling an alcohol addiction or uncontrollable alcohol cravings, be sure to seek an addiction program through your local hospital or the organizations listed in Resources. And be sure to look into nutritional programs that address the brain chemistry and blood sugar issues that play a part in all addictions. The clinics using these approaches have now been shown to offer far higher success rates than 12-step programs (up to 80 percent as opposed to 10 to 25 percent). It's a shame they don't combine both approaches, as they are quite complementary! The cofounder of Alcoholics Anonymous himself—Bill Wilson—experienced unprecedented freedom from physical agitations that remained long after he became sober from a nutritional therapy (high-dose vitamin B3), but he was opposed by his medical board when he tried to include it in his famous programs.

BEVERAGE UPGRADES AT A GLANCE

Following is a quick reference guide to help you find a pro-beauty beverage upgrade for each beauty-robbing choice you may be drinking. You'll also see the immediate and long-term benefits of upgrading your drinks. After reviewing this chart, you may want to revisit your notebook and write down the various upgrades you'd like to try. Then, note the beauty rewards you have coming.

YOUR BEVERAGE MAKEOVER

UPGRADE YOUR	FROM	TO	BEAUTY INCENTIVES
Caffeine Fix	• Coffee • Caffeinated sodas • Caffeinated teas, including commercial iced teas (see also Sugar Fix upgrades)	• Teeccino • Green tea *Energy Alternatives:* • "Green" drinks, such as Perfect Food, Green Vibrance, or Emerald Balance • "Whole" green vegetable juices (see Beauty Detox Elixir recipe, p. 71)	• Diminished skin breakouts and inflammation • Plumper, smoother skin • Decreased rebound cravings and mood swings • Alleviated fibrocystic breast pain • Better sleep • Increased energy over time • Diminished under-eye puffiness • Healthier bones
Sugar Fix (Sugar includes honey, corn syrup, high-fructose corn sweeteners, grape-juice concentrate, dextrose, and other sweeteners)	• Sodas • Most bottled iced-tea drinks • Sweetened smoothies and shakes made with bananas or juice • Fruit juices • Sugar-sweetened drink mixes	• Smartly sweetened spritzers (see recipe, p. 60) • Bottled drinks (or diluted bottled drinks) with fewer than 5 grams of sugar (see Better Bottled Drinks, p. 66)	• Slimmer body • More refined face shape • Clearer skin • Decreased fungal-related afflictions, such as dandruff, and sinus and yeast infections

(continued on next page)

UPGRADE YOUR	FROM	TO	BEAUTY INCENTIVES
Sugar Fix *(continued)*		• Berry-based (not juice- or banana-based), smartly sweetened smoothies • Lemonade made with healthy smart sweeteners	• Victory over cravings • Restored alkaline balance • Prevention of wrinkles and brown (age) spots
Soda and Diet Drinks	• Sodas • Diet sodas • Powdered diet drink mixes • Caffeinated diet drinks and sodas (see also Caffeine Fix upgrades)	• Teas and lemonade made with smart sweeteners • Spritzers (see recipe, p. 60) or seltzer • Unsweetened or smartly sweetened bottled drinks (see "Better Bottled Drinks," p. 66)	• Stronger bones • Fewer sugar cravings • Possible elimination of methanol-related ailments, such as headaches and vision problems (see also Sugar Fix Beauty Incentives)
Thirst Quenchers	• Sweetened iced tea • Tap water	• Teas and herbal infusions, smartly sweetened • Purified water • Spritzers or seltzer	• Healthier skin • Improved body ecology and decreased digestive problems • Reduced chlorine risks

UPGRADE YOUR	FROM	TO	BEAUTY INCENTIVES
Creamy Drinks	• Milk • Commercial frozen coffee drinks • Lattes • Cocoa • Sweetened smoothies and shakes made with bananas	• Organic or raw milk or goat's milk • Unsweetened hemp or nut milk • Organic steamed milk with a chai tea bag • Lattes and frozen smoothies made with Teeccino or smartly sweetened cocoa • Smoothies, smartly sweetened (see Build a Perfect Smoothie, p. 74)	• Clearer skin • Stronger bones • Better digestion • Diminished under-eye circles and allergic responses • More stable energy and blood sugar

IT'S NOT ABOUT PERFECTION; IT'S WHAT YOU DEFAULT TO

What matters more than never doing bad things is what you default to on a regular basis. If you set up your daily routine in such a way that you have ready access to superior choices—and thus will make them on a regular basis—then the occasional times you stray from your routine aren't as important. You may have periods of backsliding on your road to palate development around the holidays or when traveling, but depending on how you prepare, the degree of backsliding can be minimized.

Occasionally reverting to your former choices will remind you of the physical reasons you left them behind and help you appreciate how far your palate and your body have come. Eventually, the benefits will replace any desire to go back.

PRACTICAL STRATEGIES MAKE ALL THE DIFFERENCE

Your best intentions will inevitably be affected by convenience and practical limitations imposed by your daily routines and environment. These limitations, not willpower, are the make-or-break factors. Fortunately, your intentions are easily supported with a little planning. The following tips will help you to visualize and plan a smooth transition through your first round of beverage upgrades. Once the logistics are worked out, you'll be well on your way to effortless and cumulative beauty benefits.

If you work at home all day, making changes will be relatively easy once you've gathered your initial upgrade supplies, which usually entails a trip to the health food store. You need to prepare your upgrades in advance so they are as convenient or even more accessible than your old choices were. If you work at an office or dart around town all day, you'll need to give more thought to your strategies for heading off unhealthy, convenience-based decisions. For example, if your office kitchen has a coffeemaker full of java at an arm's reach all day, you will get nowhere with your coffee upgrades unless you plan equally convenient and tempting strategies of your own. In order to begin to create your own beauty-friendly beverage routines from this day forward, ask yourself these questions:

- Which satisfying thirst quenchers will I keep in the fridge?
- When will I make them?
- Which of my favorite brews could I carry in a thermos?
- Should I carry my own tea bags?
- Do any nearby delis carry any of the better bottled drinks (see the sidebar on page 66) or hot teas I like?
- Should I keep smart sweeteners with me in my purse or my desk?
- Which beverages will be on the tip of my tongue when I order at restaurants, coffeehouses, bars, or delis?
- Will I remember to order spritzers instead of soda? Tomato juice or a "Virgin Mary" instead of orange juice at brunch?
- Is there a place in town to get fresh mixed green juice I can add a little smart sweetener to in the afternoon if I need an energy boost?
- Do I want to make "whole juice" for myself at home?
- Should I buy or bring some ingredients for smarter smoothies to work to have in the afternoon when everyone else is picking at the snack tray and jolting themselves with coffee?

MAKE YOUR BEVERAGE A BEAUTIFYING RITUAL

Consider turning your beverage habits into uplifting, self-affirming rituals. Your afternoon beverage is a good place to start. If you take some of the steps below—especially at the office—it won't be you who feels deprived as you indulge in your new beverage ritual.

- Choose a special place or time for your afternoon beverage ritual.
- Keep a gorgeous mug or beautiful tall glass reserved for the ritual.
- Arrange a source for pure water at work or bring bottles from home.
- Buy a personal electric teapot for your desk or bring in a beautiful Japanese pot with matching cups. Offer tea to colleagues in intimate meetings.
- Keep your fridge (or a mini-fridge at work) filled with pure water, organic half-and-half, cold herbal and green teas, iced Teeccino, seltzer, limes, and unsweetened cranberry juice.
- Keep your smart sweetener packets in a beautiful, convenient container.

On your first trip to the health food store, it may seem like you're spending more, but if you consider what you spent on your beauty-draining drinks and what you're saving on the future costs of not being well, you may find that you aren't spending more after all. Don't deprive yourself of the stuff that really makes your reflection and your life more vibrant. The dividends are high when you drink yourself beautiful.

CHAPTER 5

RECLAIM THE JOY OF EATING

A JOURNEY TO TRUE NOURISHMENT

Every body is different. My own perceptions and eating philosophies have run the gamut over the years, with a lot of irony in the outcomes. Having become a poster child for today's overweight and diseased norm at an early age—and gotten out alive and transformed—I wanted to share an abbreviated tour of my detour-filled journey to my own perfect way to eat.

Back when I moved to New York from Michigan and was introduced to what I've come to call real food, I became an enthusiastic vegetarian, living on salads with light dressings, steel-cut oatmeal, fresh juices, soy milk, low-fat dairy products, and tofu stir-fries—and bingeing on whole wheat pastas or brown rice and grainy desserts from my health food store bakery. I thought I'd surely found the healthiest foods to eat, as I did feel a huge difference from switching to whole grains from white flour products. I also thought I'd found the best way to minimize the consequences of my eating disorder. What I didn't know was how much this eating style was actually perpetuating the crazy blood sugar issues that played a central role in my food addiction.

There were two isolated incidents that served to crack a hardened core presumption that still unconsciously affected my food choices, even after my eating disorder was gone. The first took place in a hotel room. I was doing a makeup job in L.A. and got to my room too late for room service. Knowing I had to eat something, I winced at the horrid choices in the mini bar. As a person who was into whole grains, protein, and vegetables and was turned off by fake, hydrogenated foods, I knew I wouldn't be eating a candy bar for dinner. The only alternative was the jar of nuts. The concept of making a meal of nuts at the time was radical. If only there'd been an oatmeal cookie or a bran muffin in that minibar! Whole grains were my comfort zone. I opened the tall glass jar thinking I'd eat just a few nuts, and wound up eating most of the jar because I was truly hungry, accepting, but not fretting, about what would probably be the consequences the following day. The next morning, as I was getting dressed, I stopped and realized that my abdomen was flatter than it had been in *years*. And after almost a whole jar of nuts! I actually stood still thinking about this for a moment. I had dropped a lot of weight over the previous year after my eating disorder had fled, but I'd always had a bloated abdomen. Well, that morning the bloat was startlingly deflated. I wondered if it was something about the nuts, never giving thought to the concept that it might have been caused by something I *didn't* eat the night before (like my usual whole grain bread or pile of brown rice). Though I didn't understand what happened or jump to any conclusions, I never forgot that incident.

The second, and defining, incident was later that year back in New York one morning. I'd just made my weekly homemade loaf of flaxseed bread (I ground the grains myself). It didn't turn out well. Rather than throw the heavy brick out, I decided to toast a piece and maybe even butter it (something I never did) to see if it could be made palatable. It tasted good enough, so I wrapped up the remainder of the loaf and went on with my day. Within an hour I felt something different but couldn't put my finger on it. As lunch approached, it struck me that I wasn't as hungry as usual, even though I'd had only one piece of bread instead of my usual two. I thought the butter might have had something to do with it.

The next day, I actually buttered both sides of one piece of bread, just to see what would happen. I plunged into my day, but again, was struck by that same new feeling. By late morning it hit me. It wasn't so much something I was feeling as it was the sudden absence of the way I'd always felt after and between meals; that subtle lift, then the drag leading up to lunch. I had thought I'd left all those swings behind along with my eating disorder. But, while they were nothing like those post-binge knockouts I used to feel, I realized that day that even my so-called healthy whole-grain foods were still drugging me. I also noticed that my abdomen had deflated substantially again, after just two mornings of eating half the bread and much more fat. That was the day I stopped eating grains for breakfast and started an experiment with weaning off them completely, gauging my body's response every step of the way. Sure enough, the fewer I ate, the better I felt. When I did eat them, I learned to always eat them with or after fat or protein, and never on an empty stomach.

I soon stopped eating any low-fat dairy and started eating things like cheese, nuts, avocado, almond butter, thick Greek yogurt, and even half-and-half in my Earl Grey tea. And after seven years as a vegetarian (for what I thought were legitimate health reasons), I introduced some red meat back into my diet; and an unanticipated reaction to it told me that my body needed it again. The immediate boost in well-being was clear. In response to this evolution in my way of eating, I experienced a profound reduction in what I never realized was subtle swelling throughout my body. I had already become a very different-looking person from overcoming my eating disorder, but over the several months of eating this way, it was like another seven years peeled away. In all the years since, I have looked better and felt better than before my eating disorder developed in my teen years.

The miracle of being free of my eating disorder was still like a daily fantasy (it always will be), and yet this new level of peace and deep satiety and the ability to burn through fat—even after having trashed my metabolism— was a surreal thrill: like learning that Santa Claus existed after all. I could not explain this to others, but I couldn't easily dodge their questions about why my body and face were changing. I remember doing makeup for a photo shoot for the top fitness magazine in the world and trying to explain this to the nutrition editor. It was the early nineties, mind you. She was so disturbed by my then unheard-of views that she couldn't even talk to me for the rest of the shoot.

The typical breakfast served on photo shoots echoed this ingrained bias in thinking. Every day I watched models and editors pick incessantly at the pastry tray and fruit salad, never really satisfied. I sometimes had to resort to sneaking chunks of cream cheese or drinking half-and-half just to get any fat (there were rarely any eggs or unsweetened yogurt, which would have been great) while escaping the consequences of crazy-making sugar and flour.

These were not fat cravings but a *requirement* for fat I was feeling because, by that point, I was burning through it like rocket fuel. Whatever amount of it I ate, my hunger would always adjust itself automatically to what I needed at the next meal—I never counted calories or had to tell myself when to stop eating, and I never put on an ounce. If someone had seen me eat the cream cheese or drink half-and-half, they might have thought I was a freak, especially since I was pushing a size four. And as someone with formerly high triglycerides, it was incredible to see those levels way down at my first testing after eating the most fat I'd ever eaten in my life. My cholesterol even dropped to 112 at one point, which is a little too low, long after I started eating much more fat. For more than a decade, I have lived in complete freedom from worry about cravings, weight, fat grams, portion control, or calories.

My mirror seems to have stopped reflecting the signs of passing years. As I proceed to my forties, I am mistaken for someone in her twenties, someone who is one of those "naturally slim" people (like the ones whom I used to not like so much).

SEEKING SCIENTIFIC VALIDATION: HOW COME I FELT SO GOOD?

This dietary evolution—along with critical nutrient supplementation—completely freed me from what looked as though it would be a tormented, substantially shorter life. I wondered *why* it had done this, when all the nutritionists and government guidelines purported that my way of eating was harmful. I wanted to share what I'd learned with others, but not if it was dangerous or just a fluke!

A couple of years after overcoming my eating disorder, I watched Dr. John MacDougall and Dr. Barry Sears duke it out in a debate about their respective popular diets. Hearing MacDougall's low-fat recommendations was like a flashback to my compulsive past. For more than a decade, my cupboards were stocked with "damage-control" diet foods like fat-free soups and shake mixes, air-popped popcorn, and rice cakes. Throughout the 1990s, after my recovery, I started to see this all-you-can-eat-of-nothing approach—which I resorted to out of desperation from my disease—being recommended by registered dieticians everywhere as an ongoing way to eat, as if it were *healthy*.

Like clockwork, America's fat consumption went down for the first time in the eighties and nineties, and obesity, diabetes, and pre-diabetes skyrocketed as much as 70 percent in certain age groups. I knew exactly what was happening. The more desperately people clung to fat- and calorie-reduced foods to avoid their own obesity, the more ravenous they were becoming for true nourishment.

I eventually came across several areas of research that resonated with aspects of what I'd experienced. One was the findings of S. Boyd Eaton, MD. His research showed that pre-agricultural humans were free of modern diseases and lived on nuts, seeds, plants, some meat, and little or no grains. When hunting and gathering ended and grain, bean, and potato cultivation began, the health of humans declined. Though my approach differs on several counts from the Paleolithic diet, I suspect that it works for some of the same reasons. Another great find was the work of Weston A. Price, whose famous research on the healthy tribes of the world consistently revealed a traditional diet that included lots of natural fats and even animal fats. I learned from this body of research what I had suspected: that even butter has some amazing benefits, and that the way dairy and meat are produced makes all of the difference as to their fatty acid profile and how they are digested. Still, my eating approach differs in important ways from the traditionally modeled applications stemming from Price's work, not because those are inherently unhealthy (I only wish I'd grown up on such food!), but because the food addiction, weight, and metabolic issues I had developed required my evolution toward more specific strategies to avoid perpetuating them.

In the mid-nineties, I learned about the late Dr. Robert Atkins' diet. I was deeply grateful for his challenge to the establishment's fat-phobic status quo. Among those who knew him, it is highly debated as to whether Atkins had intended his approach to be morphed into the bacon-glorifying style of execution made so popular by his publishers, so I don't relish saying that my approach is much more health-focused and, materially, quite different.

By the late nineties, much of the published scientific literature became available online, allowing me to start piecing together support for what I already knew in my gut.

In the meantime, I had ironically risen to the upper ranks of the beauty world as a celebrity makeup artist and on-camera cosmetics company spokesperson after my weight loss. But in that capacity, I was never really able to talk about the real "beauty secrets" that had truly transformed me, and that I knew could transform many others. What made this more frustrating was the fact that the food and body issues that had made me an oddball in high school in the eighties were starting to appear in compounding numbers of people around me by the late nineties. Worst of all, the very advice that was being doled out as a solution by professionals was the way of eating that had locked in my own enslavement.

HOW THE FRAMINGHAM STUDY "FRAMED" FAT AND CHOLESTEROL

In the late nineties, I finally learned why most health professionals were promoting the false concept that fat (even saturated fat) was harmful. The famed Framingham Study, which tracked the health of residents in that Massachusetts city since the 1940s, was used by the indoctrinators of medical thought as a key validation of their cholesterol-causes-heart-disease campaign. The methods and interpretation of those study results, which most doctors refer to regularly, have turned out to be quite controversial if not embarrassing. Against glaring, more significant conclusions to the contrary, the establishment declared that dietary cholesterol consumption should be avoided based on one obscure, misinterpreted aspect of the study: the fact that overweight people who got heart disease had slightly higher cholesterol levels. But here's the unbelievable omission in the headlines: not only was higher cholesterol found to be entirely unrelated to diet, the study actually found that *people who ate the least fat and cholesterol had the highest cholesterol levels, were heavier, and were less active than those who ate the most saturated fat and cholesterol (and had the lowest blood levels of cholesterol!)*. You may find this hard to believe, as I did. But this study, which was made famous by the industries that could afford to exploit and distort its true findings for decades, should more aptly have been considered support for the statement that consumption of fats and cholesterol is not only harmless, but correlates with improved health and longevity. You can bet that this quote from the director of the study, Dr. William Castelli, in the *Archives of Internal Medicine* in 1992 was left out of margarine and cereal company press releases:

"In Framingham, Massachusetts, the more saturated fat one ate, the more cholesterol one ate, the more calories one ate, the lower people's serum cholesterol . . . we found that the people who ate the most saturated fat, the most cholesterol and the most calories weighed the least, were more physically active and had the lowest serum cholesterol levels."

DIETARY TRUTHS COME FULL CIRCLE

In summer of 2002, just as I was finishing the first edition of this book, the *New York Times* published Gary Taubes's powerful expose of the workings behind the low-fat myth, entitled "What If It's All Been a Big Fat Lie?" It caused an unprecedented ripple throughout the mainstream nutritional community by spotlighting the mounting evidence against the purported benefits of low-fat diets as well as their dangers. Among others, Taubes's interviewed Walter Willett, chairman of the department of nutrition at the Harvard School of Public Health and one of the representatives for the longest-term health and diet study ever performed. Willet pointed out that this largest-ever collection of data showed a startling and clear correlation between America's marked reduction in fat intake and the unprecedented rise in diabetes and obesity.

The natural food industry was a step ahead, already stocking low-carb foods, and was soon trumped by the convenience of low-carb aisles in supermarkets. But these new foods soon oversaturated the market and encountered distribution problems. Many of the companies went out of business for reasons never widely understood, with only a few online sources remaining. One reason may have been that low-carb foods are simply not as profitable because they do not resell themselves as well as addictive, empty foods do. Their very point is that they wean you off cravings and you automatically eat less of them. People who craved chips, for example, could buy low-carb chips and soon forget about them in their cupboard. Selling addiction-curing foods is like a doctor healing people: a very foreign concept to industries dependent on repeat business. Low-carb foods were no more profitable for food companies than they were for the medical industry.

In the meantime, the USDA, the American Dietetic Association, the American Heart Association, and every other medical establishment pelted the low-carb concept with disparaging commentary. Their continued, unsubstantiated health warnings actually succeeded in resuscitating the food and sickness industry-friendly fat phobia myths in spite of strong emerging science to the contrary.

In 2004, after the first edition of this book was published, I came across the work of Dr. Ron Rosedale, author of *The Rosedale Diet* and one of the foremost experts on insulin and the lesser-known hormone leptin. His research was the most revelatory validation of exactly what my eating evolved to; it was literally the scientific explanation of why I instinctively came to eat even more fat than "high protein" diets allow. It did not surprise me, once I learned of the uncanny similarities in our dietary approaches, that Rosedale's renowned clinic routinely reversed type II diabetes in less than a month with the same diet I'd arrived at. It turns out that any diet that halts blood sugar and insulin spikes also allows the cells to regain their sensitivity to the powerful anti-aging, weight- and hunger-regulating hormone leptin. But it is almost impossible to derive this effect without *generous amounts of fat in the diet*.

Flash forward to March 2007. After years of glorification of low-fat diets, the results of the only long-term study ever done comparing high-, moderate-, low-, and very low-carb diets was published in the prestigious *Journal of the American Medical Association (JAMA)*. "Very low-carb" eating (in this case, Atkins) had beaten out all others (including Ornish) for both weight loss and health outcomes in 311 post-menopausal women.

SHEDDING THE DEEPER LAYERS OF FAT PHOBIA

I've no doubt you've come a long way in your understanding of the benefits of "good fats" like omega-3s, olive oil, and nuts. But I'd like to take your fat myth shedding process a few steps further. Those of you who are vegetarian will find plenty of ways to implement my approach, but for those of you who avoid animal fats or saturated fats because you think it's the healthy thing to do, please consider these facts:

- **Higher fat intake correlates with weight loss.** Both of the afore-mentioned Framingham and *JAMA* dietary comparison studies—among many others—have shown a correlation between weight loss and higher-fat, low-glycemic diets. The body fat percentage and waist-hip ratios were better in very low-carb dieters than that of low-fat dieters in the *JAMA* study.
- **Unsaturated vegetable fat "clogs arteries"—*not saturated fat*.** Unsaturated and polyunsaturated vegetable fats make up 74 percent of what clogs arteries, according to a study published in the *Lancet*.

- **Dietary fat intake does not correlate with heart disease,** according to the 2006 Women's Health Initiative study of 48,835 older women. This was also echoed in the Framingham and aforementioned *JAMA* dietary comparison studies, which found improved blood lipid levels and reduced triglycerides in the higher-fat dieters.
- **Low cholesterol in the elderly correlated with dramatically higher death rates** as compared to those with high cholesterol in a study published in the *Journal of the American Geriatrics Society.*
- **Dairy foods reduced breast cancer risk in post-menopausal women with estrogen receptor-positive tumors** in one study, and it was higher intake of vegetable fats—not animal fat—that correlated with breast cancer, according to a large Swedish study.
- **Repeated large-scale studies** (including a 2002 study of 12,553 men published in the *American Journal of Cardiology*) have failed to confirm that dietary cholesterol (such as eggs) increases blood-cholesterol levels or heart disease. However, high-glycemic foods were shown to cause obesity and raise triglycerides, posing much more danger to your heart.
- **The inhabitants of Crete, who consume 10 percent more fat than any other Mediterranean people, have the least heart disease,** and elevated cholesterol did not correlate with those who had heart disease, which has led researchers to suggest a paradigm shift in the cholesterol theory of heart disease.
- **America's reduction of animal fat intake and increased hydrogenated vegetable fat intake correlated with the sharp rise in heart disease starting in the 1920s,** and with the heavy marketing of margarine and other hydrogenated foods.
- **Eating eggs for breakfast made overweight women crave and eat less** until lunch the next day, according to a study published in the *Journal of the American College of Nutrition.*
- **Adding red meat to a high-carb diet lowered blood pressure** in an Australian study.
- **Saturated fats are not merely "inflammatory" fats in the body.** To the contrary, they are critical to both anti-inflammatory and inflammatory functioning as needed in the body. They assist conversion of

healthy essential fatty acids (EFAs) in the body. Even arachidonic acid, often called a "bad fat," is completely critical for health and well-being.

One could fill an entire book with jaw-dropping evidence that the dietary-saturated-fats-are-bad myths are as fictitious as the decades-old, die-hard myths that eggs cause heart disease or that margarine is a heart-healthy food.

So, Why the Vendetta Against Fat?

Trade. Imagine the kind of power an industry must have had to convince us for a quarter of a century that (deadly) trans fats were healthier than (expensive, perishable) butter. Just like eggs and tropical oils, beef and animal products are fresh, whole food and therefore do not fit into the fake, processed, unlimited-shelf-life business model that makes the most profits for the food industry and even the personal care product industry. The cereal industry funded studies that wrongly distorted our view of eggs by using an adulterated form of egg powder in the "research." The trans fat industry used the same shenanigans in its "study" of incredibly healthy tropical oils, actually selling your mother on a better-living-through-chemistry killer that literally embalmed our food and our bodies in a free-radical bath for decades.

Population studies are notorious even among scientists for interpreting conclusions to benefit trade. A recent study linked meat eating with breast cancer, for example. Previous research had been inconclusive, and researchers admitted that other lifestyle factors common in meat eaters might have influenced the study results. It should also be noted that grain-fed, hormone-treated, and over-cooked or processed meats are much more commonly eaten than gently cooked, unprocessed, grass-fed meats. Well-done and processed meats have indeed been linked with increased cancer risk. It is unlikely that anyone will test unprocessed, properly cooked, or grass-fed meat's effects on health.

It's even more unlikely that they would study them in the context of a low-sugar diet. There would not be a population base to study! But it's worth mentioning that fats act very differently in the context of a sugar-, flour-, and trans fats-laden diet than they do in their absence. Take-home message: your trepidation regarding all those "bad" meats, eggs, salt, tropical fats—and even vitamins for that matter—comes almost invariably from the study of adulterated or processed versions of them.

I rest my case for fat with these bizarre thoughts: What if there were no bad fats in nature? What if the only bad fats are oxidized, hydrogenated, or otherwise adulterated fats? What if even basic pro-inflammatory, omega-6-laden, bleached, commercial corn oil were not inherently "bad" in its pre-adulterated, natural, virgin, cold-pressed state (we do need some omega-6 after all)? What if you were to find out that ALL unadulterated, natural, fresh fats—tropical, saturated, animal, or otherwise—are good in the right balance and that the only major correlation ever found between fats and disease was from fats that had been degraded or chemically altered by man?

My best advice for becoming impervious to the tiring mantras of archaic health advice is to develop your own "nonstick surface" against antifat ignorance and other types of "Better Living Through Chemistry" propaganda. It was only by *rejecting* every commonly held piece of dietary "wisdom" we are pounded with—to avoid animal fats, dairy, eggs, tropical oils, butter, chocolate, and supplements, and eat lots of whole grains—that I was finally able to achieve the only complete freedom I have ever known from obesity, disease, skin, and mood problems. Let my drawn-out, dangerous journey be your shortcut to the truth.

MORE IS MORE

I'm not focused on tricking myself into
eating fewer calories, but on finding ways
to give my body more.

People want to know what I eat on a daily basis. Ironically, one would think that someone who turned around a life of out-of-control bingeing and food obsession might have become a master at restraint and self-deprivation. But that is what got me into trouble in the first place. Today, I have no use for depleted or low-fat foods. I view each meal as therapy for both my senses and my body on a cellular level. I'm not focused on tricking myself into eating fewer calories, but on finding ways to give my body more. Why stop at luscious Greek yogurt when I can add berries and nuts and maybe some whey protein or pure cocoa powder? Why stop at a dark green salad, when

I can cover it not only with olive oil but also with goat cheese, blueberries, red onion, and walnuts? Why limit yourself to a certain number of eggs per week or cook them without the yolks or butter when there is zero scientific support for doing so? Why avoid salt if the salt you're using actually gives your body minerals, rather than depleting you and throwing your fluid balance out of whack? Why go out to dinner when you can bond with your family or your "inner alchemist" in the kitchen? Why not serve far more beautifying foods at home, such as quick, aromatic sauces made with organic ingredients over grass-fed meats, uncontaminated fish, or healthier pastas or pilafs made from foods that no restaurant even offers? Why not enjoy "special occasion" treats, like dark chocolate fondues and exotic berries or nut butters on a regular basis? And finally, why would you not want to give up foods that harm, deplete, and interrupt your thriving process—forever?

Because my body is so well nourished, it is no longer led by cravings and no longer compels me to eat too much (whereas that's what it once *demanded* I do). I have no need to measure my portions or tell myself to stop eating; it just happens. I don't feel "full" after a meal, even though I eat all I want. Full-fat foods no longer feel heavy or too rich to me like they did when I was overweight and eating lots of breads and grains. I burn through them easily now, even though I exercise far less than the hours and hours per week I did during the years when I couldn't burn any fat to save my life. For more than a decade now, satiety has been a kind of amazing, comfortable, non-sedating, nonbloating, great feeling that carries no sensation in my stomach other than total contentment. You know that this is not coming from one of those "naturally thin people with a high metabolism." I shot my metabolism long ago. Every meal drugged me and made me heavier for most of my life. This is a miracle. And I want you to experience it!

A precious few doctors and nutritionists are aware that such a state—with no "shoulds" or ongoing self-discipline to avoid weight gain—exists even in "normal" people. Boot camp-style reality shows whose ratings thrive on portraying the eternal self-discipline and emotional strength required for beauty and slimness are also unlikely to feature a smarter approach, where the science of nutrition does the transforming on a cellular level with only a change in strategy, and without a lot of drama.

SAVE YOUR BEAUTY AND YOUR SANITY: MY LOW-IMPACT APPROACH

In today's blood sugar-spiking, caffeine-jolting, cortisol-pumping, high-impact world, part of the needed sanctuary from harm to ourselves—and the only way of eating that ever gave me biochemical "peace" and turned my self-destruction around—is a nutrient-rich, non-blood sugar-spiking diet that never kicks the "pendulum" into swing. It's what I call "low-impact" eating.

Low-impact eating is the perfect antidote to a high-impact world. No self-respecting doctor would deny that it's never a good thing to spike one's blood sugar. One of my key food principles is avoiding the consequences of addictive "high-impact" foods, while strategically satisfying cravings for them in revolutionary new ways. Beyond minimizing impact on blood sugar, what distinguishes my approach is its focus on deep nourishment and the true resolution of cravings. It blurs the line between health and indulgence in some very unique ways. It also does as much for your mind and spirit as it does for your body and looks. Low-impact eating, along with targeted nutritional supplements (more on that to come), completely freed me not only from my "incurable" health and skin problems, but from every last negative issue I had with food.

On the other hand, a high-impact (blood sugar-spiking) diet—particularly when coupled with inadequate nutrients—not only guarantees weight, skin, and premature aging problems (a scientific connection was recently made between insulin spikes and shorter lifespan!); it leads to increasing energy swings and very real-feeling, unsettled emotions and cravings. If such imbalances progress as they did in my case, they can lead to deficiencies in the "feel-good" brain chemicals like serotonin and dopamine. Blood sugar swings are even associated with several addictions. Low-fat diets are often similar to high-impact, high-glycemic diets, since reduced fat invariably means increased carbs and protein. On the mental health front, low-fat diets were associated with psychological problems, including depression, violence, fatigue, and even suicide, in a study published in the *Lancet*.

This is not to say that some people don't feel just fine eating low-fat diets and lots of whole grains. Anyone who is very physically active or has an unspoiled metabolism (meaning they weren't raised on sodas and white flour) may do fine, and may find that they have more latitude in the eating guidelines ahead. But even if you believe you fall into that category, I strongly recommend you try my purest approach for at least two weeks to see how you feel. If you're like most people you will discover you were actually addicted to your rice, grain, and other high-impact fixes after all. And if you currently "get spiked" (peak, then crash after eating) on a regular basis, I will wager that the physical and quality-of-life rewards you'll reap by going low-impact will be as powerful as any step you've ever taken toward physical self-transformation.

FEELING VS. COUNTING: GIVE UP THE FALSE SECURITY OF NUMBERS

Many people expect to be conscious of calories, fat, or carb grams for the rest of their days. I once had "calories per serving" committed to memory for just about every food you could think of, but I haven't counted calories for over a decade. You may be familiar with the term "low-glycemic." The glycemic index (GI) is the measure of a food's, impact on blood sugar levels in the body. The obvious high-glycemic foods such as pasta, starchy vegetables (such as potatoes and corn), and conventional candies, desserts, and baked goods, include white flour or sugar. Low-glycemic foods cause a slower rise in blood sugar than do high-impact ones and tend to be low in sugar and higher in protein, fat, fiber, and nutrients that satisfy the body longer and more authentically. So why don't I just call my approach low-carb or low-glycemic eating? Because adhering to a daily total carb limit or sticking with low GI-rated foods will not protect most people from blood sugar spikes, and says nothing of how well you are nourishing yourself. I don't memorize the GI ratings of various foods, much less the tricky calculation of "glycemic load." These things have great value in research, but I find that they can be misleading if applying universal guidelines for people. Blood sugar spikes happen at different thresholds for different people. Many factors, from your cells' sensitivity to insulin to the combination, order, and even speed at which you eat or drink foods, can affect how foods impact your blood sugar. What really matters is the impact a given food or meal has on YOU, and your ability to recognize when that threshold of being "spiked" has been crossed; and you can only do that if you relearn how it feels to be free of those reactions for at least a week or two. Reinforce this process with deep nourishment and incredible taste and you have a combination that is nothing short of miraculous.

There's something very powerful about being so free of mood and energy swings that you learn to instantly recognize—and no longer like—the old feeling you were once addicted to. Once you have reached this point, with proper nutritional reinforcement, you will be home free, and your calorie- and fat gram-counting days (and your days of feeling and looking like something that was never intended by nature) will be over.

THE "CLOSE, BUT NO CIGAR" DIETS: PROLONGING CAPTIVITY

Many so-called low-glycemic approaches still allow for frequent spikes in blood sugar with grains, starchy vegetables, beans, sweet fruits, and natural sweeteners such as honey. For most people, these diets prolong the low-grade, continued agitation of what I call "threshold eating," where the sugar pendulum never fully stops swinging, and thus keeps low-grade addictions and biochemical impediments to fat-burning alive and well, even if you don't have major food or weight problems.

It's key to understand that people with healthy metabolisms (a shrinking minority now in America), who did not grow up eating junk or drinking soda, may do okay on these plans, but those who will likely fall victim to the close-but-no-cigar, so-called low-glycemic diets are those who have weight, food, or even subclinical metabolic issues (which are common, even in thin people). For those people, each blood sugar spike is like a reintroduction of a drug they need to kick, putting the pendulum into swing again, effectively requiring a restart of the "sugar detox" process. The person might feel much better in comparison to eating a junk food diet, but will never achieve the level of peace I'm talking about.

I remember making that shift to whole grains, even during my eating disorder, and it was amazing how much better I felt. But I still had no idea what complete freedom was or that even those "healthy" whole grains, beans, and brown rice would soon come to replace the more obvious drug-foods I'd cut out of my diet. It was only once I was off the "drug" (sugar spikes) completely that I understood what freedom, effortless slimness, and the perfect relationship with food really were. Again, those who need sanctuary from blood sugar–spiking (B.S.) foods the most are the very people who tend to exploit the loopholes in the close-but-no-cigar diets in order to get their "fix." With my strategy, these foods are not only omitted, but sneakily upgraded with amazing, little-known foods that "scratch" the same "itches" without the biochemical consequences.

Any approach that allows for ANY blood sugar spikes on other than very rare occasions will keep you struggling with continued cravings and progression (though perhaps more slowly) toward metabolic disease. The rebound effects of these spikes also make weaning off your desire for druglike foods much harder than it needs to be, while keeping you burning primarily sugar and storing fat. Endocrinology 101, as Dr. Rosedale calls it. The close-but-no-cigar diets keep you searching for cravings control and energy fixes. With my approach, keeping energy up becomes a nonissue. You will finally understand what it's like to be free of energy dips, thoughts of food between meals, weight gain, and other discomforts many of us take for granted as "normal."

IS THIS ONE OF THOSE "EXTREME" DIETS?

If extremism is measured by how far we deviate from the diet thrust in front of us today, than I am certainly extreme. But the food choices your doctor should panic about are the seemingly "normal" choices the average "healthy" eater makes every day. Before the dawn of the last century, man never had to dodge the constant arm's-length convenience of liquid sugar, cheap vegetable oils, and heaps of grain-based foods all day, every day. The real extremism of my approach is in the total sanctuary it provides from constant assaults and depleted foods we humans were never meant to endure.

Of course, anyone with a health condition should talk with his or her doctor before making any dietary changes. I encourage you to weigh the scientific support for any eating plan you adopt (do see the medical references and educational resources at the back of this book, and show your doctor if he questions what you've learned here). Medical opinion is often based on scant nutritional study and a healthy dose of industry bias. I've heard a lot of parroted health mantras, such as "cutting out grains could hurt you," which has been proven false by history (humans were healthier before grains were widely eaten). Presumably, this alert is sounded because some people would get no fiber if it weren't for whole grains. But there are so many wiser ways to get fiber, which brings me to another equally ridiculous myth: that eating a very low-glycemic diet means you must not be eating any carbs. It is the "fiber carbs" that have historically made up the majority of the human diet (before processed foods and degenerative disease were introduced). Fiber carbs are central to my approach because they have the least impact on blood sugar and because they include so many tasty super-foods you may not even have tried, such as hemp seed and salba (tasty grainlike seeds), or konjac root pasta (great for Asian dishes with zero impact on blood sugar). More familiar fiber carb beauty foods include low-sugar fruits like berries and coconut and dark greens, among many other nutrient-dense vegetables. When accompanied by plenty of first-rate fats and proteins, they're even more nutritious. You've probably been eating many of these things already. The biggest difference here is what you won't be eating—or missing—at all.

THE LOW-IMPACT PRINCIPLE WILL UPGRADE ANY DIET

A heightened vigilance against blood sugar spikes can optimize the benefit from almost any diet, whether vegan, macro, raw, blood type, gluten-free, dairy-free, you name it. Even the official diets for heart disease and diabetes were found to be inferior to very low-glycemic diets in the aforementioned *JAMA* study. Low-glycemic diets are widely believed to be the optimal diet for epilepsy and polycystic ovarian syndrome (PCOS) as well.

Show me anyone who pooh-poohs these principles, and I'll show you someone who is either sick and getting sicker, someone who rarely ate bad foods growing up (and has an intact metabolism), or someone who obsessively disciplines themselves over their own food cravings and prides themselves on their boot camp routine at the gym.

Why am I so intense about this low-impact thing? Because any beauty approach that overlooks this aspect will deprive you of the most powerful opportunity to transform your reflection and your quality of life.

ARE YOU READY TO GET OFF THE RIDE?

I call it the pendulum. You can call it the roller coaster, the merry-go-round, or the Matterhorn. The important thing is to get off it. Once you do, you'll find yourself on a new continuum toward the potential nature truly intended for you. I propose you give yourself one, or better yet, two weeks off the pendulum, so you can feel what its like, regain your basic "food sanity," and come fully to your senses about what is good for your body.

I promise you this: there is not anything I will encourage you to deny yourself in terms of taste or types of food experiences. But I will show you how you can upgrade the foods you love, so that they don't hurt you anymore, by converting the old druglike, beauty-robbing foods into far more satisfying, body-loving indulgences.

CHAPTER 6

YOUR KITCHEN CABINET MAKEOVER

In this chapter, you won't find any rigid rules or absolutes, and there will be no need for self-denial (giving up empty or fake food for real treats is not self-denial). This is a chapter about giving yourself more. My approach with you—because it was the only one that finally worked for me—is to appeal to a long-neglected instinct deep within you: the ability to spontaneously make the wisest, most satisfying, and most beautifying food choices in any given situation, based on what your body tells you it really wants once you allow its true signals to return. You're about to learn how to cultivate a joyful, love-love relationship with food that will beautify your body, awaken your senses, and feed your soul with each upgrade you make.

But before we get to the exciting food upgrades ahead, let's quickly review the top food assaults to shed.

DEAD MATTER THAT STEALS YOUR VITALITY

Sugar and White Flour

You know all about sugar's cruel but seductive cycle of cravings, crashes, and weight gain, so I'll summarize the other little stones along the sugary trail to beauty devastation: Sugar causes insulin resistance. Sugar feeds cancer cells, which thrive on glucose. Sugar can cause varicose veins. Sugar feeds candida yeast. Sugar compromises your immune system for hours after you eat it. Sugar wrinkles your skin and ages your entire body. Sugar causes inflammation and

---

MERRIAM-WEBSTER ONLINE'S DEFINITION OF FOOD:

1 **a** : material consisting essentially of protein, carbohydrate, and fat used in the body of an organism to **sustain growth, repair, and vital processes and to furnish energy; also : such food together with supplementary substances (as minerals, vitamins, and condiments) b** : inorganic substances absorbed by plants in gaseous form or in water solution

2 : **nutriment** in solid form (FYI, here's the definition of nutriment: **something that nourishes or promotes growth, provides energy, repairs body tissues, and maintains life**)

3 : **something that nourishes, sustains, or supplies**

---

fluid retention. Sugar raises your triglyceride levels. Sugar depletes nutrients in the body, such as chromium, which keep you lean and stabilize your blood sugar. In fact, sugar is what makes sugar fattening. I think you get it now. White flour is readily converted to sugar in the body. Many people who claim they don't have a sweet tooth satisfy their sugar addiction with white flour-based breads and pastas, which cause the same devastation as sugar.

Hydrogenated Fat (Trans Fats)

By now I'm sure you know that trans fats are bad stuff, but it's worth noting the scenario under which we were misled, so as not to be so easily fooled in the future. For decades before the FDA finally required food manufacturers to list trans fat content on food labels, they assured us that margarine was heart-healthy food. But the American Heart Association had been informed that trans fats were more dangerous than butter (butter is not actually dangerous, by the way) but continued to put its stamp of health approval on them. Several other countries had outlawed them up to a decade earlier.

In case you didn't know, trans fats give your body a free-radical bath every time you eat them and block precious essential fatty acid (EFAs) uptake in the cells—wreaking havoc on hormone activity and causing inflammation, according to Udo Erasmus, PhD, author of *Fats That Heal, Fats That Kill*.

Unfortunately, the new required labeling honors trans fats with the implication that they are actually food; but there is no safe level of daily intake of trans fats.

Additives, Preservatives, and "Excitotoxins"

Additives won't be much of an issue once you start to make the food upgrades in this chapter, but a little added incentive to avoid them during the weaning process can't hurt. Additives can trigger allergic reactions, headaches, and even long-term neurological problems.

Sulfites, commonly found in wines, dried fruit, and salad bar foods, are sometimes used to preserve food at restaurants, where the law requires a posted notice of its use, although this law is often unheeded. Sulfites trigger mild to severe reactions in sensitive people, as can monosodium glutamate (MSG), known as an excitotoxin because it can overstimulate brain cells and trigger migraines, according to Russell L. Blaylock, MD, author of *Excitotoxins: The Taste That Kills*. "Hydrolyzed vegetable protein" is just another alias for MSG and is found in canned and prepared foods and gravy mixes. Aspartame is another well-known excitotoxin. Nitrates in bacon and other cured meats are carcinogens. Red dye #3, used in maraschino cherries, fruit cocktail, and some baked goods, has been shown to cause thyroid tumors in rats, according to a 1983 review committee report requested by the FDA.

If it never goes bad, it can't make you beautiful.

The healthiest, most revitalizing foods spoil the quickest. If it never goes bad, it was never good to begin with. And it can't make you beautiful.

BECOME A FOOD SNOB, FOR BEAUTY'S SAKE

Now you know. Food is not beauty's enemy. Empty, fake food is. "Virtual food" that has had oils and nutrients stripped, oxidized, or cooked out of it deprives your body and desensitizes your tastes while sensitizing your skin, sapping your vitality, and creating cravings that can't be satisfied. Stop eating "light" and start eating *well*. And if demanding real food is being "high-maintenance" or makes you a "food snob," then by all means, become one! It's one of the most

MYTH: *A calorie is a calorie.*

TRUTH: *It's not the calorie count; it's the calorie kind.*

The mantra that a calorie is a calorie, or even that calorie intake vs. calories burned is the ultimate determiner of your shape, is shockingly false. To explain away the weight loss most people experience when they stick with low-glycemic foods, most medical professionals will tell you that it's because people eat fewer calories on low-carb diets. And while most people (especially food addicts) will lose their cravings and binge less, and indeed eat fewer calories on a low-impact diet, several studies have shown that more than calorie reduction is at work here. Several studies have shown that groups of subjects lost more weight while eating equal, or even *more* calories (in the context of a low-glycemic diet) than their study group counterparts who ate fewer high-carb calories. In Dr. Barry Sears' classic book, *The Zone*, he refers to a landmark study published in the *Lancet* nearly fifty years ago showing that patients eating high-fat diets lost significant weight, while the high-carb eaters on *the same number of calories* lost none. A 2003 study of adolescents published in the *Journal of Pediatrics* was even more shocking, in that those in the 12-week controlled trial who ate *50 percent more low-carb calories* lost more weight than the lower-calorie consuming low-fat diet eaters. Yet another controlled trial that same year, published in the *Journal of Nutrition*, found that in two groups of women who ate an almost equal number of calories and fat, the group that ate higher protein and fewer carbs lost more weight. The *kind* of calories we eat, and their hormonal effects (namely on insulin and leptin), are the real determining factors not only in our predisposition for weight gain, but also in our cravings, energy, premature aging (via glycation), and quality of life.

beautiful things you can do for yourself. Real food should be just as accessible as a restroom and running water, and you should assert your need for it without apology.

MYTH: *A nutritionist is a nutritionist is a nutritionist.*

TRUTH: *Nutritionists who are focused on calories and fat grams won't address your deeper issues.*

Clinical—as opposed to holistic—nutrition still largely discounts the role of food, and especially supplements, as healing tools. It continues to downplay the distinction between fresh, whole foods and dead foods containing harmful ingredients like poor-quality vegetable fats.

Is your nutritionist hip? If you're getting talk about calories, egg-white omelets, fat (and even saturated fat) avoidance, RDAs, or the Food Guide Pyramid and not much else, you're not getting the information that can heal you. If statistics are any indication, most of you reading this would not do well on many of the foods on the average registered dietician's "eat more of . . ." list. Conventional wisdom, such as "everything in moderation," will not work for the pre-diabetic majority.

Once you become accustomed to true sustenance, your body will crave it, and then be utterly satisfied. It fulfills a deep need like no brightly packaged, hydrogenated piece of technology ever could.

SHIFT MORE OF YOUR BEAUTY BUDGET TO BEAUTIFYING FOODS

There's no doubt that beautifying, life-enhancing foods are more expensive than beauty-robbing ones. While my top recommendations in this book are to know about and buy the best foods you can afford, there's no need to break the bank in the process. The most important initial goal, even if you can't buy everything organic, is to get off the sugar pendulum and start evolving your palate. The money-saving benefits will start to roll in from there. I do recommend that you reallocate some of your beauty and health spending to the area where you will really see a result: what goes into your body. Deeply nourishing food is one of the few beauty splurges that actually works. Here are some considerations:

- *By eating higher quality food, you will wind up eating less food, because as nourishment deepens and blood sugar swings are halted, cravings diminish.*
- *Low-impact snacks you bring from home can save you the money and the sickness bills typical convenience snacks will cost you.*
- *Your alcohol craving will only diminish from here. This will save money, not to mention your looks, your vision, and your health.*
- *Cooking more often and eating out less equal money saved to buy better food.*
- *You'll save money on new clothes because your weight will be lower and more stable.*
- *Eggs save money over cereal; they're the best nutritional bang for the buck.*
- *Full-fat products save money over reduced-fat ones because they are filling.*
- *Homemade spritzers save money and health over sugar-packed juices.*
- *Dehydrate your own flax crackers for an inexpensive snack. Use the herbs you like.*
- *Forego a new lipstick for three bottles of good culinary oil.*
- *Find a better wireless plan so you can switch to organic.*
- *Trade an expensive outfit for half a year of home-delivered wild seafood or grass-fed foods.*
- *Use canned organic tomato instead of prepared tomato sauce for a big savings.*
- *Frozen organic berries are often cheaper and riper than fresh. Keeping berries frozen until you need them saves waste.*
- *Bulk raw nuts are cheaper and fresher than those in cans. Mix in a few roasted or tamari almonds to give them more than enough flavor.*
- *Pumpkin seeds are cheaper than nuts. Toast a bunch in the oven on foil with a little oil, spices, and good salt, like Real Salt, until puffy. Keep in the fridge and sprinkle on salads, or carry them during travel and eat them at the movies instead of popcorn. (Sneak in your own flavored seltzer as well and you've saved six bucks right there!)*
- *Hemp seed is a terrific all-purpose extender for meals and leftover sauces.*
- *Making large batches of favorite low-impact meals saves time and money.*
- *Sidestepping diabetes and lifelong skin, weight, and food issues: priceless.*

MYTH: *A beautiful body means deprivation and the end of decadence.*

TRUTH: *A beautiful body means the end of deprivation and the beginning of a new kind of decadence: pure, real food.*

Many people think of decadence as "letting go" and bingeing on fake foods that start their bodies and moods on a roller coaster of biochemical cravings and emotional guilt. They consider a full plate of full-fat, nutrient-dense, freshly prepared food off limits or extravagant. But every person—and every *body*—deserves such treatment. And you won't believe what it can do for your looks, your spirit, and your relationship with food.

Here's a taste of decadence: plump blackberries in organic, full-fat yogurt; sugar-free Belgian dark chocolate; delicate organic baby lettuces or locally grown, hand-picked heirloom tomatoes drizzled with walnut oil; exotic mushrooms and fresh herbs; arugula and goat cheese with slices of exotic pears; crisp wedges of Granny Smith apples dipped in raw, organic almond butter; organic black mission figs covered with thick Greek yogurt; free-range chicken sausage with sage and apples; ripe avocado slices, laced with Scotch Bonnet Hot Sauce, on moist, sprouted, nutty hemp seed bread; grass-fed cheese fondue with chunks of pear or midnight chocolate fondue with sour cherries. I hope I'm making your mouth water. I defy you to wolf down foods such as these. They make you slow down. I've been known to moan with delight while eating these foods. Eating the old empty foods— *that* was deprivation. Treat yourself to the most decadent foods in the world. Giving up the old empty foods and their consequences will easily offset the cost.

UPGRADE YOUR BREAKFAST TO RESET YOUR WHOLE DAY

Upgrading your breakfast to a low-impact one is one of the most powerful ways to transform how you look and feel in the short and long term. Upgrading juice and breads to eggs, or smartly sweetened yogurt with berries, or the Perfect Smoothie (see page 74) can put an end to the energy swings that dominate many peoples' lives and choices. Eggs, for example, have not only been vindicated of their supposed relationship with heart disease, they have also been found to cause people who eat them for breakfast instead of high-impact foods to eat substantially less food (up to forty percent fewer calories) until lunch the next day.

In addition, a 2006 study found that the pigments that contribute to the color of the egg yolk, called lutein and zeaxanthin, increased skin hydration 38 percent when taken as a daily 10 mg supplement. Lipid levels and elasticity of the skin also significantly increased, while oxidation of the skin lipids was inhibited. The lecithin and phospholipids in egg yolks also happen to be amazing for the skin, arteries, and the rest of the body. All this and eggs will never spike your blood sugar. Never overcook them. Order them soft and a little wet, never with golden brown edges. Poaching or hard-boiling are healthy ways to eat them. I eat nearly a dozen eggs a week.

IS ORGANIC FOOD WORTH THE PRICE? WONDER NO MORE.

It's proven now. Organic produce offers greater health benefits than conventional equivalents. Confirmation of what most people suspected came in March 2007. Organic kiwi—grown side-by-side with conventional kiwi in a controlled study by researchers at the University of California, Davis—was found to have "significantly higher" levels of polyphenols, vitamin C, and other antioxidants. Similar results were found with organic tomatoes. In 2002, the USDA standardized the requirements so that all products labeled as organic must be produced without hormones, antibiotics, pesticides, synthetic fertilizers (including sewage sludge), irradiation, or genetically modified ingredients. Organic meat must come from animals that eat only organic feed, meaning it hasn't been treated with hormones or antibiotics. The animals must also have access to the outdoors with protection from excessive heat and cold when needed. In other words, they must be treated humanely.

Six More Reasons to Buy Organic

No Pesticides

In 2006, researchers from Emory University in Atlanta found that eating an organic diet "provides a dramatic and immediate protective effect against dietary exposure to organophosphorus pesticides." The study found immediate rises in urinary concentration of metabolites with two common organophosphate pesticides, a class of chemicals known for their neurological effects on humans. As stated earlier, if you eat meat and dairy products and can buy only a few organic items, make meat and dairy products the ones you buy organic, as pesticides collect in animal fat. Whether your produce is organic or not, always use a "veggie wash" spray from the health food store to clean them. Rinsing isn't sufficient.

No Growth Hormones

The problems associated with meat and dairy are man-made, not inherent to naturally raised products. A prime example is the Recombinant Bovine Growth Hormone (rBGH), a genetically modified drug, which has been injected into conventional dairy cows since it was approved in 1993 despite warnings against such approval by the General Accounting Office; the Consumer Policy Institute of the Consumers Union, the nonprofit group that publishes *Consumer Reports* magazine; and countless other consumer and environmental groups. A more recent study correlated mothers who ate the most conventionally raised beef with sons who had lower sperm counts. The researchers from the University of Rochester Medical Center pointed to the growth hormones the cows were treated with as a possible reason for the outcome.

IGF-1, a key growth hormone that has been linked to breast and prostate cancers, may have a greater presence in hormone-treated meats and dairy. In addition to the unknown risks to humans, there are known consequences of rBGH on both the cows and the foods we eat. Because one of the common side effects of rBGH is mastitis (udder infection), additional antibiotics must be used in conventional milk production. The antibiotics and pus from the infection are commonly introduced into milk as a result of the infections. I'll bet that extra dollar you didn't want to pay for organic milk doesn't sound so unreasonable now.

No Antibiotics

In the early 1990s, *Consumer Reports* tested milk samples and found fifty-two different antibiotics commonly used to treat mastitis in cows. The Union of Concerned Scientists, a nonprofit group in Washington, D.C., estimated that more antibiotics are used to treat healthy animals in the United States than sick humans. Antibiotics are also widely used as growth promoters in conventional meat production and—many farmers believe—as a substitute for sanitary conditions and thorough inspections. This practice is of great concern among scientists and government agencies because such overuse of antibiotics can give rise to strains of drug-resistant bacteria.

For more information and documentation on antibiotics and rBGH in dairy, poultry, and meat production, contact the Consumer Policy Institute of the Consumers Union (see Resources).

No Irradiation

Foods are irradiated to kill microorganisms and stop the ripening process. Irradiation has been shown to

- Reduce nutrients in food
- Halt enzyme activity in food, which the body needs
- Form toxic byproducts, such as benzene and formaldehyde
- Cause chemicals used on the food to form completely new, foreign chemicals called unique radiolytic products (URPs) with unknown effects

No Sewage Sludge

Instead of the compost used in organic farming, conventional foods in the United States can be grown in a mudlike byproduct from sewage treatment plants, which, because it was considered hazardous, was banned by the government in the early 1990s from being dumped into oceans. Aside from the sheer disgustingness of the concept, the problem is that industrial and domestic hazardous waste and chemicals survive the sewage treatment process. In 1990, the EPA stated that sewage sludge "may include volatiles, organic solids, nutrients, disease-causing pathogenic organisms, heavy metals, inorganic ions, and toxic organic chemicals from industrial wastes, household chemicals, and pesticides."

No Genetically Modified Organisms (GMOs)

In March 2007, the first independent research on a GMO corn product approved for humans revealed "signs of hepatorenal toxicity" (that's liver and kidney toxicity). Researchers stated that "with the present data it cannot be concluded that GM corn MON863 is a safe product." Unlike the citizens of most other countries, Americans are largely unaware that much of the food they eat contains GMOs, particularly because GM corn is ubiquitous in processed foods and soft drink sweeteners. Field and lab tests reported by the Organic Consumers Association show that:

- GMOs have caused farmers to use two to five times more herbicides than in conventional seed farming.
- GMOs have created antibiotic-resistant genes. These genes are found in all GMOs. A study by researchers at the University of Newcastle-upon-Tyne showed that GMOs can transfer DNA into the bacteria of the digestive tract, so animals and humans ingesting GMOs are likely to incubate increasingly virulent pathogens as well as antibiotic-resistant organisms. (Until this recent study, the makers of GMOs denied this possibility.)
- GMOs have been found to yield herbicide-resistant super-weeds in Canada.
- GMOs have shifted delicate ecological balances, so formerly minor pests are becoming major problems. In 1999, researchers at Cornell University found that pollen from genetically modified corn was poisonous to monarch butterflies, while in a British study, rats fed genetically modified potatoes suffered damage to their vital organs and immune systems.

Not All Organic Is Really Organic

Starting around 2004, there has been a great change in the organic industry, with big companies entering the scene. Some have lobbied successfully to loosen standards, so industry giants could meet lower organic standards and still earn the seal on their labels. The best way to avoid supporting organic companies that actually threaten the cause of organic is to buy from companies that support independent farmers (rather than their demise) such as your local organic producers, as well as cooperative companies made up of networks of family farms such as Organic Valley. Supporting true organics is important. Learn more about who is and isn't true at the Organic Consumer Association's highly respected website www.organicconsumers.org. Its free newsletter is a must-read and one of the most important on the state of our food supply.

UPGRADE YOUR FISH TO SAFE AND SUSTAINABLE

According to the Council for Responsible Nutrition, at least 40 percent of American adults are deficient in omega-3 fats. Deep-sea, cold-water fish—if you can avoid contaminated varieties—is rich in omega-3 EFAs, which are great for your heart, your skin, and everything in between. Salmon is one of the foods highest in omega-3 fatty acids. In *The Perricone Prescription*, Dr. Nicholas Perricone asserts that the DMAE in salmon firms the skin by raising levels of key neurochemicals.

Cold-water fish such as salmon, mackerel, herring, and sardines are great beauty food, but avoid farm-raised fish, which are not a good source of EFAs and are rarely pure. Farm-raised fish are often artificially colored with feed additives, treated with antibiotics because of unsanitary conditions, and higher in pesticides. A 2007 study found persistent organic pesticides (POPs) in contaminated fish to be correlated with increased risk of insulin resistance, a precursor to diabetes. There is also the concern of mercury contamination. A 2005 Finish study actually found that middle-aged men who ate the most fish had added risk of heart trouble, and men who had the most mercury in their hair were found to be eating at least two times the fish of the men with normal mercury levels. Ironically, excess mercury can cause hair loss.

Environmental groups count wild Alaskan salmon (not Atlantic salmon, which is usually farmed), sablefish, sardines, anchovies, and halibut among the most sustainable, least contaminated high-omega-3 varieties, while shark, swordfish, Chilean sea bass, and orange roughy are high in mercury or PCBs and often overfished. Fish sustainability is very fragile and ever-changing, so it is important to ask questions at the fish market and be wary of culinary trends that could wipe out certain species. Fortunately, the fish oil supplement industry has little impact on fish population because it utilizes small fish, like sardines, and comprises only 2 to 3 percent of the global supply. You can find up-to-date information on sustainability and contamination levels of a variety of fish at www.oceansalive.org. You can also have wild Alaskan salmon and other premium sustainable fish delivered to you anywhere in the country through mail-order sources such as www.vitalchoice.com or through Eco Fish retailers and restaurants near you (find them by visiting www.ecofish.com). Encourage your market and local restaurants to carry only sustainable, safe fish!

A FISHY SOLUTION: OMEGA-3-FORTIFIED FOODS AND BEVERAGES

2006 was a galvanizing year for both public and scientific acceptance of the miraculous properties of fish oil and omega-3s. But industries grow impatient with consumer trends that are not based on patented (super-profitable) technologies. So the food industry has introduced patented technologies to enable omega-3-fortified processed foods and drinks. This trend is in keeping with many experts' mantra that we should "get all our nutrients from food," which is a dubiously motivated view for some (like we should get all our iodine from stripped salt and get all our vitamin D from the synthetic vitamin D added back to nutrient-depleted, antibiotic-contaminated milk).

Processed foods—no matter how fortified they are—are never a good choice, even if they are the best thing since stripped, immortally preserved white bread for the food industry. Quality natural supplements are the only fitting complement to real, whole foods. Being lured to eat processed or dead (enzyme-depleted, embalmed) foods with omega-3s added back by the very industries that stripped nutrients from our food supply with irresponsible manufacturing and agriculture is like buying your lunch from the bully who stole your lunch money yesterday. The same irony comes to mind when you think of taking a fish oil—a natural, food-based substance—as a prescription drug. It was the medical industry that collectively disparaged the use of supplements such as fish oil for decades after it was proven to work. Now they'd like you to flock to the "superior" prescription version they scrambled to patent (adulterate), once they knew the benefits of fish oil could no longer be suppressed. Please be aware of this prevalent line of thinking. It is the essence of why natural products and whole foods seem "alternative" to you, when in fact they are the holy grail of where health comes from—and every industry knows it, but doesn't want you to.

I highly suggest that you stick with eating uncontaminated, sustainable fish or grass-fed foods, and supplementing with natural, highly purified fish oil from your health food or vitamin store that has been molecularly distilled, then converted back to the body-familiar, triglyceride form (see Resources for an award-winning, environmentally responsible brand).

I don't love fish, so I personally take four or five fish oil capsules a day (cod liver oil during the winter) and try to eat grass-fed dairy and some grass-fed meat weekly. More of the miraculous beauty and body benefits of fish oil and omega-3 fats are discussed in coming chapters.

IS GRASS-FED THE NEW "FISH?"

Grass-fed is even better than organic if you're looking for the healthiest dairy and meat products. In light of all the issues with contamination in fish, as well as dwindling fish populations, it is also interesting to note that grass-fed meats boast a similar omega-3 fatty acid profile to fish! Not all organic animals are grass-fed, nor as nutritious. Not only have grass-fed foods been found to contain much higher amounts of nutrients—such as beta-carotene and antioxidants—than their grain-fed counterparts, but also five times the amount of CLA (conjugated linoleic acid), which has been shown to promote fat loss and possibly prevent cancer. CLA supplements even diminished cellulite and decreased thigh circumference when used in conjunction with certain herbal combinations in one study.

COULD GRASSLAND "CARBON FARMING" REVERSE GLOBAL WARMING?

Contrary to the misconception that devoting land to raising livestock degrades the environment—which is only correct if you're talking about conventional practices—grass-fed (the way meat was meant to be raised) actually creates superior topsoil that absorbs CO_2 from the air. In fact, this topsoil is widely believed to be the only carbon-absorbing material in nature that is voluminous enough to potentially capture all the excess carbon in the atmosphere. Some figures, such as those from Allan Yeomans, author of *Priority One: Together We Can Beat Global Warming*, suggest that if organic matter in the topsoil of the world's agriculture and grazing lands were increased by as little as 1.6 percent, the levels of CO_2 in the atmosphere would be reduced to pre-industrial levels. Visit www.CarbonFarmersofAmerica.com to learn more. In the meantime, delicious grass-fed products can be delivered to your door by one of the *New York Times's* preferred sources, U.S. Wellness Meats (see Resources).

RALLY YOUR RESOURCES FOR ORGANIC, WILD, AND GRASS-FED PRODUCTS

If your local grocery or health food store doesn't offer organic produce, or if you're having a hard time finding wild fish or grass-fed products, don't despair. First, I'd wager you'll uncover some local gems you never knew about by visiting www.localharvest.org to find out about farmers and farmers' markets in your area. In addition, a handful of standout companies deliver these things just about anywhere in the country (see Resources).

WHEN YOUR BODY TREATS A FOOD AS A TOXIN

There is one last consideration to take into account before embarking on your food upgrades: you may know about your food allergies, but what about your food sensitivities? In his book, *Your Hidden Food Allergies Are Making You Fat* (Prima Publishing, 1998), Rudy Rivera, MD, explains that when left undiagnosed, hidden allergies produce a much wider range of subtle symptoms, including weight gain. According to Dr. Susan Lark, edema (fluid retention) and even fat accumulation can result from eating foods you are sensitive to. She recommends that we note typical signs of sensitivity, which include headache, increased heart rate, diarrhea, bloating, and low energy. She also recommends eliminating typical sensitizing foods such as wheat, dairy, corn, soy, and eggs, and then adding them back one by one over a couple of weeks to determine your sensitivities. See the Resources section for information on the ALCAT test, one of the most sensitive blood tests for determining food sensitivities.

YOUR KITCHEN CABINET MAKEOVER

A makeover of the contents of your kitchen cabinet (and refrigerator) is like a sculptor acquiring a new set of tools and raw materials. Your final creation of yourself can be an entirely different work of art. The Kitchen Cabinet Makeover is a series of pro-beauty food upgrades that, once in place, will effortlessly begin to transform your body and your skin while delighting your tastes. The idea is to find practical, accessible upgrades that suit your palate while giving you maximum nourishment and taste with minimum impact on blood sugar. Remember, if you have a health condition, get approval from your doctor before changing your diet.

Your first goal should be to identify and upgrade your favorite staples—your most frequent, autopilot choices. As you upgrade your foods, moving from depleted and high-impact foods to deeply nourishing, low-impact ones, you'll notice that a big part of the initial shift will be shifting the bulk of your foods from your cabinets to your refrigerator. For example, prepared and processed foods or breads that can be kept at room temperature should all be upgraded with fresh, unprocessed, low-impact versions I'll outline in a moment—all of which must be refrigerated or frozen.

RE-SENSITIZE YOUR TASTE BUDS GRADUALLY

Remember, the best upgrades are the ones that don't feel like substitutions after only a few days. Don't deny your tastes. For example, if you like milk chocolate but dislike dark chocolate, I suggest you buy a smartly sweetened (never sugar-sweetened) milk chocolate, but you should anticipate that your taste buds will be in a very different state only days after you cut out sweet beverages and starchy foods. Before you pass final judgment on any food's flavor, your taste buds may need a few days to recover from years of over-stimulation by over-salted and over-sweetened foods; so don't write any new foods off too hastily. Once resensitized, your taste buds will regain their appreciation for the subtle flavors in real foods. In the meantime, there's a healthy way to satisfy every craving. Your changing sensibilities and bio-chemistry will soon compel you to choose foods you may never have dreamed you'd come to prefer.

DITCH THE DRUGLIKE FOOD CULPRITS FIRST

Assuming that you've already upgraded your beverages to the same effect, I strongly advise you to begin your Kitchen Cabinet Makeover by clearing out the sugar (you will never, ever need it again), flour, crackers, chips, rice-cakes, pasta (even whole grain, unless you want to serve it to your kids), and refined *anything*. Say your good-byes to juices, syrups, honey, typical candy, fat-free dairy, and artificially sweetened foods. Save your beans for your kids at this point, although the one exception is soybeans, which are the lowest-glycemic bean out there. Eden Foods makes an organic canned black soy bean to upgrade to.

Now, unless you are naturally thin and athletic and have never struggled against weight gain, throw out even your whole-grain breads (again, unless you want to feed them to your kids), and start clean with all low-impact upgrades (see Upgrade Your Grain Foods chart on page 121). You may go through a brief withdrawal period (it can be almost painless if you stock up on your upgrades and take blood sugar–stabilizing supplements discussed later). This is a critical step because the "carb claws" won't loosen their grip unless you part completely with grains and even beans at least for one and preferably two weeks. Remember, convenience and strategy really count. Stock up, plan ahead, and anticipate logistical challenges.

The above step, when executed along with your beverage upgrades, will afford you changes in the mirror in only a few days. The next step is to stock up on—and stick with—your low-impact upgrades for every high-impact

---

LINDA: CRAVINGS LIFTED IN ONE DAY

This letter is from a woman who came to one of my programs where only low-impact foods were served from breakfast until late afternoon two days in a row:

Dear Kat: I attended your workshop this past weekend. Preceding the workshop, my sugar addiction (my "demon") was out of control. I was bingeing continuously but couldn't do anything about it.

I went to the grocery store on my way home from day two and had no interest in any baked goods, candy, or sweets. I realized that I had no cravings at all. The only way I can explain it is that the quality of the foods we were served over the weekend chemically removed my cravings. My body was so ready for this! I haven't had a craving since, and I am enjoying delicious meals and snacks following your principles and have tremendous energy. It seems like a miracle to me. I also plan to continue my transformation beyond my diet. I am taking supplements and will change out my skin care, hair care, and makeup products at my first opportunity. Thank you for showing me the way to my own transformation.

—Linda Q.
Atlanta, Georgia

choice. As you read on, jot down in your notebook the upgrades you'd like to try in place of each high-impact choice you normally make. Then consider my JumpStart Menu and recipes in the next chapter before creating your shopping list.

UPGRADING YOUR BREADS, BAGELS, AND BUNS

Once you've given yourself the chance to experience a week or two without grains or flour of any kind. I still recommend that you upgrade any whole-grain breads to super-low-impact bread. The hemp seed bread from the award-winning French Meadow Bakery was tested by the Glycemic Research Institute to have the lowest glycemic index rating of any bread I've found. It is still best to eat these breads with fat or protein, such as almond butter, coconut oil, avocado slices, or olive oil.

CARBS THAT COUNT: FIGURING "EFFECTIVE CARBS"

"Effective carbs" is a term that refers to the carbs a food has that actually have impact on blood sugar. Sugar alcohols (polyols, such as erythritol and xylitol) and fiber are considered minimal-impact carbs because they pass through the digestive tract with little effect on blood sugar. You can determine the number of effective carbs by subtracting both fiber and sugar alcohol grams from the total carb count of a food. I find this especially helpful when I'm considering the value of newly introduced foods, such as some sugar alcohol-sweetened protein bars, which may appear to be high-carb, but are not once this valuable calculation is made.

HEMP SEED AND SALBA: MY AMAZING NEW UPGRADES FOR GRAINS AND RICE

Because I want to avoid any sense of deprivation in people who attend my programs, I was very excited to discover grainlike hemp seed soon after it was legalized in the U.S. in 2004. Hemp seed is a miraculous, low-glycemic food that looks and tastes similar to a coarse couscous. It boasts a near-perfect ratio of omega-3, -6, and -9 fats. As if that weren't enough, hemp seed requires no cooking and can be used as a grain just by sprinkling it

UPGRADE YOUR GRAIN FOODS

These are good times for people who seek to limit the consequences of grains in their life but are occasionally nostalgic for the old munchie and carb-y comfort food experiences. Surprisingly, you will lose your cravings for things such as chips, pastas, and breads, but low-impact versions should always be on hand anyway. Hemp seed is my most recommended stand-in for grains, which I hope you'll use all the time. It's best served instead of a bed of rice, under any dish with a sauce. It is a miracle food and won't spike you because it is packed with protein and good fats. Coconut flour is the only tasty low-impact upgrade for flour to bake with. Resistant starch and phaseolamin-containing flours are being developed, so keep an eye out. The breads, chips, and pasta—some I've mentioned by name—are one-of-a-kind products that are unmatched in taste and are the lowest available in terms of glycemic impact. I want to stress that it is possible to overdo even these low-impact chips, bread, or pastas, which is why I'm suggesting you introduce them only after one or two weeks of being clear of all spikes, so you can easily adjust your intake and how you eat them to prevent any subtle effects from them. Always serve them with fat and protein, getting some bites of those foods first.

Before	After
Grains	Organic shelled hemp seed or salba
Flours	Coconut, hemp, or nut flours
Pasta	Resistant Starch pasta, such as Dreamfield's
Asian cellophane noodles	Shirataki (konjac fiber flour) noodles
Crackers	Flourless herb and flax crackers
Breads and tortillas	Hemp seed products by French Meadow Bakery
Chips	Organic soy and flax corn chips by R.W. Garcia
Cereal	Flax, nut, hemp, and coconut-based smartly sweetened cereals

into any finished dish. I use it in pilafs and stuffed peppers, instead of bread-crumbs in meatloaf, in soups and chili—even in desserts. Hemp flour is another exceptionally unique product in that it's a low-impact, gluten-free, high-protein flour that can be used in combination with the coconut and nut flours listed in the Resources section for supernutritious and blood sugar-safe baking. Finally, hemp is one of the most eco-friendly and versatile agricultural products there is, requiring no pesticides in the growing. Find it in pouches at health food stores.

Salba is another amazing low-impact grain upgrade that even surpasses hemp seed nutritionally, though it is far pricier, and so I use it less often.

FINALLY, A SEMOLINA PASTA THAT IS LOW-IMPACT

Some (though not all) Italians can eat al dente semolina pasta without harm-ful consequences, but that's because most Italians have not been exposed to a lifetime of constant, serious blood sugar and insulin assaults. The pasta is still spiking their blood sugar, but their progress along the track to metabolic disorders is exponentially slower than a typical American's. Dreamfield's pasta is the first truly low-impact pasta I have found that tastes virtu-ally indistinguishable from Italian white semolina pasta (because it is made from semolina, not rubbery soy). With special fiber added to create a flavor-less "resistant starch," it has more fiber than whole-grain pastas but tastes much better and is far lower-glycemic. It has only 5 grams of effective carbs, compared with the blood sugar-spiking 28 to 40 grams you get with even whole-grain pastas.

Shirataki is one of the few other pastas that are truly low-impact. It's an Asian translucent pasta made from konjac root, which is a nutritive fiber that has been found to lower cholesterol and blood sugar in diabetics. Remember to always cook pasta al dente (firm), which keeps the glycemic index lower, and add virgin olive oil or cream and a protein. Pesto works well. Again, I advise taking a complete break from pasta and all other grain foods the first couple of weeks. When you do reintroduce them (many people choose not to), you'll want to be stocked up with the special low-impact versions I rec-ommend and have a strategic supplement plan going to help you to continue to recover your optimum nutritional balance and minimize your vulnerability to any blood sugar effects.

UPGRADE YOUR SWEET FIX

As you progress along your series of upgrades and start to choose less-sweet drinks and smartly sweetened treats, you'll find your taste buds will resensitize. If you preferred milk chocolate before, for example, you may find a new taste for dark chocolate—the ultimate health indulgence. Work your way darker and darker!

Denatured or Depleted Choice	Pro-Beauty Choice	Body-Decadent Splurge
• Standard ice cream, cookies, cakes, and pastries • Typical fruit salads • Fat-free, sugar-free cocoa • Cheap chocolate and candy	• Smartly sweetened chocolate • Smartly sweetened coconut flour or almond flour cookies • Berries with cream • Full-fat yogurt, smartly sweetened with berries and a sprinkling of unsweetened Uncle Sam cereal or Flax Z Snacks • Smartly sweetened cheesecake or pumpkin pie with coconut flour crust	• Organic smartly sweetened dark chocolate fondue • Smartly sweetened home-made ice cream made with real vanilla, chocolate, or coconut milk (see recipes) • Smartly sweetened home-made hot chocolate made with organic whole milk and real cocoa. • Berry parfaits made with any of the above or Greek yogurt

QUICK HOMEMADE LOW-IMPACT ICE CREAMS AND MORE

The Vita-Mix is an industrial-strength blender that can turn rock-hard frozen peaches or berries into super-smooth sorbet in seconds. This has revolutionized my beverage and dessert horizons by doing a lot of things my blender could not. I can make much healthier "whole-juice" blends, the smoothest nut milks (sweetened my way), confectioner's "sugar" out of granulated xylitol (which makes it last twice as long), and even tahini out of sesame seeds. It makes soups without a stove,

(continued on next page)

puréeing vegetables and soup ingredients to a boiling point in four minutes just by running the machine. Most importantly, unlike any other food processor, it liberates nutrients from the cell wall and seeds of produce that would normally never be available to the body. So, my raspberry ice cream (see my basic 4-Minute Ice Cream recipe with endless variations on page 145) renders the amazing nutrition both within the cell walls of the fruit's flesh and even from the seeds. Recently, the nutrients in seeds and seed oils have made health news headlines. The seed extracts of raspberries and cranberries have been found to show powerful antioxidant and skin benefits.

The machine is expensive, but I have saved so much time, made so many things I never would have otherwise enjoyed (no way I'd break out the ice cream maker twice a year, let alone twice a week!), and avoided so much wasted produce (I just freeze overripe fruit for ice cream later) that it paid itself off easily (see Resources).

BEAUTIFYING BERRIES

Fresh berries in season are not only a luscious splurge but perhaps the most impressive fruits of all when you consider their low glycemic impact, high nutrient density, high fiber content, taste, and versatility. Try throwing berries into yogurt or even over a salad. Berries contain phytochemicals that beautify the skin and also inhibit cervical and breast cancer in cultured cells, according to a May 2001 study reported by the USDA Research Service.

ANCIENT "NEW" SUPERBERRIES

The following is a sampling of what are considered some of the most antioxidant-rich, nutritious foods in the world. Some are newly available in America, whereas some familiar ones have recently become "hot" again. While the food industry uses the words "functional food" for high-tech foods that incorporate ingredients that have been proven in a lab to have various health effects, you're not likely to read the following information on the labels of most of these true superfoods. That, according to the FDA, would make the food a drug. Nonetheless, these foods have been preventing disease and making humans vibrant long before being tested in a lab. Stick with whole fruit or supplements to avoid getting spiked by juices.

Acai fruit, or Brazilian palm berry, not only tastes like slightly chocolaty berries and has ten to thirty times the anthocyanidin antioxidants of red wine, it also contains an unusually high content of the antioxidant catalyst SOD (superoxide dismutase) which makes it a true standout at quenching free radicals. Recent studies suggest it has skin and digestive benefits. The unsweetened purée (avoid the sweetened one) comes frozen in packets from health and gourmet store freezer sections. Perfect for smoothies.

Blueberry: Supplements containing pterostilbene, a phytochemical found in blueberries, inhibited colon cancer in rats in a 2006 study done at Rutgers University in New Jersey. In Ayurvedic medicine, pterostilbene is used

UPGRADE YOUR FRUITS

Get adventurous with fruit, but watch its glycemic impact if you're eating it alone or on an empty stomach. Fruit salad will tend to spike the blood sugar, while a bowl of blueberries with cream or Greek yogurt will most likely not. To avoid these spikes, eat fruit sparingly in green salads with lots of fat and protein, or submerse it in full-fat yogurt. Use only berries in smoothies.

Denatured or Depleted Choice	Pro-Beauty Choice	Body-Decadent Splurge
• Canned fruit • Fruit juices (see beverage upgrades for taste-evolving alternatives) • Dried fruit	• Fresh, whole, nutrient-dense and deep- or brightly colored fruits, such as blackberries, blueberries, raspberries, cranberries, strawberries, cantaloupe, papaya, plums, peaches, and mangoes	• Organic fresh or frozen berries: acai or goji. • Fresh Black Mission figs dipped in organic, full-fat, or Greek yogurt • Red currants, champagne grapes, exotic pears, pomegranates, or papaya with fresh mint

to balance blood sugar and lipid levels. USDA researchers have dubbed pterostilbene the "multi-tasking antioxidant." It should be noted that the Rutgers study was published just weeks after the "news" broke that antioxidants didn't work . . .

Camu Camu berry is considered a "whole food vitamin C" supplement, with the highest amount of vitamin C ever found in whole food. It is accompanied by a broad spectrum of amino acids and minerals to provide the best possible absorption. Buy it in powder form and add to smoothies.

Goji berry, from the Tibetan and Mongolian Himalayas, is a favorite food of a region of China that boasts an unusual number of centenarians. The gorgeous red-orange color of the dried berries comes from their super-high concentrations of beta-carotene and zeaxanthin, which translate to great skin food. They've also been shown to protect blood lipids from oxidation and raise levels of the body's own antioxidant enzymes, like superoxide dismutase (SOD). Mix them into full-fat foods to avoid a spike. Makes an incredible-looking ice cream or shake.

Sour cherries were recently found in animal studies to reduce pain from inflammation and gout with natural cox-2 inhibitors ten times stronger than aspirin. Sour cherry contains melatonin, which assists sleep rhythms, among other health benefits. Growers are not allowed to tell you about these benefits on their own websites or literature because that would make sour cherry a drug, the FDA says.

Sugar is what
makes sugar fattening.

GET GLOWING WITH MORE RAW

Beauty tip: If you really want to glow, eat some raw vegetables at each meal for the enzymes, which fight inflammation, allergies, and skin flare-ups. Cook-

UPGRADE YOUR VEGETABLES

Stay radiant by steering clear of starchy vegetables and stick to those in the center and right columns below. Use lots of herbs, like garlic, ginger, or lemon wedges, as well as toasted nuts and high-quality finishing oils, such as roasted sesame, walnut, or chili oils, for ethnic variation and to make your vegetable dishes savory and aromatic. If you love mineral-rich seaweed, you're lucky because it may be the healthiest vegetable of all.

Denatured or Depleted Choice	Pro-Beauty Choice	Body-Decadent Splurge
• Iceberg lettuce • Canned vegetables • Potatoes and corn	• Fresh spinach or romaine lettuce—the darker the better • Fresh peppers, parsley (tabouli made with hemp seed instead of bulgar wheat is the best way to get more of this), broccoli, sugar snaps, snow peas, asparagus, tomatoes, garlic, avocados, and onions • Frozen organic vegetables (if the fresh vegetable is not in season)	• Frozen green vegetables (if the fresh vegetable is not in season) • Organic mesclun greens • Organic baby spinach, arugula or watercress; organic yellow and red peppers; seaweed (nori, dulse) • Shiitake and other exotic mushrooms • Fresh herbs

ing and pasteurization kill vital enzymes in food. One way to start getting more raw food is to fold prewashed baby spinach, raw nuts, avocado, or shelled hemp seed into just about any dish just before serving. My Beauty Detox Elixir is another great way to get some raw. A smoothie is a perfect raw breakfast option. My Decadent Meal Salad at lunch is another enzyme-packed boost. A frozen berry ice cream is yet another raw treat. With these kinds of treats, it's easy to fool yourself into eating mostly raw!

UPGRADE YOUR OILS, DRESSINGS, AND CONDIMENTS

Infuse foods with herbs and the finest oils for rejuvenation and sensual indulgence. Major-brand corn, canola, sunflower, and safflower oils are generally bleached and oxidized and may contain hexane residues. For cooking, you want oils that don't break down with heat. For high-temperature cooking, such as stir-frying, the healthiest oil may be grape seed, which doesn't peroxidize at higher temperatures and raises the "good" and lowers the "bad" cholesterol.

Denatured or Depleted Choice	Pro-Beauty Choice	Body-Decadent Splurge
• Common bleached cooking oils • Hydrogenated shortenings • Margarine • Bottled salad dressings, spreads, and dips • Soy sauce • Extra virgin olive oil	• Organic canola oils • Roasted sesame and chili oils • Organic butter (or ghee for the lactose-intolerant) • Bragg's Liquid Aminos instead of soy sauce *For high-temperature cooking:* • Grape seed or macadamia nut oil • Unrefined virgin coconut oil	• Exotic cold-pressed finishing oils: sesame, walnut, Austrian pumpkin seed, and truffle-infused olive oil • Hemp seed oil (the only oil high in GLA) eaten only raw in salads or smoothies • Virgin red palm oil for high-temperature cooking. Loaded with carotenoids!

DESIGN A DECADENT MEAL SALAD

Forget iceberg lettuce, hydrogenated croutons, and bottled dressing. This truly decadent salad is a higher sensory experience and a whole meal in itself: many find that keeping meal salad ingredients at the office is an ideal way to make a perfect lunch each day and even to serve a great in-office business lunch.

- Dark, organic greens, such as arugula, baby spinach, or mesclun greens
- Red onion sliced super-thin
- Tart fruit such as Granny Smith apple or pear slices, dark berries, or pomegranate seeds or tart cherries
- Fresh blue cheese, feta, or Gorgonzola or alternative protein choices such as avocado, goat cheese, hard-boiled eggs, chicken, or tuna
- Toasted or raw walnuts or other nuts or seeds, such as pumpkin
- Cold-pressed gourmet oil, such as extra virgin olive, walnut, or pumpkin seed oils, lemon, and just a touch of balsamic vinegar
- Optional: a sprinkle of herbs from your spice rack, such as basil or tarragon

Greens and Your Bones

Greens may be even more effective than dairy at building bones. Vitamin K, found in large amounts in greens, was once primarily thought of as a blood-clotting agent, but now it has been discovered to be a major contributor to bone health. Oils and fats on your salad enhance the absorption of vitamin K.

LOW FAT DAIRY AND FERTILITY

A 2007 Harvard study published in *Human Reproduction* found a diet high in low-fat dairy products to substantially increase fertility problems. Of the 18,555 women of childbearing age surveyed in the Nurses' Health Study II, many were, in effect, following the USDA's recommendations to consume two or three servings of low-fat dairy per day. Over an eight-year period, it was exactly those compliers who ran into trouble. Those who consumed that amount had nearly twice the risk of infertility as those who consumed low-fat dairy less than once a week. Conversely, high-fat dairy eaters (one or more servings a day) were 27 percent less apt to be infertile than those who had one or fewer servings of high-fat dairy per week. In short, the researchers found intake of low-fat yogurts and frozen yogurts vs. whole milk and ice cream to be strikingly correlated with high and low rates of infertility, respectively.

UPGRADE YOUR DAIRY

Dairy tips: Unlike U.S. cheeses, most European cheeses do not contain growth hormones and antibiotic residues. Experts on mad cow disease advise the avoidance of meat and dairy products wherever rendered animal parts have been used in livestock feed (including the United States and Great Britain). Grass-fed meats are safe.

Denatured or Depleted Choice	Pro-Beauty Choice	Body-Decadent Splurge
• Conventionally produced milk and milk products • Nonfat dairy products • Sweetened yogurt • Processed cheese	• Organic whole plain yogurt • Kefir • Natural cheese • Organic whole milk	• Grass-fed dairy products • Greek yogurt • Organic sour cream and cottage cheese • Goat milk or raw milk • Organic butter • Biodynamic yogurt • Organic or grass-fed cheese

NUTS AND SEEDS: THE ULTIMATE BEAUTY FOOD

Nuts and seeds are "it" for providing health, taste, and beauty benefits for the skin and body. A handful of Brazil nuts pack a day's worth of selenium. Almonds and sesame seeds are high in calcium. Almonds and walnuts both lower LDL cholesterol. Walnuts raise serotonin levels. The omega-3s in flax and walnuts add luster to the skin and hair. Hummus and sesame tahini are full of calcium. Instead of bread with your hummus, try flourless flax or herb crackers, which taste surprisingly good (see Resources). Choose raw nuts whenever you can. The newly required pasteurization of all raw almonds in 2007 has called the "rawness" of even almonds labeled as raw into question. Since then, I have raised my consumption of other nuts, which are still undebatably raw. This irradiation of raw almonds removes an important nutrient source from our food supply. Some groups are challenging this unfortunate law.

I now buy a bag each of raw walnuts, Brazil nuts, and tamari-roasted almonds (since truly raw almonds no longer exist) at the health-food store.

UPGRADE YOUR PROTEIN

Eating protein at every meal is one of the best ways to keep yourself off the pendulum. The great thing about the chips and grain upgrades I'm recommending is that they are far higher in protein, fiber, and good fats than their junk-food counterparts (high-protein mini-meals are the best type of snack).

Denatured or Depleted Choice	Pro-Beauty Choice	Body-Decadent Splurge
• Conventionally raised or cured meats and poultry • Frozen breaded or fried fish • Canned or processed roasted nuts and seeds • Hydrogenated, processed peanut butter • Canned refried or baked beans	• Free-range meat and poultry • Fresh, omega-3 fat-rich fish, such as salmon • Avocado • Fresh unroasted nuts: walnuts, almonds, Brazil nuts, and soy nuts • Pumpkin and flax seeds • Natural nut butters • Sesame tahini • Canned organic soybeans • Free-range chicken sausage and ground turkey	• Wild Alaskan salmon • Free-range, nitrate-free bacon (or turkey bacon) • Protein-based low-impact bars, cereals, and munchies • Grass-fed meats • Organic raw nuts • Organic raw nut butters • Coconut flour baked goods • Hemp seed and hemp flour foods

SAFER GRILLING WITH STRATEGIC MARINADES

Grilling meats can form carcinogens called heterocyclic amines (HCAs); however, some eye-opening studies comparing sweet Western barbecue sauces with Asian antioxidant-containing marinades showed that the Western honey-based marinades increased dangerous HCAs (sugar does it again!), but Asian and tumeric- and garlic-based marinades *reduced* HCAs. Also, note that consumption of green tea helps block HCAs. So don't give up the barbecue; just do it smarter!

Just those few spicy almonds make the whole mix tasty while keeping it mostly raw. You can also toast some of the walnuts (it makes them smell and taste a little like popcorn) and add your own herbs, or even cinnamon and smart sweetener for snacks, salad toppers, or desserts. Pumpkin seeds are also great for this. Be sure to store nuts or pumpkin seeds in tightly sealed containers and refrigerate them so they don't oxidize, which produces byproducts that are aging to the body and skin.

WHY COCONUT IS KING

Coconut is a food without flaw. It's actually hypoallergenic, contains one of the most healthy and slimming oils on earth (if it's virgin and fresh), and is not only extremely low-glycemic but an antifungal as well. If you make a point of putting two tablespoons of virgin coconut oil into your smoothies, stir-fry, or dressings (I use it in chocolate fondue), you will benefit from its documented slimming, energizing, thyroid-stoking, and cholesterol ratio-improving effects. In 2005, Bruce Fife, MD, the author of several books on the health benefits of coconut, published *Cooking with Coconut Flour*, which introduced an extraordinary new product. Miraculous light-textured coconut flour can actually, for the first time, produce fluffy, yet no-spike high-protein baked goods that taste great. It has opened up a new frontier of blood sugar-safe baking that has revolutionized my program menus! It's equally exciting for both diabetics and gluten-free eaters. Both the cookbook and the coconut flour are irreplaceable (see Resources).

COOKING MAKES LIFE MORE BEAUTIFUL

I used to think that cooking was "work" that I had to take a break from living to do. Now I know that cooking is part of the essence of life that I get to live between stretches of work! Creating aromatic, mouth-watering food improves your quality of life on many levels and takes much less time than you might think. Much less than eating out. Consider cooking at home and celebrating savory, healing foods with family and friends more often. Express your creativity and passion for cultivating your own—as well as your loved ones'—vitality through amazing food. For years, I've been cooking for my lifestyle programs, and I've learned that it's hard to go wrong with real, fresh ingredients and a few key herbs. In chapter 7, I offer a core 6-Day JumpStart Menu with my favorite low-impact "throw-together," endlessly adaptable creations.

SPICE IT UP: INDULGE YOUR SENSES AND YOUR BODY

Nothing elevates a dish to gourmet, mouth-watering status more easily and healthily than herbs and spices. Two of my favorite tricks are adding sautéed fennel seed to ground turkey to give it that savory Italian sausage taste and adding a pinch of tarragon to my scrambled eggs or cream cheese for a touch of buttery sweetness. Just about every herb studied has been found to have unique health properties, including antibacterial and antifungal actions. In hot climates where refrigeration is scarce, people of many cultures, such as those in India, have depended on spices like curry to preserve food. (Please don't try that at home!)

- **Garlic** is a potent antibiotic that has been reported to lower cholesterol in some cases. It is sulfur-rich, which supports the skin.
- **Cayenne,** eaten in large amounts, has been shown to increase satiety and reduce calorie intake.
- **Ginger** improves digestion, eases nausea, improves circulation, and is being researched as a heart tonic.
- **Turmeric,** a component of Indian curry, has shown potent anti-inflammatory, anticancer, and liver-protective benefits in numerous studies. It is a natural

(continued on next page)

---

cox-2 inhibitor, blocks the absorption of estrogen-mimicking chemicals, prevents breast cancer metastasis, and even blocks radiation to varying degrees. I take turmeric every day in supplement form.

- **Cilantro,** in a study using cilantro pesto, has been shown to detoxify heavy metals by carrying them out of the body.
- **Cinnamon** has shown antibacterial activity, and one of its active components demonstrated improved sugar metabolism in a USDA study.

These tidbits are just the tip of the iceberg. Stunning benefits are just now being identified and studied for nearly every fresh herb, cold-pressed oil, and spice you can think of.

CLEVER COMBINING FOR LOW-IMPACT, HIGH-SATISFACTION MEALS

Once you have gotten through your first week or two without a blood sugar spike, you will know exactly when foods spike you, since you'll have resensitized to their effects. Although I suggest you skip all breads and grain foods and get on blood sugar-stabilizing supplements the first week, you may decide to introduce the special grain foods (see Upgrade Your Grains) once all your cravings are gone. This is when the concept of low-impact food combining can help you make better meals in all kinds of situations. Understanding that what you eat first (preferably fat or protein), as well as the combination of foods making up your meal, can greatly influence its overall glycemic impact, is key. This will allow you to enjoy certain moderately low-impact foods by making extra effort to precede and balance them with impact-buffering foods such as fat, fiber, or protein. In this way, you can combine occasional "borderline" foods along with these foods to create a low-impact meal. An example of what happens when you increase the ratio of low-impact foods to create correspondingly lower glycemic-impact meals was shown in a 2007 study published in the journal *Metabolism*, where the more almonds were added to high-glycemic meals, the more of a glycemic-impact lowering effect was found.

Clever combining takes a little trial and error, but because you'll be experimenting after your initial week off any and all blood sugar spikes, you will quickly come to recognize foods, ratios, or combinations that spike you, and you can eliminate, upgrade, or adjust the balance of fat, fiber, or protein accordingly. In this case, believe it or not, it is much safer to add more fat to something than you think you need to keep the meal from spiking you. It is very hard to overeat fat when you're not eating it with carbs, by the way, because the body starts to burn fat for fuel, and your hunger will be true to what you really need. Once you master this principle of clever low-impact combining, you will have a valuable intuitive tool that you can use in all situations to minimize future food assaults, even when you are not in control of the foods being served.

The incredible thing is that low-glycemic combinations make meals and snacks more satisfying. Think avocado or raw, grass-fed cheese melted over your low-impact chips, Greek yogurt and smartly sweetened dark chocolate in your berry parfait, organic cream in your tomato sauce, or even almond butter with your low-impact hemp seed bread French toast. Pure decadence! It's hard to believe, I know, but once you are not spiking your blood sugar, these low-impact combinations will actually keep you healthy and slim and much more sane around food.

UPGRADE YOUR FAST FOOD CHOICES

Ideally, fast foods will be infrequent choices you make on the road when you are stuck. I have found that the very fastest foods—and the least expensive—are the ones you bring with you. But everyone finds themselves stuck without their usual stash of smart foods now and then, so I want you to be prepared with these solutions:

Drive-through picks:

- **Chili:** Cheese and onions on top, extra sour cream (consider taking a phaseolamin-based supplement to buffer the potential spike from the beans).
- **Taco salad:** Skip the shell, add extra guac (again consider taking a phaseolamin-based supplement as a preemptive measure for the effects of the beans).
- **Chef salad or Chicken Ceasar:** The grilled chicken strips, blue cheese, and hardboiled eggs are great. Choose an un-sweet dressing. Skip the croutons. Add nuts from your travel stash to the salad if you can.

Travel food

Nuts, low-impact, natural protein bars or nut balls (see Resources), the above fast foods, or eggs or egg salad at the airport restaurant or deli will keep you off the pendulum. It's wonderful to eat things your body thrives on even when life is hectic. Bring along jasmine teabags and the aroma and experience will transport you even before you arrive at your destination. It's sad to see people subject their bodies to airplane foods just because someone handed it to them on a cardboard platter!

Take the Two-Week Plunge to Freedom

I hope these past few pages have inspired you to set the highest criteria for what you put in your body. In a couple of weeks or even less, you could be free of the "biochemical bondage" that has kept you from glowing and thriving. With the help of your pro-beauty food and beverage upgrades, the creative boost from my JumpStart Menu and recipe collection, and tips in the chapter ahead, you'll soon be off the "ride" and well on your way back to your untapped, glowing potential.

CHAPTER 7

YOUR 6-DAY JUMPSTART MENU AND RECIPES FOR TRANSFORMATION

Consider your kitchen to be your beauty artisan's workshop: one of the key places where you cultivate yourself with the tools and raw materials you've so passionately researched and gathered. From the recipes in this chapter, you'll be creating more transforming foods than you will ever find in the finest French cookbook. And rather than aspiring to become a chef, you'll soon become something far more important: a true connoisseur of the vitality and quality of life you are creating with food for yourself and those you love. And without one dreaded "diet food" in sight.

WHAT THIS MENU CAN DO FOR YOU IN TWO WEEKS

These recipes are designed to benefit people who use them in the context of completely weaning off sugar, flour, and grains (other than the super-low-impact grain products featured, to be introduced in the second or third week). While these recipes will be pleasing to just about any taste, they may not result in weight loss for those who are still eating high-impact foods or sweetened beverages throughout their day. You'll only reap its most exciting rewards and completely shake cravings if you keep all of your foods low-impact across the board, which is the point of the dawn-to-dusk menu and list of snack options. As always, if you are being treated for disease, ask your doctor before making any dramatic change in your diet.

Here's what you can typically expect in two weeks as you halt the "ride":

Day 1 As you incorporate a low-impact breakfast, upgrade all high-impact foods, and take your supplements faithfully, you should feel less craving and more energy in your very first afternoon, as your pendulum quickly loses momentum and rebound energy swings are noticeably reduced. You could see a reduction in facial puffiness as soon as the next morning if you are getting off sugary drinks and white-flour foods.

Days 2–3 Cravings and energy dips in the afternoons and evenings have improved dramatically, as the pendulum slows further. Bloating has greatly reduced. Taste buds have begun to re-sensitize, and real food starts to take on a new taste-appeal. Dark chocolate tastes less bitter and starts scratching a deeper "itch" than milk chocolate can.

Days 4–6 These are the days where most people who had been eating low-fat and blood sugar-spiking foods realize that they are starting to seriously transform; looser clothing, incredible energy, stable moods, calmer, clearer skin, brighter eyes, improved digestion, and even more comfortable joints are among the common experiences.

Days 7–14 Most people have lost several pounds at this point. Skin is usually much more comfortable and any redness is reduced. If you were eating a lot of B.S. and low-fat foods before, you probably feel better than you've felt in years at this point. If you've achieved a solid week without any blood sugar spikes at all, you have likely stopped the pendulum completely and become familiar with that amazing feeling of stable energy and zero cravings.

Once you are resensitized to feel the wrong foods' druglike effects, yet you no longer crave them, you may be able to introduce small amounts of the special, super-low-impact breads, chips, and pastas I've discussed without interrupting your new fat-burning fuel efficiency. Many people no longer desire these things. If you do reintroduce them, the important thing is to start with small side servings, and always have fats (a dollop of Greek yogurt, almond butter, cream, or avocado) with them to avoid any spikes.

MAKING IT HAPPEN

Choose a day on which you'll begin your two-week stretch free of druglike foods and drinks. Give yourself a few days to stock up on your food upgrades and supplements, and strategize (on paper!) how you'll anticipate and head off each craving by putting a low-impact upgrade in place for each treat you nor-

MYTH: *You shouldn't lose more than a pound a week.*

TRUTH: *Any eating approach that cuts out blood sugar spikes (and thus insulin spikes) and bad fats and steps up good fats will quickly reduce inflammation.*

Inflammation goes hand in hand with excess water weight (edema) and makes up much of what is perceived as fat in obese people. If I'd had my approach handed to me on a silver platter and did not have to stumble on each piece year by year, I'd have done what many of my readers and program participants have done: lost most of my weight in a matter of months, rather than years. If you are inflamed (swollen) with excess weight and then start eating the way man was designed to eat, you will experience weight loss that is much faster than the expert's recommended pound a week. And keeping it off will require little effort.

mally crave. Plan to make these new upgrades convenient by keeping your new sweetener, supplement, beverage, and snack upgrades in your purse, at your office, and otherwise close at hand. Do this, and you've conquered the bulk of any challenge here.

However, if you don't think this out and instead leave circumstances to chance, your transition to becoming a fat-burning machine could needlessly take weeks, months, or even years. Each high-impact assault kicks the pendulum into swing, renews cravings, and halts the fat-burning state. Stopping it completely is the only way to enter the magical land of no cravings. In that place, druglike foods actually become a nuisance that turn you off, rather than tempt you. That's when you are truly home free, and effortless, dramatic transformation is underway!

Transform your kitchen first. Once you have stocked up with berries, organic eggs, dark greens, real butter, herbs, cream, quality cooking oils, Greek yogurt, nuts, dark, smartly sweetened chocolate, and other ingredients, your sense of freedom and adventure in the kitchen will flourish. Be sure to have low-impact upgrades for each of your favorite foods and beverages.

Remember, even if you don't have organic or grass-fed products on hand, you can still reap the most important initital benefits just by making sure to stop the blood sugar spikes. For long-term health, however, I encourage you to upgrade conventional products to organic (starting with animal products) as soon as you affordably can. Some of the other products are more critical, however, such as the special sweeteners, hemp seed, and coconut flour (without which I do not recommend baked goods at all). The hemp seed breads, special chips and resistant starch pastas named in these recipes (the only of their kind) are also critical in the second or third weeks if you reintroduce such foods. If other brands are used, I can't be as confident of the outcome you will have.

Get your supplements and fiber going (see chapter 9) with a blood sugar-stabilizing formula and fish oil for starters, and you'll have much added support for issues that may be magnifying your cravings, weight gain, or moods. This will speed your transformation. In fact, it enabled mine, where diet and exercise alone could not. Do this before you make any commitment to yourself to stick with only low-impact eating (especially if you are challenged by weight or cravings issues). It's especially important during the introduction of foods you haven't been eating to up your fiber, incorporating plenty of dark greens and berries right up front, and even fiber supplements. My Beauty Detox Elixir is another great way to add fiber and step up energy during your sugar detox.

To drink or not to drink: This menu will not have the quantum benefits you could see unless you take a complete initial break from alcohol, which impedes the goal of freedom from the pendulum and is usually at the heart of beauty problems for those who find it hardest to abstain. Yeast and blood sugar issues compound the difficulty in weaning off, as the body tends to rebel initially, but your food and beverage upgrades and a basic supplement regimen will dramatically reduce the desire to drink, as blood sugar issues are part of alcohol cravings. As previously mentioned, if your drinking is out of control, please seek help. See also Joan Matthews Larson's terrific book *Seven Weeks to Sobriety* in Suggested Reading, as its nutrition principles overlap with some of those in this book, and have resulted in some of the best recovery statistics at her clinic in Minneapolis.

Prevent setbacks with strategy: Rarely are setbacks due to cravings. It's the circumstances, such as birthday parties, bar nights, and other celebrations, that make B.S. foods enticing, particularly while you're still addicted to them. If this work is important to you, you may want to find (or make) a two-week stretch where no such events are planned. For the first week or two, avoid activities you strongly associate with druglike foods or drinks, such as movies if you "must" have popcorn, or bars if you "must" drink. Give your body a chance to wean biochemically, and then you will easily enjoy these activities without harming yourself. In the future, eat some protein and fat before attending such events, or you can bring your own low-impact munchies and drinks, like roasted pumpkin seeds, smartly sweetened chocolate, coconut flour brownies, or flavored spritzers. Your supplements (especially phase 2, which you'll read more about later) will also help you to avoid harming yourself in the name of celebration. Rally your family's support. Make them the homemade ice cream recipe in the pages ahead to get them in the spirit. Tell them you'll continue to share your creations if they do not sabotage your efforts! Making meals with a family member or friend who wants to eat the same way is a great way to spend time together. Remember, this isn't diet food. Your family will want to partake in the food you'll be eating.

USING THIS 6-DAY JUMPSTART MENU

This at-a-glance menu is designed to creatively springboard you into your own unique world of beautifying menu creations. Because I want to offer you the best chance to duplicate the kind of transformation I (and others) have had, I have included here my favorite core low-impact recipes from my Total Transformation® programs, which I've created and honed for nearly a decade.

I love cooking, but dislike rules and measurements, so I never exactly duplicate anything I make. I love "throwing things together" and have been true to that spirit in this collection. These are not full recipes you need to "play chef" to create. Rather, they are simple compilations that always taste amazing because they start with simply amazing ingredients. When you incorporate such beautiful, colorful foods, your cooking becomes a visual art as much as a culinary one. And with my endless variations you could use only this collection for years and never get in a rut. I know that, like me, you'll abandon the measuring spoons and develop your own take on whichever recipe you enjoy. The joy of throwing great dishes together is rivaled only by eating them.

YOUR 6-DAY JUMPSTART MENU AT-A-GLANCE

	DAY 1	DAY 2	DAY 3
Breakfast	Tarragon Scrambled Eggs and Organic Chicken Sausage	The Perfect Smoothie	Huevos Rancheros with Black Soybeans and Salsa
Lunch	Decadent Meal Salad with Herb Flax Crackers	Portobello Pizzas	Grass-fed BLT with Favorite Cole Slaw
Dinner	Grass-fed Meatloaf and Creamed Spinach	Wild Salmon with Dill and Baby Greens with Crumbled Stilton, and Grass-fed Bacon	Southwest Hemp Seed Pilaf Over Avocados
Dessert	Coconut Flour Brownies and 4-Minute Ice Cream	Greek Yogurt with Berries and Chocolate	Midnight Chocolate Fondue with Jicama and Lime
	DAY 4	DAY 5	DAY 6
Breakfast	Organic Whole Yogurt with Berries and Nuts	Poached Eggs and Smoked Wild Salmon	Coconut Flour Pancakes with Greek Yogurt and Acai Topping
Lunch	Dilled Egg Salad with Flourless Herb Crackers and Mixed Baby Greens	Organic Chicken Sausage with Hemp Seed Tabouli	Turkey Chili with Black Soybeans and Low-Impact Chips
Dinner	Turkey Tomato Fennel Sauce over Hemp Seed	Cheese Fondue with a Baby Spinach Salad	Grass-Fed Filet Mignon or Thai Fish over Hemp Seed with Arugula Salad and Berries
Dessert	Goji Berry Shake	One-Minute Chocolate Mousse	Cherry-Chocolate Float

Note that you needn't follow any one day's selections or even use these recipes at all if you have your favorite recipes to convert to low-impact. No need to reinvent any wheels here. Your Aunt June's meatloaf or your dad's Super Bowl chili are the best starting points for a menu you will truly stick with. By immediately upgrading any high-impact ingredients (sweeteners, flours, starches, beans, and grains) to low-impact equivalents, you'll soon be enjoying far more beautifying versions of foods you love and make already. You'll learn to upgrade any recipe you love to a low-impact, pro-beauty creation. You can receive additional recipes through my newsletter at www.informedbeauty.com.

Day 1 – Breakfast

Tarragon Scrambled Eggs with Chicken Sausage

My favorite scrambled eggs are organic and whisked together with tarragon and a little onion-flavored Real Salt and pepper, poured into a layer of melted organic butter, and scrambled quickly over medium-low heat. Tarragon gives the eggs a fantastic, creamy-sweet flavor. Any organic chicken sausage cooked as directed makes a quick, yet special accompaniment. For a crunchy, herb twist, crumble some Lydia's Flourless Curry Crackers into the eggs.

Day 1 – Lunch

Decadent Meal Salad

Follow recipe on page 128

Day 1 – Dinner

Grass-fed Lamb Meatloaf

Using a meatloaf recipe you prefer, upgrade the crackers or breadcrumbs you normally mix into the meat with French Meadow Bakery's hemp seed bread, coarsely ground with any additional herbs you want to add in a blender. The meat upgrade I suggest is grass-fed ground beef or the ultimate, grass-fed ground lamb (available from US Wellness Meats). Upgrade any ketchup with tomato paste. Ramp up the herbs. I am particularly fond of a lot of sage in meatloaf but have been known to go crazy with fennel, rosemary, and lots of chili powder. I have even put raw cocoa nibs in my meatloaf. Meatloaf alchemy is quite an artistic release!

Suggested side, creamed spinach: Sauté a good spoonful of minced garlic in a couple of tablespoons of sizzling butter for a minute or so. Add a splash of heavy cream and a sprinkle of tarragon and some Real Salt and bring back to a simmer. Throw in a large fistful of rinsed and dried fresh spinach (remove stems and grit first, of course), and cook down for a few minutes until it looks like creamed spinach (the spinach will shrink dramatically; it's fun to watch!). Adjust your cream or spinach ratio and salt to your preference. For a nice presentation and a ricelike feel, serve the spinach over a bed of hemp seed. Variation: Makes a terrific stuffer for roasted red peppers.

Day 1 – Dessert

Coconut Flour Brownies

This recipe is a variation from Dr. Bruce Fife's revolutionary cookbook, Cooking with Coconut Flour. The amazing thing about coconut flour brownies is that they taste like great, deep chocolate brownies, but your body just thinks its perfect, high-fiber health food. Coconut flour is a baking miracle that doesn't spike you! No other flour tastes like this without consequences. Suggested complement: 4-Minute Ice Cream made mocha-style with Teeccino herbal coffee.

 1 cup xylitol (such as NuNatural's)
 3/4 teaspoon Real Salt
 8 squares unsweetened baking chocolate
 6 organic eggs
 1 cup coconut flour (available through Simply Coconut)
 2/3 cup of unsweetened coconut milk
 2 teaspoons of vanilla flavoring
 1-1/2 cups of organic butter
 Optional: 1 cup crushed walnuts

Blend butter and chocolate over low heat. Remove from heat and let cool. Mix together eggs, xylitol, salt, coconut milk, and flavoring. Stir in chocolate mix-

ture and flour until smooth. Fold nuts in if desired. Pour into a large greased brownie pan and bake at 350° for 20–25 minutes or until knife comes out clean.

4-Minute Ice Cream

Any ice cream recipe you already make can be made low-impact by upgrading sugar to a smart sweetener. Using a Vita-Mix saves me so much time that I know it is the only reason I make ice cream at all. You won't believe how much like coffee ice cream the Teeccino Maya Café makes this variation of my basic 4-Minute Ice Cream. See below for endless variations.

> Pint of organic half-and-half sweetened with eight drops of vanilla stevia liquid (such as Nunaturals)
> Pint of Teeccino Maya Café made double strength (follow brewing instructions)
> 2 ice cube trays
> 1/2 cup of organic heavy cream
> Flavoring options, listed below

Pour half-and-half and prepared, cooled Teeccino into ice cube trays and freeze solid. When ready to serve ice cream, empty cubes into the Vita-Mix (not filling more than half full) and add half of the heavy cream. Add any additional desired flavoring listed below. With the lid on, using the machine's included tamper to force the cubes into the blades, process on high speed, stopping the machine if the cubes get stuck. Add remaining cubes and additional splashes of heavy cream if needed to process the cubes, but the less liquid and the quicker you can pulverize the cubes, the thicker and more scoopable your ice cream will be. Check the sweetness and adjust with smart sweetener to taste. That's it! You'll never miss sugary ice cream again! Serve over coconut brownies. (Although I have even stirred the brownies into the ice cream at my programs. No words can describe it . . .)

Endless variations: Make plain vanilla or add any of the following: several heaping spoonfuls of organic chocolate powder (such as Dagoba's unsweetened cocoa powder); 1 tablespoon matcha green tea powder (for green tea ice cream, or combine with cocoa for matcha-mocha ice cream, probably my ultimate favorite); one drop of food-grade peppermint essential oil (it's very concentrated);

a tablespoon of goji berries (the color is unbelievable); a packet or two of unsweetened frozen açai fruit (such as Sambazon's); a cup of fresh or frozen organic blackberries, blueberries, strawberries, or tart cherries. Courtney Holden, profiled on page 212, suggests a "strawberry cheesecake" combination of frozen strawberries and a package of organic cream cheese. We've only scratched the surface!

Day 2 – Breakfast

The Perfect Smoothie: See page 74 for recipe

Here's the No-time Shortcut. Nutiva makes an award-winning hemp shake mix with acai fruit that with a few ice cubes, milk, or yogurt—or even just stirred into yogurt—makes a quick but very hearty treat. No sweetener needs to be added.

Day 2 – Lunch

Portobello Mushroom Pizzas

Heat oven to 400°. Arrange favorite pizza toppings such as unsweetened tomato sauce, herbs such as basil and oregano, parmesan cheese, and onion and garlic slivers atop overturned large Portobello mushroom caps, reserving the mozzarella cheese to add at the last minute. Place these works of art on foil or a cookie sheet and bake for 20 minutes or until sizzling and fork-tender. Top with mozzarella cheese and put under broiler until golden brown, or around 3–5 minutes. Variation: Use Greek salad ingredients, such as olives, red onion, and feta instead, or just broil or sauté the mushrooms alone after brushing them with extra virgin olive oil and balsamic vinegar, maybe a sprinkle of rosemary. Serve whole or in strips over a bed of baby greens drizzled with olive oil and a squeeze of lemon.

Day 2 – Dinner

Wild Alaskan Salmon in Dill Sauce

This salmon recipe is courtesy of Randy Hartnell, president of Vital Choice Seafood, which specializes in national delivery of sustainable, uncontaminated fish.

Suggested side: Greens with Crumbled Stilton and Blackberries

(6) 4-oz wild Alaskan salmon fillets, (available from Vital Choice)
1/2 cup organic butter
3 egg yolks
1 teaspoon grated onion
1 tablespoon vinegar
1/2 teaspoon dried tarragon
1 tablespoon lemon juice
1 tablespoon fresh or dry dill
Real Salt, to taste

Preheat grill for medium heat or use broiler. If the salmon is fresh, be careful not to overcook it. Place still-FROZEN salmon filet directly on lightly oiled grill (or broiler). Cook salmon for 6–8 minutes per side (less for fresh fillets) or until pink only inside. Remove salmon from the grill to allow it to continue cooking while away from heat. Serve with a lemon-infused dill sauce!

Dill Sauce: Heat butter in heavy saucepan until hot and foamy but not browned. In a small bowl, whisk egg yolks, lemon juice, salt, tarragon, and dill. Gradually add butter. Return mixture to saucepan and heat over very low heat until mixture is slightly thickened. Serve immediately.

Variations: Try the same recipe but with halibut or sablefish; any herb can be used in place of the dill.

Serve with greens, red onion slivers, goat cheese, and blackberries drizzled with olive oil and lemon.

Day 2 – Dessert

Greek Yogurt with Berries and Chocolate

With the consistency of a rich mousse, Greek yogurt is incredibly versatile and equally at home as a garnish to a savory meal—such as a soup or chili—or a sweet dessert or breakfast parfait. For this dessert, simply sweeten Greek yogurt (such as Fage's) with several drops of vanilla stevia, then layer with fresh or frozen berries and melted, smartly sweetened dark chocolate. There will be little conversation once this is served!

Day 3 – Breakfast

Huevos Rancheros with Black Soybeans and Salsa

Follow a basic huevos rancheros recipe (basically eggs the way you like them with salsa and avocado and cheese), but upgrade the refried beans with mashed black soybeans (such as Eden Organic's) and garlic-flavored Real Salt; add olive oil to make them creamy.

Grated cheese would be in order (the ultimate upgrade for this would be the raw, grass-fed jalapeño cheddar from US Wellness Meats). In week two, you could serve this over half of a very low-impact tortilla (such as French Meadow Bakery's Healthy Hemp tortilla). A mound of Greek yogurt and a sprinkle of scallions makes a fantastic, though optional, finish.

Day 3 – Lunch

Grass-fed BLT with Favorite Cole Slaw

The healthy BLT would incorporate grass-fed bacon (such as US Wellness Meats), cooked just tender. The first week, you'll simply wrap the bacon (optional: avocado slices) and tomato in large lettuce leaves spread generously with real mayonnaise (such as Spectrum Organic's olive oil mayo). The second or third week, try wrapping this bundle in a hemp seed tortilla from French Meadow Bakery, which you've first sautéed in butter. Additional ingredients could be baby Swiss cheese, dill pickle (such as Strub's organic), or even Granny Smith apple slices.

Suggested side, Favorite Cole Slaw: Upgrade your favorite traditional cole slaw recipe by using a smart sweetener instead of sugar and real organic mayo. Caraway seeds are always a nice touch. Cabbage is very good food for your stomach.

Day 3 – Dinner

Southwest Hemp Seed Pilaf over Avocado

This is a signature dish I developed for my programs. It is a new kind of food because of the amazing hemp seed base: a cross between Spanish rice and taco salad that will "scratch the grain itch" without spiking your blood sugar. It is also largely raw (hemp seed requires no cooking), gluten-free, and full of healthy fats. Serves 4–8 as side dish or entrée. Vary recipe by adding ground free-range turkey or topping with chicken strips.

2 roasted red peppers (see Roasted Red Peppers recipe below)
5 tablespoons high temperature cooking oil such as Mac Nut or grape seed oils
1 medium roughly diced onion
1 cup raw pumpkin seeds
2 teaspoons minced garlic
1/2 teaspoon Real Salt
1/2 teaspoon cumin
1/2 teaspoon coriander
1 large can drained, canned organic roasted tomatoes (such as Muir Glen's)
4-1/2 cups shelled hemp seed (such as Nutiva's)
1/4 cup washed and chopped fresh cilantro
1/4 teaspoon ground cayenne pepper
1/3 cup chopped scallions or green onions
2 cups organic baby spinach (pre-washed, bagged kind is easiest)
2 avocados cut into 3/4" pieces
Optional: 4 tablespoons lemon olive oil, or the juice of half a lemon to garnish
Optional: 1" piece of finely chopped jalapeno pepper

Sauté onion and pumpkin seeds over medium heat in oil until pumpkin seeds start to snap and pop. Add garlic and sauté another minute (mixture will be golden brown). Add tomatoes, spices, and salt and heat until simmering. Remove from heat. Stir in roasted red peppers, hemp seed, cilantro (jalapeño if desired), and scallions. Place spinach in a large serving bowl. Pour hemp seed mixture over top and gently fold into spinach. Arrange avocados on top and drizzle with oil.

Over-the-top garnishes: a dollop of Greek yogurt and low-impact tortilla chips such as those by R. W. Garcia (for scooping).

ROASTED RED PEPPERS: A VERSATILE STAPLE

This is an incredibly tasty, versatile ingredient to dramatically heighten the taste of salads, soups, and just about any other dish. You can do this using either your broiler or a gas stove. Place the entire washed (uncut) pepper on low flame or under broiler and turn every few minutes. The outer skin will turn black and it may blister. Once the whole pepper is black, remove from heat (carefully, with a long utensil) and rinse it under cold water. Once cool enough to touch, rub off all charred material under cold running water. The remaining pepper is sweet and tasty. Remove the inner seeds and white pith and cut into 2″-long strips or leave whole for stuffed peppers. Use immediately or store in olive oil in a glass jar in refrigerator (lasts at least a month if entirely covered). Peppers can be stuffed with many of the recipes here, including Hemp Seed Tabouli, Creamed Spinach, Grass-fed Meatloaf, Southwest Hemp Seed Pilaf, or even the BLT with Avocado.

Day 3 – Dessert

Midnight Chocolate Fondue
Served with jicama and lime

Follow a classic chocolate fondue recipe, but be sure to start with unsweetened dark chocolate, add a couple of tablespoons of virgin coconut oil (such as Nutiva's), and sweeten smartly. I was excited to experiment with different lesssweet dipping options and found that jicama, a large root vegetable with a nonsweet, watermelonlike texture, was divine, particularly when saturated with in lime prior to dipping. Jicama is loaded with vitamin C and doesn't brown once it's cut (because of the lack of sugar).

Other low-impact dipping choices include Granny Smith apples, blackberries, and strawberries. Make it exotic by adding ground cinnamon and a bit of ground cayenne pepper to the fondue. Herbs such as rosemary and tarragon are another chocolate chapter altogether...

Day 4 – Breakfast

Organic Whole Yogurt with Berries and Nuts

Use unsweetened organic whole yogurt, add smart sweetener, berries, and then swirl in nut butters or sprinkle on raw or toasted nuts according to your whims. After the second week, you could experiment with sprinkling on a low-glycemic cereal such as Uncle Sam's or Flax Z Snacks; just eat a few bites of the yogurt before you take a bite of the cereal.

Day 4 – Lunch

Dilled Egg Salad, Flourless Herb Crackers

Served with mixed baby greens

   Boil a dozen organic eggs for three minutes and place under cold water. Remove from shells and cut eggs in large, uneven chunks. Sprinkle generously with Real Salt and pepper and fold in enough real mayo to make very creamy, without mushing up the yolks too much. Add fresh or dry dill to taste. Add a touch of paprika as a garnish. Serve with flourless herb and flax crackers, such as Lydia's Organics, over a bed of greens or with roasted pumpkin seeds.

Day 4 – Dinner

Turkey-Tomato Fennel Sauce Over Hemp Seed

This is also one of my signature sauces, and the credit for its mouthwatering aroma and taste goes primarily to the fennel seed, which gives it a sweet, sausagelike taste that is amazing. Folding in baby spinach right at the end is the way to give the dish a wonderful color contrast and get in an entire salad's worth of greens without eating what seems like a salad.

   3 tablespoons high temp. cooking oil, such as grape seed or mac nut oil
   1 tablespoon fennel seeds
   1–4 cloves garlic, minced (I buy the pre-minced to save time)
   1 medium diced onion
   1 pound ground turkey (such as Shelton's Free Range ground turkey)

1 large can whole organic tomatoes, (such as Muir Glen's), drained
1/4 teaspoon cayenne pepper
1/2 teaspoon Real Salt
Black pepper to taste
1/3–1/2 cup organic heavy cream or half-and-half
Optional: 1 roasted red pepper, diced or sliced in small slices
Optional: 2 cups organic baby spinach

Sauté fennel seeds in oil over medium heat until they become fragrant and golden. Add onion and garlic and sauté briefly. Add ground turkey to pan, mixing well with fennel, onion, and garlic. Brown lightly until all pink is gone. Add tomatoes, salt, pepper, and cayenne and simmer another five minutes or longer. Add one-third to one-half cup of organic heavy cream or half-and-half to make a pink sauce. If desired, add roasted red pepper and/or fold in some prewashed baby spinach. Serve over a bed of hemp seed (such as Nutiva's).

Starting in week two, you can serve this as a sauce over very low-glycemic pasta (such as Dreamfield's) or over a hemp seed bagel (available from French Meadow Bakery), Sloppy Joe-style. Serves 4–6.

Day 4 – Dessert

Goji Berry Shake

This is a spectacular-looking treat, due to the intense red-orange carotenoid pigments of goji berries, which makes them incredibly nutritious. I love this recipe because it minimizes any chance of spiking from goji berries, which are a dried fruit. Follow my 4-Minute Ice Cream recipe using half-and-half ice cubes. Add a heaping tablespoon or more of soaked, drained goji berries (cover in not-quite-hot water for several hours to plump, then drain, to enhance flavor and mixability). After processing, add a little extra milk or half-and-half to turn the ice cream into a shake. Variations include adding a touch of vanilla extract or vanilla whey. Blend all ingredients on high speed until smooth. Rather have goji ice cream? Just omit the extra liquid step. Garnish with lightly toasted walnuts or raw cocoa nibs.

Day 5 – Breakfast

Poached Eggs with Smoked Wild Salmon

Poached eggs are about the healthiest way to cook eggs; there is little direct contact with scorching heat since water is used. You can either use a poacher or drop the eggs gently into vinegar-tinged boiling water "freestyle" from a shot glass, then gently maneuver and "unite" the egg as it cooks. I love the primordial look of a poached egg done this way. Complement the eggs with smoked wild Alaskan salmon. Capers are a nice garnish. If you dislike salmon, consider grass-fed bacon as an accompaniment.

In week 2, you can serve two eggs with one half of a lightly toasted, well buttered, very low-impact hemp seed bagel from French Meadow Bakery.

Day 5 – Lunch

Organic Chicken Sausage with Hemp Seed Tabouli

Prepare sausage as per package. For tabouli, follow any traditional tabouli recipe, but upgrade the bulgar wheat or grain with raw hemp seed. For a major shortcut, use prepared tabouli mix packets such as Simply Organic's. An alternative short-cut accompaniment to the chicken sausage is a side of real, organic, sulfite-free sauerkraut (such as Strub's). Sauerkraut is amazing for digestive health but sulfite-free is hard to find. Variation: Use hemp seed tabouli to stuff Roasted Red Peppers.

In week two or three, you could use French Meadow Bakery's hemp seed tortilla to wrap around chicken sausage and either the tabouli or the sauerkraut. Sauté the tortilla in butter first.

Day 5 – Dinner

Grass-fed Cheese Fondue

I love this kind of dinner because you feel like a kid making and eating it. You also wind up eating a salad's worth of vegetables or fruits. You can either wing this (it's hard to get into too much trouble melting cheese) or follow a fabulous traditional recipe combining fontina and Swiss cheeses, a little white wine, maybe some beef or chicken stock (or a bouillon cube as a shortcut), and maybe a dash of nutmeg and onion-flavored Real Salt. If possible, upgrade conventional cheese to raw, grass-fed cheeses (such as US Wellness Meats). Dipping options include radicchio chunks (love the bitterness against the cheese), Granny Smith apples, large berries, button mushrooms, blanched asparagus, sliced cooked chicken or grass-fed sausage, tomato chunks, or—in the second week—French Meadow Bakery's Healthy Hemp bread (cubed). This is a good example of good low-glycemic combining, as the cheese greatly lowers the impact of the bread.

Day 5 – Dessert

One-Minute Chocolate Mousse
Combine full-fat organic Greek yogurt (such as Fage) with a few drops of vanilla stevia and unsweetened organic cocoa powder (such as Dagoba's). Healthy enough to eat at any time of the day (heaven plus antioxidants for breakfast!). Vanilla whey protein powder, nuts, raw cacao nibs, nut butter, and berries are some possible variations. A touch of almond, cherry, walnut, or vanilla flavoring are all wonderful, too.

Day 6 – Breakfast

Coconut Flour Pancakes with Greek Yogurt and Acai Topping
You've never had pancakes like these. Miraculous coconut flour makes them spike-free. Greek yogurt (optional) and acai fruit make them truly exotic and decadent. Use berries if you don't have unsweetened frozen acai. This recipe was adapted from Cooking with Coconut Flour *by Bruce Fife, ND.*

> 2 eggs
> 2 tablespoons virgin coconut oil or butter
> 1/4 teaspoon vanilla extract
> 1 packet de-bittered stevia (such as NuStevia by NuNaturals)
> 1/8 teaspoon Real Salt
> 1/3 cup unsweetened coconut milk
> 1/8 teaspoon baking powder
> 3 tablespoons sifted coconut flour (available from Simply Coconut)

Blend together eggs, coconut oil, vanilla extract, coconut milk, stevia, and salt. Combine coconut flour with baking powder and thoroughly mix into batter. Heat 1 tablespoon of coconut oil or butter in a large skillet. Spoon batter onto hot skillet, making pancakes about 2-1/2 to 3 inches in diameter. Makes 8 to 10 pancakes.

Açai Topping:
1 frozen packet unsweetened açai purée from Sambazon
3 teaspoons water
Xylitol (such as NuNatural)
Maple flavoring (such as Frontier Natural Flavors)
1/2 teaspoon guar gum (thickening agent) from the health food store
Optional: Greek yogurt (such as Total by Fage)

In a saucepan, heat water to boil and add guar gum, xylitol, and maple flavoring, stirring until thickened. Turn off heat and add açai packet to melt. Stir to combine. Heat just until warm and drizzle over buttered coconut flour pancakes topped with Greek yogurt. A dusting of cinnamon or nutmeg makes a great plate garnish.
Variations: Use frozen blueberries or blackberries in place of the açai. Enhance the depth of flavor with a drop of food-grade tangerine, lime, or nutmeg essential oil (such as Young Living).

Day 6 – Lunch

Turkey Chili with Black Soy Beans and Low-Impact Chips
Starting with your favorite chili recipe, upgrade any beans to super-low-impact black soybeans (such as Eden Organic) to avoid a spike. Then upgrade the meat with free-range ground turkey (such as Shelton's). Use organic tomatoes (Muir Glen's canned are affordable). For a shortcut, use an organic chili seasoning mix (such as Simply Organic). For an extraordinary touch, add a bit of cinnamon to your recipe. Eliminate any sweet ingredients, such as molasses. Use low-impact tortilla chips (such as R.W. Garcia's Spicy Flax and Soy Tortilla Chips).
Variations: Add cheddar cheese and chopped raw onions on top; add a dollop of Greek yogurt or sour cream on top; pour over hemp seed; add guacamole,

avocado slices, or red pepper and roasted pumpkin seeds; poach a few eggs and add them to the top.

Day 6 – Dinner

Grass-fed Filet Mignon

The grass-fed filet mignon (available from US Wellness Meats) is a great source of healthy omega-3s. The taste is also incredible. Rub with your favorite dry herbs. When broiling grass-fed steaks check them often, as grass-fed meats cook much faster than other meats and contain more delicate fats. Never eat well-done meats, as they have been linked with both breast and prostate cancers. If you desire a medium center, remove from oven at medium rare. The meat will continue to cook for a minute or two after it's removed from heat just as fish will. Serve with the arugula salad with berries for a complete meal.

Thai Fish over Hemp Seed

  (4) 4-ounce halibut or sablefish filets (available from Vital Choice)
  Minced garlic
  Chopped onion
  1/4 cup virgin coconut oil
  Red pepper strips
  1–2 tablespoons curry powder (or prepared curry paste, such as Seeds of Change)
  1 small can water chestnut slices, drained
  1/2 cup toasted sesame seeds
  1 can unsweetened organic coconut milk

  Sauté the garlic and onion in butter and oil in a medium saucepan. Add red pepper strips and continue sautéing lightly. Add coconut oil and blend in curry powder or paste to taste. It can be extremely spicy, so add incrementally, tasting along the way. Add coconut milk and drained water chestnut slices, simmering the sauce on medium heat. Coat fish with sesame seeds and grill or broil, taking care not to overcook fish, then top with sauce. A side of lightly sautéed snow peas finished with toasted sesame oil and a squeeze of lime would make a nice complement. Serve alongside Snow Peas with Sesame oil.

Day 6 – Dessert

Chocolate-Cherry Float

See the 4-Minute Ice Cream recipe and make the chocolate variation. Scoop chocolate ice cream into a deep drinking cup. Fill with Steaz Diet Black Cherry Soda (the only diet soda sweetened with stevia). If you can't find Steaz Diet soda, don't use the regular; use cherry-flavored seltzer or plain seltzer water with cherry flavoring and liquid vanilla stevia added. Also consider adding the brand-new supplement/food hybrid, cocoa extract (by NuNaturals) to the Steaz Diet, or cherry seltzer water over homemade vanilla 4-Minute Ice Cream.

MORE UPGRADE IDEAS FOR SPECIAL OCCASIONS

Upgrade Your Brunch Favorites

Better Eggs Benedict

Follow any hollandaise sauce recipe and poach your eggs (organic, preferably), but skip the English muffin. Use hemp seed instead the first week, or French Meadow Bakery hemp seed bagel halves starting the third week. *Florentine variation*: Sauté organic baby spinach in butter and a squeeze of lemon and place under eggs (over hemp seed or bagel half) before covering all with hollandaise.

Transformed French Toast (starting week 2)

Again, follow a traditional French toast recipe, upgrading any sugar with a smart sweetener. Use French Meadow Bakery's hemp seed bread instead of regular bread. This actually makes the final result lots tastier and heartier. Add a heaping tablespoon of melted virgin coconut oil to the beaten eggs you dip the bread into to lower the impact and add a wonderful taste. Add vanilla to the egg mixture. Saturate the bread completely with the egg mixture before you cook it in butter. This is key for creating a low-impact result. Top with a maple flavoring-spiked, smartly sweetened purée of dark berries or acai fruit. A dollop of Greek yogurt and a sprinkle of cinnamon complete the picture. As long as you've gone that far, maybe some crushed walnuts? I have also topped these with homemade cranberry sauce. Unbelievable, and leftover toast actually makes a fantastic portable snack.

Suggested Brunch Beverages:

- Teeccino Lattes (Teeccino is made for both coffee and espresso brewers)
- Virgin Bloody Marys (just add lime, spices, and a celery garnish to tomato juice)

Upgrade Your Holiday Traditions

Savory Smart Stuffing

Upgrade the croutons to homemade low-impact ones created from French Meadow Bakery's hemp seed bread. Just butter slices of bread and sprinkle on your favorite stuffing herbs, such as sage and rosemary. Bake until crisp and cut into croutons. Follow your stuffing and bird recipes as usual.

Perfect Pumpkin Pie

Go crustless, or make the crust with coconut flour. Sweeten smartly. Use cream instead of condensed or evaporated milk.

Excellent Eggnog

Start with a traditional eggnog recipe but use organic eggs; upgrade the sweetener to a smart one. Either use a little rum, or no rum and rum flavoring instead; don't forget the nutmeg.

Clever Cranberry Sauce

Just use real cranberries with a little water and plenty of smart sweetener. Add your favorite touches, such as cinnamon sticks, orange rinds, or my favorite: pomegranate seeds. Mulling spices also make a great sauce.

Merrier Mulled Cider

Start with a 4:1 ratio of water to unsweetened pure cranberry juice. Sweeten smartly to taste, then simmer with mulling spices, such as prepared mulling spice packets by Simply Organic.

Suggested Snacks

A snack that isn't worthy of being a meal is probably not fit to be a snack. With these meal-worthy options, you'll never be at a loss for taste or satiety in a pinch. Just remember to keep them in your purse and at the office.

- Free-range turkey jerky such as Shelton's
- A few squares of low-impact chocolate
- Low-impact chips (see Resources) with salsa or guacamole
- Raw nuts with a few roasted or spiced nuts mixed in for taste
- Crunchy baked cheese snacks, like Just the Cheese, "Popped Cheese," or Kitchen Table Bakers' gourmet cheese crackers (flourless)
- Olives and sliced cheese
- Very low-impact energy bars, such Paleo bars or Think Bars
- Half an avocado with hot sauce or salsa
- Flourless herb/flax crackers with egg salad
- Bites of Greek yogurt
- Plain kefir or Plain Yo-Goat (a goat milk yogurt drink), smartly sweetened or flavored if desired
- Roasted pumpkin seeds
- Spoonfuls of almond butter
- Low-impact pumpkin pie, smartly sweetened (crustless or coconut crust)
- Coconut flour brownie
- A piece of Transformed French Toast

CHAPTER 8

WHEN FOOD IS YOUR DRUG

It's often the most self-disciplined people
who skip meals or starve themselves,
who fall victim to compulsion.

Most of us use food for comfort now and then. But more and more of us—at least thirteen million in this country—use food more like a drug. As someone who is completely free of any negative issues with food after a twelve-year, heroinlike addiction to it eventually endangered my life, I'm not here to tell you what you already know about psychoanalytic or pharmaceutical approaches to food addiction. I'm much more compelled to fill in some glaring informational blanks that could have saved me enormous struggle and a serious health crisis, had someone shared them with me.

First, if you believe you have an eating disorder, I strongly urge you to seek medical supervision, keep an eye on your health, and address your emotional issues. I will share the emotional considerations that helped me here, but more importantly, I'll outline the crucial biochemical and nutritional factors that are too often overlooked in conventional treatment, which made all the difference for me and for many others when all else failed. Even if your relationship with food is relatively healthy or only mildly addictive, the insights that follow may help you resolve or avoid negative food issues altogether.

Many people who have followed my approach have found themselves free of issues with food they never even knew they had.

SIZE HAS LITTLE TO DO WITH IT

You don't need to have an eating disorder to get fat, and you certainly don't need to be fat to have an eating disorder. People often make the mistake of assuming otherwise, and even the medical world may overlook a person's eating disorder because that person is a normal size. Thin people with eating disorders can suffer terribly, thinking of food every minute, and destroying their metabolisms by starving for days after a binge. This can be worse for your health than getting big by overeating gradually.

ARE YOU ADDICTED TO FOOD?

Here are ten signs—both mild and severe—that you may be using food as a drug:

- You need a sugar or caffeine fix to get you from lunch to dinner.
- You think about food a lot when you're not eating.
- You regularly reward yourself with large amounts of food and then feel guilt or shame.
- You feel the urge to binge when you are upset.
- You skip meals purposely and then gorge in one sitting.
- You get a buzz from food.
- You salivate over food advertisements.
- You prefer to eat alone, so you can eat all you want in peace.
- You obsess about your next meal, even while full from the previous one.
- You deal with out-of-control appetite by having nonfat frozen yogurt, huge plates of vegetables, or fat-free chips.
- You worry about not getting enough food when you have to share.
- You continue to eat even after you experience physical discomfort from an overly full stomach.

HOW CRAVINGS BECOME COMPULSIONS

Food obsession falls under the form of self-sabotage I call compulsive self-sabotage, the hardest kind of self-destruction to shake. Unlike lack of information or incessant marketing cues, which lead to unwitting or culturally-assisted self-sabotage, food addiction—like other forms of compulsive self-sabotage such as smoking, drinking, and even hard drug abuse—is fed by much stronger roots: your biochemistry and emotions intertwined. Compulsive self-sabotage can be as serious as a full-blown food addiction or as seemingly innocent as your coffee or juice fix, your fourth glass of wine, or that twinge of torment you feel as you scan the pastry selection and rationalize that "healthier" whole grain muffin, while waiting in line for your green tea (sugar–saturated) Frappuccino. Even if this little vice never escalates, it is still likely taking years off your life and adding years to your looks.

But what starts out innocently enough can become a growing need. For example, a person may feel a "crash" an hour or so after eating a sugary or starchy meal and then reach for sweets, chips, or caffeine around 11 a.m. and 2 p.m. to relift their blood sugar and even their feel-good brain chemicals. The problem is, *the more we eat, take, or drink things that spike these "feel good" brain chemicals, the more we cause their depletion in our natural brain chemistry.* Sugar and alcohol binges, for example, are shown to spike dopamine (the same neurotransmitter that gives cocaine its pleasurable effect) and, over time, reduce our natural receptors for it. They also deplete serotonin. This can lead to seriously handicapped function of the brain's feel-good responses, diminishing our sense of well-being and making us vulnerable to deeper depression and more serious cravings in between "fixes." And when a person can no longer ride out a low without getting their fix again, they have officially become an addict.

Now you may still believe that willpower is the best protection from these lures. But *it's often the most self-disciplined people who skip meals or starve themselves, who fall victim to compulsion.* If they are made vulnerable by common brain chemical imbalances, heredity, or common hidden nutrient deficits (and many thin and athletic people are), there are certain compulsions that not only defy willpower but actually thrive on it.

Starve Your Vice of Its Support Through a Process of Shedding

The principles of shedding were the essence of what freed me. They can lead you steadily toward true freedom from any kind of compulsive self-sabotage because they systematically starve the emotional and chemical roots that feed it, until it loosens its grip and lets go.

The Three Ingredients of Food Obsession

When food is used as padding from our pain, our challenges, or a life we cannot fully embrace, it becomes a drug. And make no mistake: food—like drugs—can have strong chemical effects. It can produce a serotonin rush and can even cause the body to release natural opiates by triggering chemical reactions in the brain. In some cases, fermentation in the stomach can raise one's blood-alcohol level and cause an intoxicating effect similar to alcohol, or one may develop the dopamine-spiking pattern I mentioned earlier. I call this buzz the "elation and sedation effect." People aren't born with this chemical relationship with food; they develop it.

An addictive relationship with food requires three factors:

- The emotional need for the "drug" (food)
- The biochemical relationship with food that helps you use it as a drug
- The druglike foods themselves and their prevalence in your life

The combination of these three factors is the key to both the development of food obsession and complete freedom from it. Dealing with one aspect of the problem alone, such as emotional issues or better food choices, is never enough. Only when we address all three aspects at once will the demon finally flee. But too often the approach people take to deal with their food issues does not address any of these factors.

IS CONQUERING OUR EMOTIONS A PREREQUISITE OF CONQUERING FOOD OBSESSION?

I learned, to my own great surprise, that focusing on only emotional issues as a starting point, while sound in theory, set me up for a decade of needless struggle that might have been partially or even entirely avoidable if I'd only looked at my biochemical issues first. I cannot credit my years of intense emotional work with freeing me from my disease. Even those emotional breakthroughs I did have, which I will share in a moment, were not at all fruitful until I finally addressed my biochemical addiction to food through food and food supplements themselves. And because I have shared this hard lesson with many others for years, I have watched them escape what appeared to be inescapable odds and achieve incredible, healthy transformation that greatly lifted their emotional struggles as an end result, rather than a prerequisite. I've included some of their stories in chapter 10.

CONVENTIONAL TREATMENT OFTEN LEAVES CORE BIOCHEMICAL FACTORS UNADDRESSED

The clinical approach to eating disorders typically combines therapy and often anti-depressants with nutritional counseling. It also entails either learning about basic food pyramid principles. If you are a "restrictor" (anorexic or bulimic)—it may discourage you from thinking about calories at all (and encourage you to eat destructive high-impact foods). Virtually all programs will seek to help you identify the triggers behind what is viewed largely as "emotional eating." Exploring the emotional issues that make you use food as a drug is important. I did not choose therapy, but instead spent a lot of time reading self-help books and journaling. If you seek therapy, just be sure to find an experienced counselor with a successful track record with eating disorders who has not depended only on prescribing drugs. Finally, whether you undergo counseling or not, remember that it ultimately comes down to you; don't fall into the trap of waiting for the answer to come from someone else.

Critical Mood Nutrients

I would have sworn that my emotions were behind my eating disorder. Only years later would I fully understand the staggering (and deceptive) power of the biochemical influences that masquerade as emotions. The factors below are just a sampling of nutritional factors that contribute not only to eating disorders, but to other addictions and emotional balance in general:

Imbalances in the "feel-good" brain chemicals, such as serotonin and dopamine, have been directly linked to depression, anxiety, insomnia, carb cravings, and even compulsions such as alcoholism, bulimia, and gambling. Supplementation with the amino acid L-tryptophan or its derivative, 5Htp, as well as L-tyrosine have been shown in numerous studies to increase serotonin and dopamine respectively without side effects. Serotonin deficiency predicted bulimia relapses in one study. Similar malfunctions in serotonin and dopamine balance have been seen in all addictions. Addiction clinics that incorporate amino acid therapies achieve success rates up to 60 percent greater than addiction clinics and 12-step programs that do not.

Blood sugar stabilizing nutrients can stabilize the blood sugar changes that create cravings and mood swings (not to mention weight problems). Nutrients such as chromium, gymnema, cinnamon, and alpha-lipoic acid, among others, help the body use insulin and metabolize sugar more efficiently. Zinc, another blood sugar stabilizing mineral, can actually resensitize the taste buds, reducing the need for sugar and salt in order to taste real food. In one study, zinc brought appetite back to anorexics. Abstaining from sugar itself reduces cravings of all kinds dramatically.

Omega-3 fatty acids, such as fish oil, have been proven to significantly reduce just about all of the common mood disorders connected with eating disorders and other addictions, including depression, anxiety, and even anger and aggression. It also helps resensitize the cells to insulin and helps the body burn fat.

N-acetyl cysteine (NAC) has shown promising effects in reducing compulsive-obsessive behaviors and raising serotonin and dopamine, in preliminary research.

B vitamin deficiencies have been linked with both depression and many addictions. NAD, a form of niacin, caused a stop to almost all withdrawal symptoms in alcoholics within four days in a study published in the *Journal of Surgical Obstetrics and Gynecology.* Low folic acid levels have been shown in depression.

Other nutrients, such as L-theanine, a component of green tea, relora, GABA, and Holy basil, have well-substantiated antianxiety effects. One need only do a quick Internet search to access myriad published studies about natural substances that improve mood, which the average psychiatrist might never find the time to read.

These supplements helped to dismantle my druglike relationship with food. Lack of nutritional raw materials for emotional health almost guarantees what often seem like insurmountable "emotional issues." Had I not taken these strategic nutritional steps to balance these key deficiency components of my food obsession, I would have remained at war with my body, no matter how many emotional breakthroughs I had, and I would have kept blaming my own "insanity" for my problem. Science has shown that a deficient brain cannot overcome certain problems without nutrient correction. Nutrition, unlike drugs, can actually restore basic functions, rather than just temporarily making up for them (while creating new imbalances), as drugs too often do.

DON'T SETTLE FOR A WEIGHT-LOSS OR "FOOD" PLAN; STRATEGIZE A HEALTH-GAIN PLAN

If you are burdened with excess weight, don't call it a weight problem. Don't let even your doctor call it that or treat it as such anymore. Weight is just a symptom of any number of health imbalances and addictive reactions with food that may or may not be connected with your emotional issues. Even if your doctor is focused on getting your weight into the "healthy" range, you will have more success and lose weight as an exciting side effect if you set out to regain your health instead. This was the only strategy that finally worked for me.

EXERCISE SENSE

Compulsion can thrive and express itself through strict dieting and exercise programs and must be dealt with separately from weight loss. I did a tremendous amount of exercise throughout most of my eating disorder, and I'm sure it kept me from becoming even more obese, but it did nothing at all to address my eating disorder. If you feel ashamed of yourself or inadequate if you skip a workout, the overall effect is negative and will likely distracting you from the real issues behind your food issues. Don't focus on exercise as the cure for your problem, and don't feel bad if it doesn't result in weight loss.

If you are addicted to food, don't let friends or doctor convince you that exercise can solve your problem or that your problem is due to lack of exercise. Once you've switched to low-impact eating and addressed your biochemical imbalances nutritionally, you will be surprised at your desire to get moving again, and you will take joy in activity. Exercise that is properly fueled with a focus on health (not calorie burning) will have a far more positive impact than weight loss-focused exercise. Some gym cultures may be negative for someone who is challenged with food or body image issues, so I suggest you find an activity in an environment that will really lift your spirit, like walking with a friend, yoga, or dancing at home to music or a video. Even

(continued on next page)

giving a massage to a loved one or catching up on physical household chores to wonderful music can give you the activity you need, while keeping you free from self-conscious or calorie-obsessed associations. Science has now found that repeated short bursts of activity with rest in between (called interval training) is preferable to sustained aerobic activity for health and fat burning, by the way.

Plan a strategy to balance the health issues that affect you. Take comfort in knowling that by upgrading the druglike food culprits I've outlined in this book to their low-impact counterparts, you will take untold stress off just about any health issue and can literally halt one of the most important mechanisms upon which food obsession depends: blood sugar swings. Explore every nutritional angle for addressing mood and blood sugar, thyroid, hormonal, and brain chemistry issues.

MOLLY AND THE DIET DOCTORS

Several years ago, I did the makeup for a model named Molly, who told me that she hadn't been able to keep any food down, except a bit here and there, for days. At the advice of her agent, she had been taking a popular but controversial weight-loss drug.

The woman was extremely skinny, even for a model, so it blew my mind that some-one with a medical license would give her this drug, which even then—before it was found to be deadly—was to be prescribed only to the substantially overweight. As Molly walked onto the set, she told me that she had temporarily lost her sight just a few days before and that the doctor had given her another drug to counteract that side effect. As I watched her pose, I actually saw her sway. It was amazing that this stranger had just told me this without blinking an eye. She was clearly calling out for help she wasn't getting elsewhere. In between shots, I gave her a special "meal cookie" I had made at home with nuts, flaxseeds, pumpkin seeds, grated carrots, and soy flour (I use coconut flour today). Later in the day she told me that this was the first food that had stayed down in days. Once we had finished the shoot, I gave her the number of an alternative doctor in Manhattan experienced with weaning people off the drug she was taking.

A few years later, I worked with Molly again and was happy to see that she was doing well. She thanked me for convincing her to get off of that drug. She had suffered some permanent effects from the weight-loss drug that required her to take precautions, such as taking antibiotics when having her teeth cleaned, but she was grateful to be alive and well.

SHEDDING SELF-SABOTAGING EMOTIONS

Once you begin to support your biochemistry and your emotional health with deep, rebalancing nourishment, working on your emotional issues will be more fruitful. Either therapy or solitary pursuits such as journaling, yoga, self-help books, or creative projects are all potent catalysts for emotional healing. The following were some of the emotional concepts that were key for me, once my biochemical issues were addressed:

- **Uproot your emotional triggers and family legacies.** If you are able to uncover and reject anything that has been "bestowed" or projected upon you by a parent or a traumatic experience, you will begin to dispel the inexplicable shame that often propels a person toward self-sabotage. By going through this effort now, you may also spare your own children the same legacy. Mother-daughter relationships, and sometimes father-daughter relationships, are behind most of the eating disorders and other self-destructive vices I see in the women who seek my help. Sometimes those closest to us have the most invested in our staying in our old patterns, not necessarily because they want bad things for us, but because our breaking free would cause them to look more deeply at themselves. Get some physical and emotional space.
- **Get angry, and then let it go.** Don't wait for apologies or answers from others who've done you wrong or contributed to your problem. Tell them exactly how you feel. Express your anger, but keep in mind that the worse this person treated you, the less likely you are to get an

admission or an apology from him or her. Realize that by waiting for one, you could go on putting your life on hold forever. Move ahead. Only you can change your situation now.

- **Deal creatively with stress and low moods.** We all know how far-reaching the effects of stress can be, both physically and emotionally. Set aside time and boundaries to pursue a creative passion of self-expression. Use alone time to tune in to yourself (not tune out). Learn from depression and anxiety. If you're more than mildly depressed, be sure to seek medical supervision, but also keep in mind that depression may be signaling you to step back from your normal routine to reassess how you are living your life. Be sure to spend time with people who encourage you to express yourself.

- **Give up the rules, the numbers, and the scale.** Preset menus and strict food lists encourage us to give up control and skip the thinking process. Calorie counting and weigh-ins put emphasis on numbers, which are deceptive and needlessly discouraging. All calories are not created equal, and neither are pounds. Forget calories and fat grams and the scale. Numbers are distractions from the real problem, and they cause more guilt trips.

- **Give yourself emotional padding to replace the physical and chemical padding that your vice provides.** Perfectionism and harsh self-judgment are usually a part of food obsession. They are signs that we are challenged in the area of unconditional self-love, which is the only padding that can replace the padding your vice gives you from your vulnerability and pain. Failure without an excuse is a scary prospect you never have to face as long as you have your compulsion as a buffer between you and your feelings and challenges. Give yourself permission to fail at all of the what-ifs and the thin dreams that you've accumulated.

This poem offers perhaps the best example I've come across of how to give ourselves the emotional "padding" and sanctuary of unconditional self-love. At the same time, it illustrates the courage it takes to let ourselves be uncovered and to give up the protective "layers" that obscure our inner beauty. The author is unknown.

The Difference Between Strength and Courage

It takes strength to be firm, It takes courage to be gentle,

It takes strength to stand guard, It takes courage to let down your guard,

It takes strength to conquer, It takes courage to surrender,

It takes strength to be certain, It takes courage to have doubt,

It takes strength to fit in, It takes courage to stand out,

It takes strength to feel a friend's pain, It takes courage to feel your own pain,

It takes strength to hide your own pains, It takes courage to show them,

It takes strength to endure abuse, It takes courage to stop it,

It takes strength to stand alone, It takes courage to lean on another,

It takes strength to love, It takes courage to be loved,

It takes strength to survive, It takes courage to live.

STACY: ANATOMY OF A TOTAL TRANSFORMATION

"If they only knew" was what I thought as I looked at my coworkers. I am highly respected at my marketing firm. They saw a "together" woman of relatively normal weight who they knew was a freak about the "F word" (fat). Little did they know that once alone at home, I had this freakish life of torment with food. In order to protect myself from my own inevitable nightly binges, I stocked up on my special foods that allowed me to binge with minimal repercussions. Each night featured the same ludicrous scene: I'd go in and out of the kitchen, battling the gravitational pull to the box of Luna bars or the half-gallon of fat-free ice cream. "No, I should go to sleep! Am I going to do it? No . . . Yes." This was my secret hell.

I had already been to a nutritionist, who got me eating much healthier food in general. I thought it would help, but to my surprise, it had little effect on my secret problem. I began to wonder if my own emotional issues were worse than I wanted to admit. I had binged and gone through stages of purging through college, but I had figured out how to binge on completely empty foods and minimize the weight gain. My life was not my own, and I didn't sleep. My body was agitated, and I was truly obsessed with food.

My nutritionist got me to attend Kat's program, and after seeing her own history and transformation and knowing she could truly relate, I was finally convinced not

(continued on next page)

only to try to eat some fat but also to take supplements to help my cravings and moods. I started eating plain, regular, organic yogurt and berries for breakfast (instead of artificially sweetened, nonfat yogurt); drinking green tea and a great-tasting herbal coffee I brewed in the coffeemaker (tastes the same—only better) instead of coffee. I started making Kat's decadent salads for lunch, adding garnishes I would never have touched before, like nuts, cheese, and olive oil, and taking essential fatty acids, chromium, 5HTP, carb-blockers, and melatonin at night. During the first couple of days, I tried one of Kat's tricks at a staff meeting where there were only bagels and cream cheese to eat. My coworkers' jaws dropped, and even I was having an out-of-body experience, when I took half a bagel and piled on some cream cheese, so I could eat it without starting my sugar pendulum. My coworkers had never seen me eat fat. After eating it, I felt calm and free of thoughts of food, cravings, and energy slumps until lunch, while everyone else kept making trips back to the pastry tray. At lunch, one woman in the office was entranced by the arugula salad I was eating at my desk. People have a powerful response when they see real, beautifully prepared food in a setting where we so often abuse ourselves.

It has been only one month since I made these changes, and my bingeing has stopped. I don't remember when it fully stopped, but for the last couple of weeks, I have been able to sit alone in my own house and—incredibly—not have obsessive thoughts or feel that menacing pull toward the refrigerator. Those nights feel like a distant memory, though it was such a short time ago. And since I started taking melatonin and using a sleep mask, I have been sleeping through the night until my alarm goes off, which is also a first. And the sleep, along with my sane relationship with food, has really changed something in me. I have always been a confident woman and I have loved my career, but for the first time in so long, I am feeling "pretty."

I have emotional issues like everyone else, but they are much less of a factor than I had thought. Something in my head has clicked in a big way. It has affected my attitude toward myself and my definition of food, but it is more a result of what has happened than the cause. I am free of the real cause of the craziness, and I know exactly what it was now. There is no struggle and no desire to go back. I have learned to free myself.

IT'S NEVER ALL IN YOUR HEAD

Remember that whether your vice is drinking, smoking, or eating, there are biochemical reasons behind it all. The urge to binge or overeat are not signs of your weak character but of imbalances in your body. Abstaining or even emotional or spiritual work alone cannot correct those imbalances.

Don't wait for conventional medicine and clinical nutrition to point you to the only health-building, truly rebalancing, drug-free escape from the biochemical bondage of food obsession there is: unpatentable, natural supplements.

Beyond this chapter, each facet of this book will help free you from unhealthy obsessions and compulsive self-sabotage. Our subconscious picks up on each positive action we make on our own behalf. Each upgraded choice will lift your spirit higher, embolden your self-advocacy, and deepen your self-respect. As more and more desensitizing choices and physical "noise" are lifted away, you'll begin to find negative self-treatment increasingly undesirable. This is the turning point at which any downward spiral will reverse and become an upward one.

It's impossible to predict the day your "demon" will let go, but it will if you continue to shed the layers of issues that feed it. When it does, it will be merely a thrilling side effect of a much more profound transformation you have already begun.

CHAPTER 9

ACHIEVE MAXIMUM RADIANCE WITH SUPPLEMENTS

"The fruit thereof shall be your meat, and the leaf your medicine."

—Ezekiel 47:12

It's hard for me to contain my enthusiasm for supplements. As an informed layperson who saved my own health and transformed my appearance with their crucial help, I consider supplements a key component of any serious beauty and body arsenal. Changing my head played a part in overcoming my eating disorder, but using supplements to change my biochemical relationship with food is what truly freed me from food addiction and healed the other serious health issues and imbalances caused by over a decade of self-abuse. I give supplements full credit for reversing my liver disorder and many other issues I'd been told I would be stuck with for the rest of my life. But maybe you take far better care of yourself than I once did, which is quite likely. Is it possible that you have sidestepped the need for supplements by doing all the right things? Are healthier food choices, exercise, and stress management enough to protect your precious vitality? Take this quiz and find out.

Which statements apply to you?
- I don't drink coffee or alcohol, or smoke.
- I was raised on whole, organic foods.

- I had very little sugar, soda, or white flour while growing up.
- I don't live in a polluted environment.
- I am not taking any prescription drugs.
- I don't drink, or shower in, chlorinated water.
- I have never taken antibiotics.
- I eat primarily raw, locally grown, organic food.
- I do not experience energy swings from food.
- I am not under a lot of stress.

If all of the above apply to you, you might not need to take supplements, but it still wouldn't hurt.

Vitamins and minerals are naturally occurring substances that have proven to be infinitely safer than synthetic drugs (and even far safer than foods). They can interact with prescription drugs; therefore, you should work with your doctor if you are being treated for specific health issues.

While far fewer government studies are conducted on natural (unpatentable) substances than on synthetic drugs, much of the evidence supporting the supple-

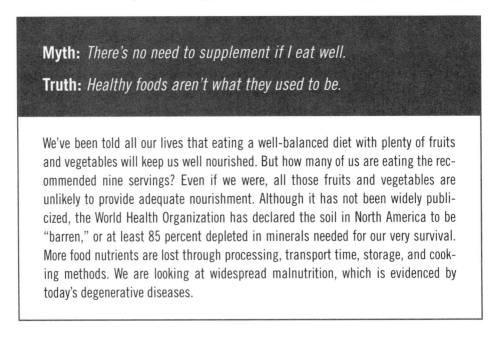

Myth: *There's no need to supplement if I eat well.*

Truth: *Healthy foods aren't what they used to be.*

We've been told all our lives that eating a well-balanced diet with plenty of fruits and vegetables will keep us well nourished. But how many of us are eating the recommended nine servings? Even if we were, all those fruits and vegetables are unlikely to provide adequate nourishment. Although it has not been widely publicized, the World Health Organization has declared the soil in North America to be "barren," or at least 85 percent depleted in minerals needed for our very survival. More food nutrients are lost through processing, transport time, storage, and cooking methods. We are looking at widespread malnutrition, which is evidenced by today's degenerative diseases.

ments covered in the following pages is far more conclusive than the conflicting science behind such accepted things as mammograms, the belief that dietary cholesterol causes heart disease, the purported benefits of low-fat diets, and many common surgical procedures thought to be necessary. If supplements such as fish oil were patentable synthetic drugs, the million-dollar TV ad campaign might go something like this: "Common side effects include relief from dry skin; silkier hair; anti-inflammatory effects throughout the body; reduced joint pain; improved immunity, hormone function, moods, and cholesterol levels; and countless other desirables. Warning: nature heals in ways we can only begin to predict."

NATURE IN THERAPEUTIC DOSES

No conventional doctor has ever warned me of the dangers of eating depleted foods. They tend to focus only on calorie intake. But the deficiencies found in most Americans of many key nutrients tested—such as chromium, zinc, magnesium and calcium, vitamins A, D, and E, and omega-3 fats—is startling. If your doctor is unconcerned with the harm and gradual malnourishment that come from eating empty foods, then he is not likely to grasp the importance of putting those nutrients back. If you don't look into what quality supplements can do for you, you are shortchanging nature's intention for you by denying yourself the most intuitive, therapeutic way to replenish yourself in this depleted and denatured world.

To put the safety of supplements into perspective, let's first consider that food kills 5,000 people a year, according to the CDC. Deaths from properly prescribed drugs exceed 106,000 deaths annually (and 2.2 million reported injuries), according to the *Journal of the American Medical Association* (*JAMA*). By contrast, only two deaths were reported in 2003 from non-iron-containing vitamin and mineral supplements, according to the American Association of Poison Control Centers. Zero deaths were reported from Chinese or ayurvedic herbal medicines; seven from intentionally abused stimulants like ephedra, ma huang, and yohimbe; two from iron poisoning; three from potassium, two from sodium, one from vitamin C, and one from vitamin B6—running neck and neck with deaths reported from plain soap, table salt, and baking soda. Most of these deaths couldn't be confirmed to be from those supplements. Considering that high-dose vitamin C increased male lifespan by six years without negative side effects in two studies published in the journal *Epidemiology*, there appears

> *MYTH: Dietary supplements are unregulated, unproven, and unsafe.*
>
> *TRUTH: Dietary supplements are both regulated and highly censored.*

The next time people tell you that supplements are unregulated, set them straight. Supplements are subject to extensive labeling requirements, including full disclosure of ingredients, nutrition information, and censorship of health-benefit claims by the FDA. Even most proven health claims, such as protection against certain cancers, reversal of dysplasia (abnormal cell growth), lowered cholesterol, decreased inflammation, relief from depression, improved insulin action, birth-defect prevention, and bone-loss prevention, for the most part, cannot legally be communicated on labels. So rather than supplement labels exaggerating, they are actually not at all representative of what most supplements are truly capable of.

According to Dr. Julian Whitaker, director of the Whitaker Wellness Institute and editor of the newsletter *Health and Healing*, more than eight thousand clinical studies attest to the protective effects of individual antioxidant vitamins, minerals, and extracts from mushrooms, herbs, and other medicinal plants.

to be an unheard-of risk-benefit ratio with such supplements. And that's just one amazing example out of thousands.

CAN MY DOCTOR TEACH ME ABOUT SUPPLEMENTS?

A doctor can only teach you about supplements if he has taught himself. This takes years of daily reading. Of all people, your poor doctor, who barely has time to see each patient, does not usually have time to do this and still keep up with the constant influx of "priority" new drug protocols. Books and naturopathic doctors are better places to turn for in-depth information. While the average doctor might know about a few supplements or suggest a multivitamin, some fish oil, or vitamin D, for example, this does not reflect a grasp of nutrition, which is not taught in medical school other than encouragement to overlook its importance. Pharmaceutical medicine, which is taught in medical school, is just that: pharmaceutical. While it is important to keep your doctor in the loop about the supplements you're taking if you are on prescription drugs or dealing with a health issue, expecting good information from him about food supplements is like asking a plumber about your home's electrical wiring. Keep in mind that the most well-known database for medical professionals, Medline, lists studies from most of the notable medical journals but does not list one of the best sources for information on nutritional supplements, the *Journal of Orthomolecular Medicine*. Orthomolecular medicine is a term coined by the late Linus Pauling, a two-time Nobel Prize laureate, who defined it as "the preservation of good health and the treatment of disease by varying the concentration in the human body of substances that are *normally present in the body*." I encourage you and your doctor to always include more than just Medline in your search for healing information. The link to free searchable archives from the *Journal of Orthomolecular Medicine* and other great sources, as well as ways to find doctors who are informed about nutrition and supplements in your area, are listed in the Resources section.

The important thing is to find a doctor who knows and admits the limits of his own knowledge and respects your desire to use prescription drugs as a last resort. You also need a doctor who does not ignore scientific proof (which means he would not fall for most headline news about supplements), buy into programmed thinking, or make sweeping generalizations about supplements. This is always a red flag of ignorance, since supplements are as diverse as foods. In short, ask not what your doctor thinks about supplements. Ask what he *knows*.

Luckily, with a search engine and a few spare hours, it's easy for any layman using a little good sense to know more about how supplements can benefit their own issues than the average doctor might ever teach themselves. Kind of sad, but that's no exaggeration.

GET GORGEOUS BY GUARDING YOUR HEALTH

Beauty and health are inseparable. What might be the best regimens for health issues like breast cancer prevention, antiaging, blood sugar issues, or eye health, are also some of the best supplements for your skin and your body. For example, alpha-lipoic acid detoxifies the body, recycles antioxidants for antiaging effects, and helps stabilize blood sugar for a slimmer body and wrinkle prevention. Both green tea and selenium have been shown to help prevent skin and breast cancer. Tocotrienols, a category of vitamin E components that inhibit human breast cancer cell lines in culture, are now believed to offer possibly greater antioxidant protection to the skin than the traditional, well-studied alpha tocopherol form of vitamin E. Dr. Nicholas Perricone notes that tocotrienols reduce redness and flaking in severely dry skin, prevent nails from cracking, and even make the hair shinier.

HOW CARMEN BECAME A CONVERT

Carmen, a bus driver who attended one of my presentations in New York, got excited when she learned about the studies that showed horse chestnut seed extract could shrink the swelling of varicose veins as well as compression-hose therapy while also actually decreasing ankle circumference in women with varicose veins (chronic venous insufficiency)—all this while improving vascular function throughout the entire body.

Carmen was so amazed and inspired by the reduced swelling and pain in her varicose veins after only a few weeks of using horse chestnut seed extract that she decided to start taking other supplements, like fish oil, quercetin, nettle, and methylsulfonylmethane (MSM). She soon noticed an improvement in her allergies and psoriasis. Her skin no longer burned in the shower and she was able to sit outside at her sister's country home in upstate New York for the first time without having an allergy attack. "I feel like these supplements have taken ten years off," said Carmen.

DO ANTIOXIDANTS WORK OR NOT?

Just as the average person has begun to grasp the impact of oxidative stress (free radicals) on the skin and body caused by such lifestyle assaults as sun exposure, smoking, grilled meats, and trans fats, some shocking headlines proclaimed that antioxidant supplements do not work. Most people are used to such controversial headlines being disproved only days later, but in case you have any doubts about the power of antioxidants—and I'm not talking about antioxidants in food but antioxidants in *supplement form*—let me give you some hard examples of their proven effects, beauty and beyond:

Milk thistle's active component, silymarin, demonstrated inhibitory effects on photoaging and skin cancer in several animal studies. Another of its components, silibinin, was shown to inhibit human breast, cervical, and prostate cancer and inhibit the spread of breast cancer.

Pycnogenol, a pine bark extract, not only reduced skin redness from UVB exposure in one study; it significantly reduced chronic leg swelling and pain up to 64 percent in women with varicose veins in another.

Alpha-lipoic acid (ALA) actually recycles other antioxidants in the body, and is protective of skin while it reduces the progresson of diabetes.

Carotenoids, such as lycopene, lutein, and zeaxanthin, have all been found to significantly improve or protect skin health. Lycopene also reduces prostate cancer risk, while lutein and zeaxanthin together reduced the risk of both cataracts and age-related macular degeneration in several studies.

Vitamin E supplementation has been shown not only to reduce dermatitis but to improve blood sugar control in diabetics and immunity in older people. Diets high in vitamin E and multivitamins failed to offer heart protection in a Harvard study, but supplements did.

In addition to its proven role in collagen formation, wound healing, and connective tissue functions, vitamin C, in combination with other antioxidants, has shown sun-protective effects in the skin. 300 mg of vitamin C per day has dramatically reduced the risk of cataracts. 800 mg per day extended lifespan (more on that in a moment), and 1,500 mg per day allowed asthmatic women to exercise without their airways closing up. High doses are now being studied against cancer.

Along with its well-known sleep cycle-regulating effects, the antioxidant hormone melatonin has shown protective effects against both UV radiation in the skin and cancer in the body.

Selenium supplementation has demonstrated synergy with other antioxidant supplements in benefiting the skin, and it also reduced cancer mortality in humans by 50 percent over ten years, in a study published in *JAMA*.

The next time you read a headline that says antioxidants or supplements don't work, you can send this—or the hundreds of research citations in the back of this book—to the editor.

BEYOND ANTIOXIDANTS: NEXT-GENERATION ANTIOXIDANT "CATALYSTS"

You may be familiar with the phrase "high-ORAC"-rated (oxygen radical absorbance capacity) foods, often used to describe the comparative antioxidant power of fruits, vegetables, and super-foods. But what looks to be a far more effective therapy against oxidative stress is emerging, and it may revolutionize our approach to fighting free radicals. Enter the antioxidant enzyme catalysts. Clinical research has shown that the body's own antioxidant enzymes, such as SOD (superoxide dismutase), can be activated by certain nutrients and are literally thousands of times more powerful than any ingested antioxidant supplement or food at quenching oxidative stress. One would literally have to consume dozens of pounds of high-ORAC foods each day to realize the antioxidant effects obtained by merely switching on these enzymes already in the body with single daily doses of these antioxidant catalysts. Some brands are listed in the Resources section.

ANTIAGING SUPPLEMENTS: FACT OR FICTION?

Just as the debate on antioxidants has continued even though thousands of studies have determined their effectiveness, "expert panels" are still debating whether supplements could possibly have antiaging effects. "More evidence is needed," they often conclude. You be the judge. Let's start with humble little vitamin C, which, at a dose of 800 mg per day, increased the lifespan of men by six years compared to men who took only the RDA amounts in a ten-year study on over 11,000 males done at UCLA in 1992. Another study of similar size and length, published only a few years later, showed a 42 percent reduction in death from all causes in those who took both vitamins C and E. According to renowned nutritionist Oz Garcia, author of *Look and Feel Fabulous Forever*, the amazing hormone-precursor DHEA's antiaging benefits are documented in well over two thousand published studies, demonstrating its ability to improve age-related stress, immunity, hormonal, weight, libido, mood, and heart issues. Garcia suggests taking salivary or blood tests under medical supervision when using DHEA.

Yet another powerful approach to antiaging is the prevention of glycation, which wrinkles the skin and ages the entire body by producing its own free radical-generating "cooked" proteins throughout the body. Animal studies have demonstrated that a dipeptide called carnosine (not to be confused with

L-carnitine) not only inhibited glycation but extended lifespan, improved brain function, and even improved the appearance of rats by keeping their fur dark and glossy and reducing skin ulcers. Similarly, a combination of ALA and the amino acid acetyl L-carnitine caused a reversal of age-related memory, mobility, and cellular decline in rats.

Do these effects translate to humans? Dr. Ron Rosedale, a renowned authority on metabolic health, had this to say: "The same genes that regulate aging in yeast, worms, and mice are found (with slight variations) in humans as well. Translating an appropriate dose for a supplement is the key challenge in achieving these effects in humans. As a general rule, any modality, diet, or supplement that reduces glycation, insulin, or leptin, or anything that enhances mitochondrial health (which determines the body's ability to convert fuel into usable energy) will extend lifespan. ALA, acetyl L-carnitine, carnosine, and many other nutrients fit that criteria."

Speaking of mitochondrial health, a 2006 placebo-controlled Japanese study published in *Experimental Gerontology* showed the incredible antiaging effects of a new more bioavailable form of CoQ10 called ubiquinol in mice. The effects of CoQ10 in preventing mitochondrial energy decline in aging cells is well known. Ubiquinol slowed the onset of aging markers 40 percent more effectively than conventional CoQ10 in mice, and produced as much as *a 51 percent decrease in biological aging* at the equivalent of late middle age (at a dose equivalent to human intake of 200–300 mg per day), compared to controls. Photos of the mice, featured in the spring 2007 issue of *Life Extension* magazine, showed decrepit features such as spinal humps, dull fur, and ulcers on the untreated mice, while those fed ubiquinol remained "attractive."

Additionally, a hugely publicized 2006 study conducted at Harvard found that resveratrol, a powerful antioxidant from red grape skins, extended lifespan, increased exercise tolerance, and protected the brains of aging mammals (among other miraculous benefits) without side effects. But as quickly as the news came, the ensuing headlines discouraged people from taking resveratrol supplements, dumbfounding resveratrol supplement makers. But having captured America's full attention, scientists assured us they were busy at work synthesizing a "better" (patentable, adulterated) prescription version of the natural substance. Then the confusion really hit when we all "learned" from headlines a few months later that antioxidants "don't really work after all."

> ## MORE BEAUTIFUL REASON TO QUIT SMOKING
> A 2002 study done by scientists at the Scripps Research Institute in La Jolla, California, found that smoking accelerates the glycation process. A nicotine byproduct caused an accelerated "cooking" as well as the formation of health- and skin-destroying glycated proteins. Additionally, a 2007 study done in Rome linked smoking with greater incidence of noninflammatory acne and reduced skin secretions of vitamin E.

CAN SUPPLEMENTATION MAKE UP FOR FLAWED GENES?

The amazing ability of nutrion to influence how or whether genetic traits translate into disease should give new hope to anyone feeling doomed by their genes. Pterostilbene, the previously discussed substance found in blueberries, can inhibit the expression of certain genes upon which the progression of colon cancer depends. Resveratrol was found to switch on genes that aid DNA repair and extend life, while switching off disease-promoting genes, thus slowing the rate of disease and aging in mammals. In the August 2002 edition of *Health and Healing*, Dr. Julian Whitaker stated that someone with a family history of colon cancer can reduce the doubled risk of getting colon cancer to that of the average person by taking 400 mcg of folic acid every day. Sometimes, even when gene expression is inevitable, nutritional supplementation can mitigate the effects of the defect by making up for its consequences. For example, genetic inability to convert omega-6 fatty acids to the anti-inflammatory gamma linoleic (GLA) can lead to eczema. GLA supplementation is believed to somewhat make up for this deficiency and relieve its symptoms, such as itching, flaking, inflammation, and dryness. These examples are the tip of the iceberg.

START WITH A HIGH-QUALITY, HIGH-POTENCY CORE MULTI-NUTRIENT REGIMEN

A high-potency multivitamin, along with omega-3s, such as fish oil, and a blood sugar formula are a good bare-minimum "American antidote" regimen to address issues of depleted food and ongoing or past assaults to our biochemistry. Green powders, high-dose vitamin D3, and a good ionic mineral supplement add another measure of basic recovery and protection. These things are prerequisites just to halt nutritional depletion so you can regain control of your cravings, moods, and energy.

All vitamins are not created equal. You get what you pay for. Avoid little one-per-day pills that have 100 percent of all the Recommended Dietary Allowances (RDAs). They're useless. One little pill stuffed with body-foreign "USP" (synthetic), isolated vitamins will do little for you. These are the substances generally found in discounted pharmacy vitamins. The point of food supplements is that they are utilized like food by the body. In order to do this, they must generally be naturally occurring nutrients from foods, mineral deposits in the earth, or plants.

RECOMMENDED DAILY ALLOWANCES (RDAS) ARE NOT ENOUGH

RDAs are archaic figures that were developed to prevent serious malnutrition or deficiencies (which we now know they do not even do). Unless you're sailing to the New World and are merely trying to avoid scurvy, go beyond RDAs if you're looking to achieve even basic health, let alone radiance. RDAs effectively limit your capacity to heal yourself or even prevent disease. For example, you'd need at least three times the RDA of vitamin C to achieve the amounts shown in studies to decrease the risk of cataracts, increase lifespan, or help keep airways open during exercise if you're an asthmatic woman. Vitamin E's major heart benefits do not really kick in until you're taking at least 800 IU (more than ten times the RDA) and only if it's the natural form. Vitamin D does not show its power to prevent autoimmune diseases like MS, bone loss, colon cancer, seasonal affective disorder (SAD), or cut breast cancer risk in half unless you take more than 2,000 IU per day (five times the RDA!). Even prenatal supplements were shown to leave mothers-to-be dangerously deficient in vitamin D. If RDAs are set for our protection, the science shows that they consistently achieve just the opposite: dangerous deficiency with false security.

The most advanced, full-spectrum multi-nutrient regimens contain therapeutically proven potencies of nutrients that far exceed RDAs. They often look like horse pills or consist of multiple capsules and oil pills (EFAs don't combine well in pills or capsules and so are taken separately). They have a distinctive odor when fresh (if a tablet) and are usually taken three times a day (although just one of these pills would likely give you more benefit than a week's worth of once-per-day little pills). Avoid cheap vitamins, generic drugstore brands, and brands filled with dicalcium phosphate, cellulose, and other fillers. United States Pharmacopeia (USP) vitamins are all synthetic. Several studies show decreased absorption or benefit in synthetic vitamins, such as dl-alpha tocopherol (the synthetic form of vitamin E), while the d-alpha natural form was more beneficial. Here are some things to seek in your multivitamin:

- Look for whole-food-based and natural forms of nutrients, which have typically shown superior absorption. Fermented whole food-based multivitamins are among the best absorbed. Organic versions have more recently become available. Some effervescent, drinkable multi formulas (the ones without sugar) are also very high quality. See Resources for some premier brands.
- Look for mixed carotenoids, such as lutein, lycopene, and zeaxanthin, along with beta-carotene. Recent studies show that mixed carotenoids work together to reduce DNA damage and protect the skin against the harmful effects of ultraviolet radiation—a major contributor to premature skin aging.
- Look for not only the natural form of vitamin E, but also mixed tocopherols, which include gamma- and delta-tocopherol and tocotrienols.
- Look for vitamin C accompanied by bioflavanoids, like quercetin.
- Look for the more absorbable calcium citrate over calcium carbonate.
- Look for phytonutrients, like turmeric, grape seed, and green tea.
- Look for the D3 form as opposed to the D2 form of vitamin D; D3 was found to be 60 to 80 percent more effective in therapies against the aforementioned array of vitamin D-related diseases than the D2 form.

NANOTECH SUPPLEMENTS: WHAT YOU NEED TO KNOW

Nanotechnology is a mind-boggling technology that holds incredible potential to revolutionize medical treatments and offer much new hope. It is a double-edged sword, however, that is unregulated and not even labeled in its current applications in foods, packaging, cosmetics, and now supplements. Using particles as small as a billionth of a meter, or about ten times the size of an atom, these particles can bypass digestion, slice right through skin and cell membranes, and even be taken up in cell receptors, which can be a mechanism for instant effects.

This concerns many scientists, as these particles could have unintended effects in the body and the environment. Unlabeled products that contain nanoparticles often claim to have rapid or timed-release effects or reach deep layers other products don't reach. But the Institute of Food Science and Technology (IFST) says that nanoparticles must be regarded as new, potentially harmful materials until they are tested. I will be avoiding nanoparticles as much as possible until more is known, and if I ever do knowingly consume or apply them, I will never use anything containing a synthetic. I'll revisit their application in skin care products in the coming chapters.

WHAT SHOULD YOU PAY FOR SUPPLEMENTS?

It depends on what you want to get out of them. You might not invest what I gladly pay for supplements, but then they basically saved my life, so I'm willing to pay a little more. As if that wasn't enough, they subsequently healed my liver and digestion, stoked my thyroid, improved my blood sugar levels, corrected the hormone imbalance that was keeping me pear shaped, and balanced the brain chemistry that had kept me obsessed with food. No exaggeration here! Every one of these issues was corrected for me by supplements when eating the best way possible and exercise made no difference. Supplements saved me from a miserable, futile, short life, and to me, that's priceless. Considering that I spend less on them than many people spend on clothes, I'm amazed at the bargain.

Okay, so you want numbers. I'd say that for a good basic "American antidote" regimen with a high-end, whole-food-based multivitamin and mineral supplement, comprehensive blood sugar stabilizing formula, a pure, high-potency fish oil (assuming you're taking 3 to 4 per day), and one other targeted supplement from the charts ahead, you should expect to pay around $80 to $100 per month. If you take this every day without fail, the benefits, both immediately and cumulatively, will be amazing and will likely save you untold doctor bills, sick days, and lost vitality and beauty in the long run. If you are faced with the recommendation by your doctor to start on a prescription antidepressant, antibiotic, or cholesterol-lowering drug, working with your doctor to first try one of the proven natural mood-lifters such as 5htp, or the proven cholesterol-lowering supplement policosanol, or one of the natural antibiotics discussed in the "Big Guns" section of chapter 14 could save your future quality of life in one quick move.

A-LIST SUPPLEMENTS WITH BEAUTY SIDE EFFECTS

The nutritional supplements listed in the charts that follow are some of the most well researched and highly regarded in the field at this writing. Volumes could be—and have been—written on each of these, as they have remained at the top of the most learned nutrition enthusiasts' lists for nearly a decade, with occasional evolutions to the recommended form of the nutrient. I know you don't have time to read page after page about one supplement when there are so many of them that you need to be aware of. So consider these pages your at-a-glance reference for powerful, synergistic cellular-level beauty and body therapy. More specific supplements for skin conditions are listed in the Skin Strategy Makeover Chart in chapter 13. Amazingly, each of these all-star supplements initiates a chain reaction of improvements that will almost certainly have head-to-toe effects. My goal is for you to get excited about the incredible quality of life and vitality to be gained from supplements and to encourage you, through the additional resources, to make your own discoveries. As far as dosages go, the high end of the dosages recommended on product labels generally corresponds with therapeutic benefit shown in studies. Information for exceptional or hard-to-find products is listed in Resources.

Important: The information in this chapter, as in the others, is not intended to diagnose or treat disease. Enlist your doctor's supervision when addressing health issues with supplements or if you are currently taking prescription medications.

Nutrient	Benefit
High-potency multivitamin and minerals regimens *Note: You may opt to add a separate liquid ionic trace mineral or seaweed supplement to increase your intake of naturally balanced minerals.*	Lowered risk of heart disease and stroke to prevention of birth defects and everything in between. **Beauty side effects:** Vary according to formula, but the first change a person usually notices is decreased cravings and increased energy.

Nutrient	Benefit
Blood sugar control formula	These formulas containing chromium, vanadium, lipoic acid, the B vitamin derivative benfotiamine, and herbs such as gymnema sylvestre and cinnamon assist insulin function and inhibit premature aging from glycation. **Beauty side effects:** Controlled blood sugar saves your shape and your skin from the ravages of glycation, inflammation, and fat storage-promoting insulin spikes.
Green powder: Such as barley grass, chlorella, spirulina, and seaweed supplements	Rich in enzymes, phytochemicals, and body-detoxifying chlorophyll. **Beauty side effects:** Beautiful, clear skin; faster healing of bruises due to enzymes and vitamin K.
Omega-3 EFAs: Such as fish, flax, borage, and evening primrose oils	EFAs improve virtually all cell processes. **Beauty side effects:** Anti-inflammatory; replenishes healing lipids to the skin and hair. Protects bones, heart, and breasts. Speeds weight loss; lifts moods, and improved blood sugar.
Probiotics: Such as acidophilus and other strains of beneficial bacteria	Rebalances the good bacteria in the gut for better digestion and immunity. **Beauty side effects:** Improved digestion clears the skin and diminishes sensitivity and some inflammatory skin conditions.
Vitamin C with bioflavanoids. 300–1,500 mg are used in many studies to achieve important protective benefits.	Boosts immunity heart protection, and fights free radicals. **Beauty side effects:** Boosts collagen formation and the skin's natural protection from sun damage.
N-acetyl cysteine (NAC)	Forms glutathione, a key detoxifying agent in the body; reduced compulsive-obsessive behavior in preliminary research. **Beauty side effects:** Increased detoxification clears the skin. Decreased compulsion clears the mind.

continued on the next page

Nutrient	Benefit
Alpha-lipoic acid or R-lipoic acid (a better-utilized form)	Recycles other antioxidants in the body and scavenges more types of free radicals than any other known antioxidant. **Beauty side effects:** Antioxidant, antiaging, and anti-inflammatory for the skin. Blood sugar-stabilizing for weight control and energy, plus wrinkle protection.
Antioxidant enzyme catalysts	Trigger a dramatic increase in SOD and CAT enzymes resulting in thousands of times the antioxidant activity of antioxidant supplements or foods. **Beauty side effects:** Dramatically decreases oxidative stress, slowing aging to skin and body.
Ubiquinol form of Coenzyme Q10 (CoQ10), absorbed up to eight times better than the ubiquinone form	A powerful antiaging, free radical-scavenging, and proven breast cancer- and heart disease-inhibiting enzyme. It is depleted by cholesterol-lowering drugs. **Beauty side effects:** Increases cellular energy and may stimulate tissue regeneration. Fights photo-aging and environmental skin effects. Slowed the aging process in mice.
Vitamin D3 (This may already be in your multivitamin in RDA amounts, but 1,000–2,000 IU are used in most studies to achieve important protective benefits.)	Reduces risk of autoimmune diseases; inhibits cell proliferation associated with several cancers. **Beauty side effects:** Prevents bone loss. May help psoriasis. 1,000 IU/day may reduce breast cancer up to 50 percent.
Carnosine *Note*: Not to be confused with the amino acid L-carnitine (below)	Extended lifespan, inhibited glycation throughout the body, and reversed the physical changes and mental decline associated with aging in rats. **Beauty side effects:** Inhibits skin and body aging from glycation.
L-carnitine, or Acetyl L-carnitine	Heart-protective, blood sugar-stabilizing supplement. **Beauty side effects:** In combination with alpha-lipoic acid, it has been shown to reverse many effects of aging. It also helps weight loss.

SUPPLEMENTS THAT HELP BALANCE WEIGHT-RELATED HEALTH ISSUES

A variety of hormonal and chemical factors you may not even have considered may be dominating your body and keeping you from losing weight.

The following supplements not only helped me change my chemical relationship with food but actually reproportioned my body shape from "pear" to normal and helped me regain my health in many other ways in the process.

But don't run out and buy them all! First, identify your issues and zero in on the support you need. If you are currently taking or considering prescription weight-loss drugs, or even antidepression drugs, ask your doctor to work with you to see if any of these alternatives might spare you the possible side effects, while actually improving your health.

Weight-Related Issues	*Proven Supplement Support*
Blood sugar support and cravings	• Chromium (polynicotinate form might have advantages over picolinate) • Alpha-lipoic acid • Vanadyl sulfate • *Garcinia cambogia* (Citrimax) • *Benfotiamine* • Gymnema sylvestre • Omega-3 fatty acids • Caralluma fimbriata extract, found in the product Slimaluma, is a proven appetite suppressant • 100 percent pure South African hoodia gordonii (beware of watered-down, uncertified hoodia products) is another proven appetite suppressant • Slendesta is a proven CCK (appetite hormone) inhibitor
Mood, stress, and anxiety	See "Critical Mood Nutrients," page 165

continued on the next page

Weight-Related Issues	*Proven Supplement Support*
Fat metabolism/absorption	The following have been shown to increase fat burning: • Green tea • CLA • Hydroxycitric acid (garcinia cambogia fruit) • Fucoxanthin • Chitosan is shellfish cartilage that absorbs fat. It also can absorb healthy fats, so you shouldn't take it when eating healthy fats or with your vitamins.
Carbohydrate metabolism *Take these supplements one-half hour before meals.*	Phaseolamin-based carb blockers, such as Carb Intercept, Ultimate Carb Control C-120X, or other Phase 2-containing supplements, block the enzymes that turn starches and grains into sugar and are extremely safe. They really help to get you off the sugar pendulum and make a difference you can feel the first time you use them. Once you stop eating blood sugar-spiking foods, you should still keep these in your pocketbook for unexpected situations and celebrations. I use them to this day, not to control my weight, but to avoid energy swings from occasional "borderline" foods.
Hormone balancers and releasers	• Pregnenelone, a hormone precursor, safely encourages the production of needed hormones in the body, including DHEA. • Chaste tree berry (vitex) can safely balance estrogen and progesterone levels that also help normalize weight and body proportion. • Kelp and L-tyrosine stoke a sluggish thyroid. • The amino acids L-ornithine and L-arginine help you release hGH, which keeps you lean.

OMEGA FATS AND BEAUTY: A LOVE STORY

My very first, leap-of-faith, life-saving supplement regimen included fish oil, which—combined with alpha-lipoic acid and milk thistle—not only healed my

HOW KELLY LOST THE FINAL TEN

When I consulted with Kelly, a petite woman at 5'2", about her weight, energy, and food issues, I found that she was already eating quality, fresh, real food that she prepared daily from scratch. But Kelly had major issues with energy that required her to take an afternoon nap to get through the day. I encouraged Kelly to cut out sugar and look into supplements and how they might increase her energy and address her energy dips. She was skeptical, but after looking at some compelling scientific research, Kelly began taking an advanced multi-nutrient regimen. After a couple of months, she added a supplement that combined CoQ10 and the amino acid L-carnitine to her regimen after reading about their proven energizing and heart-health effects. Soon Kelly's reservations about the efficacy of supplements were eliminated. She was amazed to find herself skipping her usual nap and staying productive throughout the day. Even more surprising, Kelly lost just over ten pounds over the next couple of months. "That's major," she said. "I've been trying to lose that final ten for nearly a decade." And when she stopped taking the multivitamin regimen after running out, her appetite and cravings returned. That's how much our bodies need nutrients we so often deprive them of.

sick liver (food couldn't do it, as I had already been eating the healthiest way I could) but also completely transformed my skin and my moods. This was back at the dawn of the nineties, more than a decade before fish oil became known to the general public. Today, there are hundreds of studies on omega-3 oils showing dramatic reductions in everything from anger and anxiety to depression, from risk of sudden heart attack to insulin resistance, and from joint inflammation to bone loss and much more.

On the beauty front, the skin, weight loss, and hair benefits of fish oil and omega-3s has now been confirmed in dozens of published studies, showing significant improvement in nearly all major skin diseases involving inflammation, including eczema, psoriasis, and even sunburn. More recent studies confirm that fish oil protects against UV radiation, reducing the skin's responses to both UVA (blistering) and UVB (redness) radiation. The antiaging and even damage-reversing effect from fish oil was confirmed in a study published in the *Journal of Lipid Research*.

The effect on my own skin from fish oil was nothing short of amazing. Within a couple of months of starting this regimen, my skin literally "forgot" that it had been continually irritated, prone to horrible rashes on my eyes and chin, and unquenchably dry all my life. It forgot that it needed heavy-duty lotions in order not to crawl with discomfort after every bath and shower. The space between my brows, the crannies on the sides of my nose, and my legs all failed to attend to their constant scaling. Dryness and inflammation had "left the building" along with my need for body moisturizers. I almost forgot to remember these things as they ended, but I'll never forget what it was like to take for granted that I would have those problems for the rest of my life and then learn I was wrong.

My hair was transformed dramatically from my fish oil regimen, too. It went from being super-brittle, coarse, and dull to being glossy and silky, enabling me to grow it out long (and have it actually grow downward instead of outward) for the first time since my childhood. Beyond the fact that hair is a biological appendage of the skin (which is why people with oily skin have oily hair, and people with dry skin have dry hair), there are other possible explanations for fish oil's effects on the hair. Hair health is particularly vulnerable to hormone imbalances and compromised circulation (many hair loss remedies focus on that). Stress is another cause for changes in the hair (alopecia areata, or temporary, nonhereditary hair loss, is caused by stress or trauma). Because omega-3s and fish oil have been proven to increase circulation, reduce the impact of stress, and help balance hormone activity, they offer proven benefit in each of these important contributors to hair health.

FISH VS. FLAX OIL

Several studies have compared the actions of fish oil to plant-based omega-3 oils and have found that fish oil supplementation more effectively raises the body's levels of EPA and DHA (the components responsible for most of the documented health benefits). Getting EPA and DHA from flax oil requires a conversion by the body, which many people do not efficiently make. Still, flax is better than not supplementing with omega-3s at all (so strict vegans might be able to get all their omega-3s from flax, but might also be biologically challenged in converting it to anti-inflammatory compounds). Molecularly distilled fish oils are the gold standard in supplementation recommended by more and more mainstream, as well as alternative, MDs. Avoid cheap drug store brands. Ironically, getting all your fish oil from fish could give you unwanted outcomes unless you are careful about avoiding mercury, as high mercury levels not only contribute to heart problems but are also known to cause hair loss.

I have taken fish oil for nearly two decades now, with few interruptions. And those interruptions are valuable reminders of what it was like to live in both the physical and emotional discomfort in my own skin. Fish oil is unquestionable proof that real "magic bullets" sometimes do exist.

GLA: THE GOOD OMEGA-6 FAT

If you've read about omega fats, you've likely read that we need to up our ratios of omega-3 fats to harmful omega-6 fats. The exception is GLA (gamma-linolenic acid), an anti-inflammatory omega-6 fat found in evening primrose and even more plentifully in borage seed oils.

GLA has been shown in some studies to improve inflammatory skin problems, such as psoriasis and eczema. Many people have been found to be born with an inability to convert linoleic acid (such as that from flax seed oil which does not contain GLA) into the inflammation-reducing GLA, and it was found that supplementing can help alleviate inflammatory skin conditions caused by this inherited trait. Aside from GLA supplements (I take a supplement that contains both fish oil and GLA), the only foods with meaningful amounts of GLA are the hemp seeds and hemp oil. See the Resources section for more information on these foods and supplements.

PRO-BEAUTY PROBIOTICS: FEED YOUR GOOD BUGS

Our modern lifestyle poses a challenge to the good bacteria (probiotics) that dwell in our guts. From the drugs we take to the chlorinated water we drink and shower in, our precious bugs are fighting for survival. And when they start to lose, more virulent bad bugs, like the *Candida albicans* strain, can rule over our gut and other parts of our bodies. This can contribute to a stubborn imbalance of good and bad bacteria and yeast in the gut and even on the skin, and a cascade of autoimmune syndromes and "skindromes."

Consuming probiotics and taking other steps to regain your pro-beauty ecology may help with a range of problems, including acne, poor digestion, itchy skin, dandruff, athlete's foot, allergies, and sinus and vaginal yeast issues.

The Simple Solutions

- Take a good probiotic, which you'll find at a quality vitamin store.
- Eat a lot of plain yogurt and drink kefir (always unsweetened).
- Starve your yeast of the sugar, flour, and starch on which it thrives.
- Eat loads of garlic, which kills yeast and other bacteria pathogens.
- Take a yeast-fighting supplement, such as Candex or Kolorex.
- Install water and shower filters to minimize chlorine, which can contribute to probiotic depletion in the body.

CULTIVATING RADIANT INNER HYGIENE: UPGRADE YOUR DETOX PLAN

Nourishment and its counterpart, detoxification, are the dynamic duo that create radiance.

When most of us think "personal hygiene," we think of the cleansing and deodorizing products on our bathroom shelves. But cultivating vibrant internal ecology through daily inner hygiene can make you glow in a way that all the external scrubbing, buffing, and makeup cannot. The first half of my life was my "toxic accumulation" period. My liver crisis and all of my health problems were how I ultimately paid. Detoxifying was what got me out of the woods, so I could find my path back to health and balancing my specific issues.

Detox is not just for special occasions, and it shouldn't be harsh. Once you've adopted your first round of food and beverage upgrades, you'll have already started to detox on autopilot. My way of eating—particularly when food is prepared the way I suggest in the JumpStart Menu chapter—may not taste or feel like a "detox experience," but it is deceptively effective at helping you cleanse yourself nonstop from the inside out.

As a former extremist who would do anything at least temporarily, I'm no longer a fan of fasting and juicing. These can be harmful if you have weight, food, or metabolic issues because they can lead to blood sugar swings, metabolism kinks, and even subsequent bingeing. The need to cut out solid food or fat in order to detox is an absolute myth. Once you have cut out all blood sugar spikes, your head-to-toe inflammation will diminish further than any typical juicing and brown rice program can take it. You absolutely should never do without fat once you are primarily burning it (which automatically happens when you stop getting spiked). The key is to support all of your digestive and elimination pathways, and you can do that just from how you eat and care for yourself on a daily basis. Certain fats help immensely with improving your inner ecology and actually liberate fat so it can be eliminated from the body. A couple of tablespoons of virgin coconut oil in your smoothies, lots of extra virgin olive oil or hemp oil on your salads, fish oil capsules, and avocado all actually boost detox. Even some nuts, raw eggs, or gently cooked grass-fed meats won't interfere with detox, as long as you're getting lots of fiber. However, overcooked, conventional, or processed and well-done meats or protein definitely will interfere, and should be minimized whether you are detoxing or not. Dark greens or green drinks (or the chlorella supplement below), berries, and additional fiber from flax crackers and the superior, nonharsh nutritive fiber supplements mentioned below and in the Resources section will maximize the autopilot cleansing effects of your everyday diet.

To take detox to the next level, incorporate my Beauty Detox Elixir or green drinks at least twice a week. In addition, you might consider some of the following one-of-a-kind supplements to address specific detox desires and issues:

- **Superior nutritive fibers** such as coconut fiber or food-based fibers providing probiotic or antifungal support without harsh herbs (like senna).
- **Broken cell wall chlorella** has been shown to bind with and remove heavy metals from the body (important to people who live in big cities). Great if you haven't been able to get enough greens or green drinks in your diet. Perfect for travel.
- **Complete internal cleansing kits** such as CleanseSmart by Renew Life support all of the body's channels of elimination. Do this one once you have gotten into the swing of the previous chapters' upgrades.
- **Liver cleansing supplements,** such as LiverCare from Himalaya Herbs: this is the #1-selling liver product in the world, with over a hundred clinical studies proving efficacy. Some studies show it works better than milk thistle at rejuvenating liver cells. Prescription drugs tend to tax the liver, so if you're on them or are stressing your liver, this is one to consider. I take this every day because of my past liver issues.
- **Pure seaweed supplements and baths** to assist fluid and lymph drainage and heavy metal detox and reduce swelling while delivering

ionizing, perfectly balanced trace minerals from seaweed extracts. Spa Technologies is the purest source I've found for these.

- **PectaSol** (available from several brands including Source Naturals) is a unique form of modified citrus pectin (MCP) shown to be one of the most effective supplements for removing mercury and other heavy metals from the body. Recommended by many biological dentists where mercury fillings are a concern.
- **Internal oxygenating supplements,** such as Bio-Oxygen from Bio Group, International or ChlorOxygen, a chlorophyll concentrate from Herbs, Etc. These oxygenate (and thus purify and "wake up") the colon and digestive tract for effective detoxification and energize the body.
- **Parasite cleanses,** such as ParaGone, incorporating black walnut hull and wormwood. Tackle this only after you're feeling great on all your upgrades, and when you don't have a demanding week ahead.

PROTECT YOUR BREASTS AS YOU BEAUTIFY YOUR SKIN

Certain toxins in our environment, water, and skin products have now been shown to accumulate in breast tissue and breast milk as well as prostate tissue. Breasts might even be viewed as two small (or voluptuous) microcosms of the environment you live in. You can control that environment to a certain degree by eating organic foods and organic or grass-fed animal products, installing water and shower filters and using natural body care and home cleaning products (see Resources). But eliminating your exposure to chemical pollutants completely is, of course, impossible. Luckily, there are many supplements proven to protect the breasts from the harmful hormone-mimicking effects linked with increasing environmental pollution and accumulation of chemicals in the body. Most have been found to protect the prostate as well.

Conveniently, what protects the breasts can also create beautiful skin and a healthy body. All of the supplements below have amazing body-wide effects and will help beautify your skin. For example, omega-3 fatty acids from fish oil may offer protection from breast cancer and benign breast disease. At the same time, they may help relieve eczema. Chlorella detoxifies carcinogenic substances and also helps heal skin wounds. Vitamin D3 may help alleviate psoriasis as it reduces your risk of breast cancer up to 50 percent, and so on. Nature doesn't just work on parts, like a medical doctor or mechanic.

Here are some of the best-researched natural breast health supplements that have been studied for more than a decade but are only beginning to be acknowledged for their amazing effects.

Breast Supplement Superstars	*Benefit*
D-glucarate (in broccoli)	D-glucarate has been shown to inhibit proliferative estrogens and breast tumor formation.
DIM and Indole-3 carbinol (from cruciferous vegetables)	Both DIM and I3C inhibit growth of estrogen receptor-positive breast cancer cells.
Green tea	Green tea increases the body's key detoxifying substance, glutathione. It has been shown to cause apoptosis, or cancer cell death.
Curcumin (in turmeric)	In addition to being an antioxidant and anti-inflammatory, curcumin has also been shown to block harmful estrogen-mimicking chemicals.
Milk thistle/Silibinin	Milk thistle detoxifies and regenerates liver tissue and has been shown to inhibit cancer cell replication and to make some types of chemotherapy more effective.
Melatonin	An association between decreased melatonin levels and breast cancer risk has been suggested and is being further investigated with regard to sun and sleep factors. Lower levels of melatonin have been linked with eating disorders and insulin resistance.
Tocotrienols	Tocotrienols from palm oil demonstrated antiproliferative effects on human breast cancer cell lines. Dr. Perricone recommends them for beautiful skin.
Lignans and Brevail	Lignans from flaxseed and Brevail, a proprietary lignan concentrate supplement, have been shown to decrease breast cancer risk and shrink tumors by blocking harmful estrogens from docking in estrogen receptor sites.

continued on the next page

Breast Supplement Superstars	Benefit
Fish oil	Fish oil shrank breast cancer tumors in mice, and was found to facilitate several mechanisms leading to cancer cell death (apoptosis) in a study published in the *International Journal of Cancer*.
Vitamin D3	A University of California at San Diego study concluded that supplementing with 1,000 IU of vitamin D daily might lower breast cancer risk up to 50 percent

CAN GOING "WIRELESS" KEEP BREASTS HEALTHIER?

In 1996, an unpublished study of 4,700 women supported what some doctors have suggested in the past, only to encounter mockery: bras are unhealthy for breasts. In the study, those who wore a bra twenty-four hours a day had breast cancer rates 125 times higher than those who wore no bra at all. The scientists theorize that bras restrict lymph drainage in the breast area, which allows toxins to build. Bear in mind that this study did not factor in lifestyle conditions or use controls and was not published in a respected medical journal. In the meantime, consider a bra that doesn't bind or constrict.

SUPPLEMENT SENSE

While most supplements are composed of substances that are found in your body right now, some botanicals—like any food—could cause sensitivity or, in rare cases, an allergic reaction. Keep in mind, though, that because food supplements are based on an entirely different principle—one of stimulating and balancing optimal body functioning, rather than blocking symptoms or needed functions as most drugs are designed to do—they can take anywhere from one hour to several weeks to show their effects. The benefits of quality supplementation, I assure you, are well worth it. Here's a checklist for getting started:

- Start slowly. Introduce only a couple of vitamins and only one herb at a time unless otherwise directed by your healthcare provider.
- Consider starting with a quality full-spectrum multivitamin and mineral regimen and omega-3 fatty acids, such as fish oil, as well as a good blood sugar-stabilizing formula. This regimen is a great antidote to years of food assaults and nutrient depletion.
- Be aware that combining nutrition bars, fortified foods, and meal-replacement shakes (all of which I discourage for the most part) can give you too much of some nutrients, like vitamin A and iron, which can build up in the body.
- Again, be sure to tell your doctor what you're planning to take, particularly if you are on prescription medications.
- Upgrade and evolve your supplement regimen as your needs change and your knowledge expands. See Resources for educational sources to help you stay informed.

DON'T WAIT. MAKE SUPPLEMENTS YOUR NEW BEAUTY RITUAL TODAY

One could grow old (and sick) waiting for their doctor or the five o'clock news to encourage them to rejuvenate their looks and their quality of life with the most intuitive, natural, and therapeutic gifts we've been given for healing. But don't risk your radiance by waiting. With no more discipline than it takes to brush your teeth, you can start to experience the physical and cellular vitality you were meant to have, today. Many people (including myself) have experienced the best health and looks of their life well after thirty because of the miracle of nature in therapeutic doses.

CHAPTER 10

TRANSFORMATION PROFILES

While I'm convinced that there's no more powerful teacher or inspiration than a real success story, I've learned from my own experience that transformation begins long before the body starts to change form, and it goes on long after the "after" shot is taken. And so, these are just snapshots of five real individuals who have set their own course with a boost from the principles laid forth in this book.

I want to assure you that these aren't examples of exceptionally disciplined people. Most consider themselves to be far from disciplined. And they do not attribute their transformations to "hard work" or emotional breakthroughs. These are transformations at the *cellular level*.

First there's Georgianna, who, after experiencing her own skin and body transformation, set out to save her husband's health—and their marriage. Amy, a formerly obese, food-addicted mother of two toddlers, regained control and got her life back. Then there's Betty, who undertook my program looking for skin improvement and wound up with much more. Then Rudi, whose brother handed him my book and was shocked at his unrecognizable brother four months later (though no more shocked than Rudi's doctor). Finally, there's Courtney, who learned to deeply nourish herself and let go of her deadly fear of food—even after an expensive inpatient treatment for bulimia failed. Her cystic acne cleared up, too.

GEORGIANNA SAVES HER OWN SKIN AND HER MARRIAGE

Georgianna is the president and COO of one of the largest utility companies in Texas.

When I first read Kat's story, there were a lot of resonating issues, but I was really wanting to just look and feel better. I was also pushed to the limit, work-wise, and felt like I had just forgotten myself. I remember thinking "it's now or never." My first go-around with this book changed a lot of things for me. I started cooking at home (even with my hectic schedule) and cut out flour and sugar completely. Because of all the corporate functions, I'd spent years eating take-out, but I realized it was actually faster, easier, and better to eat at home. No driving, ordering, or waiting. The meals I used to cook before were mostly potatoes and casseroles, pasta and bread. Now they are simple combinations of free-range meat, poultry, or fish, herb sauces, fresh produce, and olive oil. I also now use xylitol instead of sugar. No more sugar or artificial sweeteners for my grandchildren.

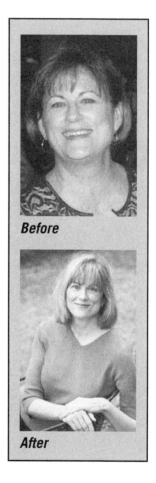

Before

After

It has done something for my spirit to be making meals again. And my food bills are half what they were. My favorite breakfast became stevia-sweetened whole yogurt and berries, when before it had been whatever pastry or bagel I could pick up on the way to the office. My lunch of choice became any kind of "decadent meal salad," which I learned to either make or compile at business lunches, even if I had to ask for extra avocado or nuts on the side. I'd intended to stock up on some of the low-impact pastas and special breads Kat recommends, but by the time I got around to it, I no longer craved bread at all. Occasionally, I might eat a piece of freshly baked bread at a restaurant, but the pleasure and temptation it used to give me are just not there any more. Most surprising is that I've lost my taste for wine. I used to think about it and have a glass first thing after coming home from work. Now it doesn't even enter my mind. I've noticed that supplements, like phase 2 and chromium, can really make a big difference in preventing the sugar swings from starting again when you do eat something that might spike you.

Now for the physical changes: From the very first week of cutting out sugar and flour I felt a powerful difference in my energy. And the weight came off. I was soon fitting into suits I hadn't worn in years. This inspired me to start doing yoga, which has added tremendously to the changes I'm experiencing. I'm now down to a size 10 from a 14, and I can tell my body wants to keep going, which I look forward to!

I also changed my deodorant soap to olive oil soap and installed a shower filter, and I could feel a difference in the comfort of my skin immediately. As time went on, the personality of my skin changed so completely that my chronic itching and flaking patches diminished and finally disappeared. I was dependant on steroid creams for my arms and hairline for patches of seborrhea, but I no longer have flare-ups. I started wearing sleeveless tops again and eventually stopped using lotions altogether. You almost don't notice these gradual changes until you step back and think about what life was like before, and it really is incredible. Around Christmas of 2006, I did add a topical seaweed serum and a drinkable collagen product from Kat's resources. The difference on my face was amazing. It was hard to believe there were no acids in it. My ruddiness improved to the point that I stopped wearing foundation. I almost stopped taking the drink after a couple of months because it was so expensive, but then I spotted some changes in my triple-strength magnifying mirror after a little over a month. My under-eye circles were diminishing. The shocker was that the age spots on the backs of my hands were getting noticeably lighter (this was what the studies claimed, but I had never expected it to actually happen). The skin there had been dry and crinkly, and it didn't look that way anymore. I would not have believed this was possible without lasers or intervention. Everyone who knows me asks what I've done. My skin is now much smoother, not just on my face, but all over my body. I'm wearing less makeup than I've worn in years. Not bad for a grandma!

Another thing: some of my health stats have improved. Glucose and cholesterol are down, and the most unexpected news is that the nodules on my thyroid are actually *shrinking*.

When you do this for yourself, you realize you're heading off otherwise-inevitable problems. My husband Dick's disregard for his health was a long-time issue between us, and his smoking was becoming intolerable to me. He knew it. And it was no small gesture when he agreed to join me for one of Kat's retreats in 2006 and pledged to quit smoking that week. He doesn't say such things lightly, so I was thrilled. I knew that eating satisfying food free from blood sugar spikes all week would be the best possible support for Dick to kick the habit. Since he was also a sugar addict and a big coffee and wine drinker, we were in for some interesting days, though nothing like the experience he had expected. He made jokes at first when Kat suggested herbal coffee as an upgrade for his black coffee, but he was humbled when he actually tried it. He knew he had never eaten so well and that his knee-jerk assessments of the "health foods" I'd been so into, which he never even tried, had been way off the mark. It was he who had been the deprived one!

He weaned off coffee in about three days. And as promised, he did not light up the entire week. His low point was the third day, when he went through a day of flulike detox symptoms and had to take lots of naps (and I endured a few fits of his grumpiness), and then after that day, he started to immerse himself in the cooking and make elaborate salads as well as cranberry spritzers for himself to have instead of his wine. To me it was amazing that he was in the kitchen joking with all the women and cooking up a storm while going through triple withdrawal from coffee, cigarettes, and wine—which I know he never could have done all at once had it not been for the kind of nourishment and satisfaction he was getting from the food. He has not smoked since. This has basically been a make-or-break development that means more than he may know. He still drinks a little wine but nothing like before. He is looking healthier by the day as a result.

Between the two of us, who knows how many years have been added. I could not picture that future together if Dick had continued his blatant self-destruction. You can't be awakened about your own health and then watch your life partner kill himself. I'm so thankful that something came along to wake me up and also get through to Dick. This may well have saved our marriage.

RUDI ETCHEVERRI WALKING AWAY FROM OBESITY AND DIABETES

Rudi had a lot of things working against him in life. He was a very rotund but active delivery truck driver whose constant physical labor didn't seem to budge his obesity. He was estranged from his wife, had become borderline alcoholic, and was on a downward spiral of self-destruction. It was a very unlikely turn of events that turned his life around.

I would never have done this had my brother not put this book in front of me. Long ago I gave up the idea that I could ever feel the way I once did. But because of Kat's pictures and story, I thought: "I'm going to trust this person."

The thing I started to say to myself once I was about thirty pounds into this wild ride was: "How is this happening? I'm not even trying." After the first two weeks, there was no feeling of giving up anything at all. I didn't change how much I ate. I did the upgrades that Kat articulated in the book. It took me a couple of weeks to line up all the replacements for my usual snacks, but once I got those going, I soon didn't even need some of them. I was clear of cravings and my body started to burn itself off nonstop. My clothes became loose almost immediately, and before the month was over, I was rounding up clothes I hadn't worn in years. The second month I decided to see my doctor. I had already lost around twenty-five pounds. He was shocked at the improvements in my glucose and blood pressure and took me off all my diabetes medication. He told me to keep doing whatever I was doing.

The irony is that every day I deliver Kaisers, subs, doughnuts from my truck—things that were killing me.

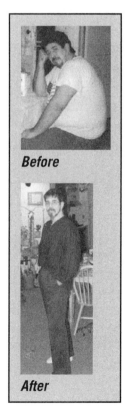

Before

After

Out of the whole crew, I was the guy who was the biggest, but now I'm the only one with no belly. In fact, I just turned fifty, and I have six-pack abs for the first time in my life, without doing sit-ups. I've been doing this delivery truck job for years, but it didn't feel like exercise because I was always dragging myself around with zero energy. In retrospect, I was lifting an "extra person" around. It was the food strategy that finally worked.

I look in the mirror now and see another person. My waist has gone from 46" to 32"! Things are renewed with my wife. My energy and my self-esteem are reborn. Friends even say I talk differently. I lost a hundred and ten pounds of attitude and gained a new life.

AMY MONTGOMERY'S PROCESS OF SHEDDING HER PADDING FROM LIFE

Amy, an obese single mother, carried her 220-pound frame around while constantly chasing two toddlers but couldn't lose an ounce.

When my sister gave me Kat's book out of concern, I weighed the heaviest I had in my life and was just beginning to admit that I needed help. I had tried all the popular diet plans and the weigh-ins but with no long-term success. I was in deep despair from losing my marriage, which was compounded by the fact that I was approaching my highest weight ever, 223 pounds. I was feeling truly hopeless. Until I read the chapter about food addiction, I did not even know that I had an eating disorder. I just thought there was something wrong with me or maybe deep inside I just didn't care about myself. It's hard to say if I treated myself poorly because I felt terrible about myself, or if I felt terrible about myself because of what I couldn't stop doing to my body. At a size 22, I was ashamed for my kids at having such an overweight mother.

I always knew my emotional issues affected my eating, but I started to learn about the physical issues that came into play, which I had had no clue about. I made a game plan for myself after reading the book. I decided to do three things: 1) I started to change any starchy or sugary food or drink choices to low-glycemic choices, which surprisingly required no sacrifice. 2) I started taking supplements to balance my blood sugar, moods, and hormone levels.

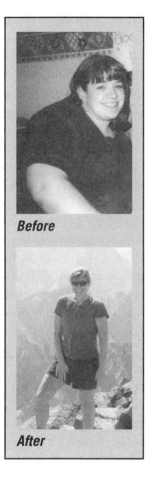

Before

After

I took them faithfully because I saw how they had worked for Kat. 3) I started dealing with my emotional issues. Reading some self-help books and spending time with supportive people. My mother and sister have been so great through this.

The changes in my body and in my psyche over the last year have been incredible. I've lost eighty-five pounds at this point. I don't have any set weight loss goal, but I think my body will lose even more as I get healthier. It's so gradual, unlike when I've lost weight before. I don't have good weeks and bad weeks where I "succeed" at depriving myself or revert to bingeing. This isn't like that. I'm not even exactly sure when all my cravings subsided or when the control that food had over me started to disappear. It just seemed that all of a sudden I did not need to have that ice cream binge in order to feel better. It was amazing to actually feel satisfied eating good food and to feel the moodiness and lethargy (and self-loathing) diminish steadily over time. I know that it's because I was finally off the "sugar pendulum," as Kat calls it. It feels like I've been released from prison. I get a little craving now and then, but the thought of bingeing on candy bars or wolfing down half a gallon of ice cream while the kids are with their father does not even occur to me, whereas once those urges dominated my mind and my life.

What surprised me the most was the effect the supplements have had in helping with my cravings, moods, and energy over time. That has been mind-blowing. Only a month or so after I started on them, I no longer needed the afternoon nap that had been interfering with my job. I'd swear I've regained a sense of emotional control as well, but again, so much of my "insanity" was actually my body's chemistry. I look back at when I counted food points, went to weekly weigh-ins, and just "cut back" on what I ate and realize I didn't understand what was happening in my body. I don't think of supplements as "magic diet pills." I've learned what each one does and I take them for specific health issues. I believe they enabled me to resist the wrong kind of foods long enough to break my addiction.

I've started exercising more again. I didn't do much during the initial weight loss, but more and more—because I feel better—I find myself wanting to spend active time, rather than "eating" time, with friends. Recently, I've gotten into hiking. Not long ago, I climbed the tallest peak in Idaho. This is not something I would ever have imagined doing a year ago!

I still have my emotional issues like everybody, but it is less destructive because I'm dealing with it and feeling it, instead of drugging myself with food. I am very proud of my new body. The fact that I got informed beyond what you usually hear and took action has given me an unexpected, new source of self-esteem and hope. I was once convinced I'd have to heal all my emotions before I could ever permanently lose weight or be at peace with food, but it wasn't true. I still have emotional issues like anyone else, but my body is simply not using food—or any substance—as a drug anymore. And I don't believe it ever will again.

> **My comments on Rudi and Amy's stories:** The typical reality show drill sergeant would have put Rudi and Amy on a treadmill and fed them a restricted-calorie, low-fat diet. Had either remained in their former biochemical state, or chosen to tackle only their external symptom (weight) just by eating fewer calories and exercising even more, they would still be tormented today, even if they'd reached their weight goals, at constant war with their biochemical imbalances. And they would still be craving the foods that were killing them.

BETTY ISENHOUR: ON BEAUTY AND ACCIDENTAL FREEDOM FROM DISEASE

In addition to doing research for her salon, Betty attended my program hoping to drop a few pounds and thought it would be good to eat healthy food for a week, meet some new people, and learn some makeup techniques. She was not expecting what actually occurred.

I attended one of Kat James's recent Total Transformation® workshops. I'm an esthetician and wanted to know what her skin approach was. Since then, after seeing tremendous changes in my own skin, I have dramatically changed the offerings at my salon.

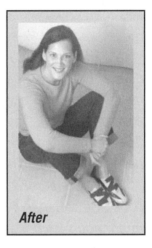

After

For years, I have been dealing with Wegener's granulomatosis, a vascular disease very much like lupus but much more aggressive when aggravated. This disease has caused changes in the structure of my nose, and at the program, it was active. One of the more obvious signs of it was having to drain my eye of fluid frequently.

Before attending the workshop my blood sugar levels were high and my doctor had told me he was concerned, and that I also needed to be on a statin drug for cholesterol. I knew I had the sugar issue, but I was off it immediately when I started the program, and I continued Kat's food strategies from the program and her book as soon as I got home to satisfy my sweet tooth without spiking myself. I also looked into some of the supplements Kat had talked about, and I started taking them.

When I returned to the doctor for a check-up, they tested the inflammation level in my body from every organ to see if the Wegener's was active. I have been meaning to write this for a long time because my doctor simply could not believe my test results. He said, and I quote, "You have less inflammation in your body than I probably do." Both my blood sugar and cholesterol levels were in the normal range, and the inflammation was less than 1 percent. This is almost unheard of in a vascular patient and especially for me. He was amazed and so was I. I never had to take the statin, and I have had more energy than I can ever remember. I am eternally grateful for her helping me live a better life.

—Much love, Betty Isenhour

COURTNEY HOLDEN: FROM THE OTHER SIDE OF BULIMIA

Ironically, it was my severe cystic acne that led me to Kat's book. I went to a dermatologist, and he said he could help me if what I had was a bacterial problem, but if my skin was the sign of something related to how I was taking care of myself, he couldn't help me. I'm sure that from how I looked (rail-thin, breaking hair) he suspected a deeper problem. Being the "neat freak" that I am, I was able to keep my bingeing and purging a secret. But my wasting body couldn't be covered up. Still, my acne was what I chose to focus on. I tried a "detox" program with an herbalist, but after months of this, my skin never cleared up. The herbalist referred me to a naturopathic clinician who mentioned Kat's book at a seminar. I opened it up looking for information for my acne, not knowing I would be telling people about my freedom from bulimia only a few months later.

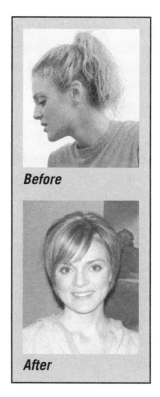

Before

After

For seven years I battled an alternating pattern of anorexia and bingeing and purging. I was extremely close to death. I got down to 90 pounds. Downy hairs covered my face and arms. I was cold all the time. I'd lost all control (bingeing and purging 3 to 4 times a day) and my dad begged me to admit myself into an expensive eating disorder treatment facility known for its 90 percent success rate.

I was told by the doctors at the clinic that, if I survived, I would fight my eating disorder every day for the rest of my life. My meal plan consisted of the highest daily recommendations for each group in the food guide pyramid (which included eleven servings of grains a day). Pizzas, brownies, and ice cream were frequently on the menu. We were served a sugary synthetic vitamin drink if we didn't eat. I was always bloated, and I suffered from acid reflux, nervousness, severe acne, and an irregular heartbeat. I entered treatment without medication, but I left with a bunch of pharmaceutical drugs to manage my problem including Lexapro (an antidepressant), Prevacid (for acid reflux), Seroquel (to sleep), and Ortho Tri-Cyclen (hormones to control my acne). I struggled not to purge at this facility because of the astronomical price my father paid for me to be there.

Throughout this process, I was encouraged to search for mishaps in my life that may have led me to use food as a release. I soon believed my eating disorder was a product of my emotions that would remain with me unless I could learn to find inner peace and forgive those who had influenced it. It made a lot of sense. I also had a lot of strained, unresolved relationships that were made worse by my disease, and my emotions felt like insanity at times. I got through each day with prayers. At the end of the program, I was sent home on a rigid meal plan based on a version of the food pyramid.

Unfortunately, the clinic didn't work. My first binge and purge happened within two months from returning from the treatment facility. My stepmom had been preparing all of my meals to the letter, so I didn't have to deal with food choices and prep, which I knew I couldn't handle. She went out one night, and I had to prepare my own dinner. When I attempted to make something in the kitchen, my anxiety got the best of me, and I found one of my favorite calming drugs (in this case, shortbread) and ate until my body became numb. I immediately purged, and this started the vicious cycle again, which continued for four more years, with many periods of holding on for survival. Then I was introduced to Kat's book.

A few weeks before attending Kat's program, I was well into trying some of the supplements and food upgrades in her book. I started taking fish oil and blood sugar stabilizers, and I'd started upgrading some foods. But I modified the fat issue to my liking because using the butter and cream, I decided, was not going to work for me. I binged less but still had the urge leading up to the program. Once there, I initially panicked at the thought of eating the fatty foods but was comforted by Kat's living example, and I was determined to "eat along with her." If she had not gone through exactly what I was going through, there's no way I would have eaten those foods (or kept them down). I ate these otherworldly, full-fat foods day in and day out, always feeling my body just drop its chatter at each meal, as if it wanted to just be still to savor something it hadn't been getting. The food never gave me the feeling I thought it would. I kept waiting for my urge to binge, which would inevitably be followed by a purge, but the urge never came. This was a shock that continued each day until I'd gone through the week without even the urge to binge or purge. It was a security blanket to have the food prepared by someone else, but by the middle of the week, I was in the kitchen helping and even creating some dishes of my own. I had never prepared and savored food with such joy.

When I got back home, I was incredibly excited but still a little concerned about preparing the foods on my own. Kat had told me to channel my perfectionism into deeply nourishing myself. I realized after the program that I had never known what that meant. I flawlessly upgraded my entire kitchen (even "borderline" foods were thrown out). I ate only what I brought into my home. I cooked exactly the dishes that were made at Kat's program, always wondering if "this is the meal I will feel like bingeing on or purging after," but I just kept on following it to the letter.

Many changes happened to my body, most of them within the first few weeks of eating this way. I started sleeping through the night without medication. I started thinking more clearly and much less obsessively. Amazingly, I actually like the bit of shapeliness I have gained. It's very different from what I put on at the clinic. My stomach is still flat, and my digestion is better than ever. No bloating. No nervousness or heart flutters. That's all been gone since the program.

Most unbelievable to me: my body had not been able to have its own cycle for the past two years without using the Nuva Ring (a contraception method). This ring determined the exact date of my period. After only two weeks of eating this way, my body decided to have its cycle on its own.

There has also been a significant change in my acne. By Christmas, all of the cystic knots under my chin were completely gone. This is without any use of expensive products and after the herbal regimen and contraceptive pills had failed. The first time I saw my family after the program, you should have seen the way my father looked at my face. He said, "Court—you look ... (moment of silence)...HEALTHY!"

Then I had my usual appointment with my medical doctor, who had a lot of questions for me once she learned about the return of my cycle. My body temperature was also up, and my pulse was normal. I had obviously put on at least ten pounds. When she asked me what I thought about my current weight (they always ask that one), I told her I didn't own a scale anymore. Then she asked about my caloric intake. I told her I had no idea. Then she asked, "What are you doing for your skin now? It has improved significantly." She went on for a few more minutes, and we were near the end of my appointment, so I thought she would schedule me for my usual follow-up appointment in two to three months. Then she said, "Courtney, I'll see you in a year, and I don't see the need to do labs." A one-year follow-up? It was an emotional moment for me.

Before I saw my doctor, she had had no hopes for my improvement, which was obvious from her past notes to my insurers. You can only imagine what my notes would have looked like if I told her I traded in *ativan* for Holy basil and gave up *ambien* for 5htp and melatonin. But I spared her those details. Today, I take a blood sugar stabilizer. I know my eating disorder has made it difficult for me to achieve balanced sugar levels on my own. I definitely wake up shaky until I have a nutritious, fatty breakfast. The same goes before bedtime. I have always heard not to eat before bed, but the majority of the time, my body requires it. And it makes me feel far more balanced in the morning. I take my 5htp before I go to bed. If I skip it, I seem to want a starchy snack to sleep. If I take it, I'm perfectly happy with full fat yogurt or a spoonful of almond butter. I also take fish oil because it has every health benefit known to man, and most important, it supports my moods. I have been on fish oil consistently since the start of Kat's program. Since then, not only has everyone noticed I'm completely calmed, emotionally, but we've all been amazed with the glow in my skin.

The amazing thing is that I am finally feeling and looking how I always wanted to by doing the opposite of depriving myself. There is not a taste or a rule that I am confined to except the axioms in Kat's book. It would have never entered the minds of those who tried so hard to help me to nourish me this way, and it would have never entered my mind to do it for myself.

My family situation has changed also. I am the oldest of seven children, but I've kept myself isolated from as many family social events as I could in recent years. Since my transformation, there has been a new desire to engage with family and people in general. I actually planned a trip to New York City with my sister and my stepmother, which is something I would have never done. At Christmas, I contributed a pumpkin pie with a coconut flour crust, and a homemade casserole with wild salmon, spinach, cream, and stilton cheese (I call it my wild salmon "bubbly"), rather than the diet foods I usually brought and ate by myself. Everyone devoured them. For the first time, I was thankful for food at Thanksgiving.

The trip was my best vacation ever. I had energy to walk the streets, enough of my own body warmth to survive the harsh weather, stamina, and the mental clarity to enjoy the events we attended (I actually was there mentally and not in another world), such joy that I had robbed myself of in the past. Eating was simple. If someone offered me bread or sugary foods, my stepmom would say "that's not Courtney's thing," (I'm sure waitresses think I'm "dieting," but I no longer eat for slimness, only for health).

I don't understand why it is taught that suffering is a lifestyle. This was the greatest misinformation I received. I now understand that every imbalance has a root cause and isn't some incurable plague that decided to pick me. I now know that finding peace doesn't require suffering or a daily battle. I have been truly freed of those things. If I were to go back now and trace the cycle of my eating disorder, I wouldn't have wasted so many years on looking at all the mishaps in my life. I now know that much of what my body was crying from—and for—was the truth about nourishment.

Today, six months after my final binge, I stand firmly transformed along with Kat, as another success story of the Truth. I have no doubt that I will live the rest of my life without my eating disorder.

Here's an excerpt from a letter to Kat my father has written: "It leaves you broken. You will do anything, but then you can't do anything. You wonder when she will give up and just die. I paid $30,000 to check my daughter into an inpatient clinic. It didn't work, and I just waited to lose her. Then I saw her following the program with you, and following the teachings of your book. I was speechless at the change in Courtney. The clinic said she would battle her problem for the rest of her life. But they were wrong. Goliath has been slain."

PART III

THE MAKEUP-LESS MAKEOVER

CHAPTER 11

GET BACK YOUR "VIRGIN" SKIN

More often than not, it's what you don't *do*
that makes your skin beautiful.

To go without makeup is every woman's right. To look great without it is every woman's possibility. The most beautiful skin is supple, glowing, and hydrated and shows healthy circulation. And contrary to popular belief, even "perfect" skin bears the occasional, if not frequent, blemish. We can have perfect skin, but we still have to live in an imperfect world. As someone who's been in contact with a new face—and heard a new skin story—just about every day since my beauty career began, I can often guess what a woman has been up to by looking closely at her face or at her hair. Interestingly, more and more of the skin problems I see are caused by the very regimens and treatments that are used to make the skin beautiful. The tough surface, immovable blemishes, and oily rebound due to drying regimens; the rawness from overzealous lunchtime peels; the crepey, dry tightness of alpha hydroxy acid abuse; the flaky patches from benzoyl peroxide dabbing—none of it wears makeup well. The concept of "normal" doesn't have much use in skin typing anymore. Just about everyone's skin has been rendered sensitive by today's aggressive products and treatments.

BEAUTIFUL SKIN SHOULDN'T BE HARD WORK

Good skin isn't about doing a three-part regimen twice a day or keeping your face sterile and oil-free. It's about wisdom, strategy, and restraint. The idea that you're not doing enough of this or that is nonsense. More often than not, it's what you *don't* do that makes your skin beautiful.

Healthy skin in a balanced body maintains itself with minimal fuss, renews itself at just the right pace, and glows on its own. In order to get to this point, you need to first recover your skin's full, protective functions. If your skin is already healthy, this chapter will help you avoid the pitfalls that often jeopardize good skin. But if you have found yourself dependent on a skin regimen that has left your skin more sensitive or problematic, this is the road back to "virgin" skin. These are the first steps toward a truly holistic approach to your best skin ever.

PEEL BACK THE LAYERS OF REGIMEN OVERKILL

Marketing mania has most of us convinced that nature in action is an unruly phenomenon to be neutralized or tamed. Advertisements teach us that hair follicles, sweat glands, surface-level skin cells, sebum, and all bacteria are beauty's mortal enemies. We are seduced into seeking the latest, harshest ways to show our hair, skin, and bodily functions who's in charge. We think nothing of using products that strip us of "bad" oil and peel away that "bad" surface skin because our poor bodies aren't as smart as the scientists who devise these approaches. We dab on blemish creams that kill all that "bad" bacteria while drying the skin into a drawn, lifeless state that is far removed from nature's intention. Real beauty has nothing to do with tingling, deep-cleaning, super-exfoliating products. These measures are overkill, and the costs to your skin, your hair, and possibly even your health can be considerable. Most "new and improved" (read: harsh) products and more aggressive exfoliating techniques compromise our skin's precious self-protective matrix. All of this has created a whole spectrum of new "skindromes" with equally unnatural new maintenance requirements. Before we know it, we're a slave to new skin problems and the upkeep these regimens create while we sacrifice the inherent self-protective potential as well as the natural glow our skin once had. These harsh approaches to skin care are based on the false assumption that our skin doesn't already come equipped with its own superior antibacterial, antiwrinkle, and anti-invader protection system. But a well-nourished body brings these built-in "pro-beauty functions" to the skin. The trick is not destroying them.

TREATMENT-CAUSED "SKINDROMES"

Certain skin products and regimens pose subtle, or sometimes major, irritations to the skin that compromise its ability to deal optimally with daily challenges. Just as your body must recover its original immunity after you eat sugar, your skin must recover its immunity after you treat your face with harsh detergents or toxic products. Some of us put a great deal of money and effort into fixing our skin without addressing the internal issues or external irritants that may be causing it to be vulnerable and reactive in the first place.

Common dermatological skin treatments can cause compounded problems that often make the original skin issue look like a walk in the park. One course of antibiotics for acne, for example, can destroy most of the protective

---

WEANING OFF STEROID CREAMS

Kathy received a consultation with me as a gift from her boyfriend. She had been struggling with a rash on her chin and using over-the-counter hydrocortisone ointment on it for almost a year. It always worked initially, but then the rash returned. She noticed that the patch of skin became increasingly crepey and translucent between outbreaks. When I told Kathy that steroid ointments thin the skin over time, she became interested in exploring alternatives. She was surprised that I began with a checklist of harmful habits to shed rather than leading her right to another product to replace the steroid ointment. No new cream was going to help as long as she was stripping and smothering her skin with irritating foaming cleansers and perfumed moisturizers and aggravating her skin with sugary, pro-inflammatory foods and drinks.

I advised Kathy to get a checkup with her doctor to screen the prescription drugs she was taking for their possible effects on her skin and to pinpoint any other health issues signaled by her rashes. No matter what cream I suggested (licorice, chamomile, or pyrithione zinc–based products, in this case), she would have to go through steroid withdrawal and let the rash run its course at least once before it would begin to subside and the skin could recover its immunity.

(continued on next page)

> In the meantime, she could greatly reduce inflammation and allergic responses by eliminating foods she was sensitive to and by looking into anti-inflammatory and immune-calming supplements. I showed Kathy abstracts from peer-reviewed studies on some of these substances, so she could involve (and inform) her dermatologist and make her final choices with him. Finally, I introduced her to cosmetics that could cover the redness on her face without irritating her skin. It was clear at the end of our consultation that she was blown away that no one had ever told her she was destroying her skin's future with the steroid cream.
>
> A couple of months later, Kathy told me she had not only stayed off the steroid cream but also her rash was finally gone and the redness that remained was subsiding. In addition, her use of supplements and the food and skin product upgrades had dramatically changed her entire complexion as well as other issues. She felt better all over. And most exciting for me, she was thinking about quitting smoking, an area she would not negotiate at our initial consultation. Her boyfriend was thrilled.

bacteria that keep your gut in working order, leaving you with problems that are no longer skin-deep. Next thing you know, you could be suffering from yeast infections, malabsorption, food sensitivities, and a host of other problems, not to mention a wicked relapse of the original skin problem. Recurrences are especially likely if you use topical hydrocortisone ointments, which eventually thin the skin and wear down its natural immunity.

RECOVER YOUR SKIN'S BASIC PRO-BEAUTY FUNCTIONS

Many of my past and present clients have applied a "first do no harm" philosophy to their skin issues and have been able to reverse the domino effect of skin regimens that were sensitizing and disabling their skin, wean themselves off steroid creams and antibiotics, and even drastically change—or discover—their true skin type. Chances are your own skin problems are not entirely nature's doing, and the solution for them probably isn't something you can apply to the surface. In fact, it might be what you stop applying that has the greatest impact.

Like the rest of our bodies, our skin needs a sanctuary from irritants and assaults in order to recover its pro-beauty functions and reverse the compounded problems that can get out of control once these basic functions are compromised. In order to get back our "virgin skin," we must:

- Recover the integrity of the skin's outer layer, which is called the stratum corneum
- Recover the integrity of the precious hydrolipid barrier that enables the skin to retain water, fight wrinkles, and keep out harmful chemicals
- Recover uninterrupted function of the skin's bacteria-fighting surface acidity, known as its acid mantle

Once we get back these basic components of "virgin skin," we can have a far greater success rate in identifying the real solutions for our skin—if we still need them. For some, merely stopping the assaults to basic skin function is all it takes for their skin to fully recover.

The Stratum Corneum: The Gatekeeper of Beautiful Skin

The skin's outer layer is called the stratum corneum. Since the emergence of alpha hydroxy acids in the mid-1990s, the trend in skin care has been to penetrate and break this layer to reveal plump, healthy skin. But this outer layer contains most of the skin's antiaging, antiwrinkling, and antibacterial protection, and it is the skin's primary sunscreen. Immature cells beneath the surface need the protection of this outer layer to develop properly and be healthy when they arrive at the surface. Recovering and maintaining the stratum corneum will optimize your skin's pro-beauty function and ecology. It is a necessary first step if you want a shot at perfect, low-maintenence skin.

The Hydrolipid Barrier

The skin depends on the hydrolipid barrier to retain water. It is the skin's waterproof seal that was never meant to be broken but is commonly destroyed by modern, high-tech skin care regimens. The barrier is a primary defense against foreign substances, drying, and wrinkling.

The Acid Mantle

The skin's acid mantle, made of sweat, mature skin cells, bacteria, and sebum, is the optimum surface skin environment. It sounds like something we should get rid of altogether, but the acid mantle is the naturally low-pH skin surface that protects the skin against infectious bacteria—and thus acne and other irritations. It can easily be obliterated by skin products that contain detergents, soaps, or antiseptics, and in many women—and even teens!—it is never given a chance to recover or perform its intended function. Its absence inevitably leads to skin problems that can only be controlled but never resolved until we restore the acid mantle.

THE SKIN ASSAULTS TO SHED

Alpha Hydroxy Acids

Alpha hydroxy acids (AHAs)—the popular skin-exfoliating acids that include glycolic, citric, malic, and lactic acids—are prevalent in mainstream cleansers, moisturizers, toners, and even makeup. Several prominent skin experts over the years have expressed concerns that continued use of AHAs could compromise the skin's protective functions. The FDA is currently investigating concerns that AHAs—which have never been studied long-term—might damage DNA by increasing sun exposure and promote skin cancer. In an interview with *Fashion Wire Daily*, Dr. Lynn Drake, chief of dermatology at the University of Oklahoma and past president of the American Academy of Dermatology, said, "We honestly don't know the long-term effects of alpha hydroxy acids on the skin. The body has a mechanism for rejuvenating the skin automatically. With AHAs, I'm concerned that we are going to change the normal biorhythms of the skin."

Over-Exfoliating

Over-exfoliating with AHAs as well as other physical exfoliants, such as cleansing grains and scrubs, ages and sensitizes the skin by
- Abrading, tearing, and sensitizing the skin
- Dramatically increasing the skin's vulnerability to sun damage
- Destroying the hydrolipid barrier
- Compromising the acid mantle
- Making it vulnerable to chemicals it was never intended to absorb

And while keeping acne-prone skin clear of debris is important, any irritating exfoliating product can aggravate inflammation. If full-blown acne is the issue, then working your way down to the mildest exfoliation products and removing as many irritating ingredients from them as possible will help you recover your skin's natural defenses.

To wean yourself off AHAs and other exfoliants, use antimicrobial essential oils for acne as well as gentle but effective green papaya-based masks and seaweed and other nourishing and detoxifying serums to stimulate cell renewal and collagen production for wrinkle reversal and prevention. See chapter 13 and the Resources for further recommendations.

Oil-Stripping and Drying Regimens

Virtually all soaps, foaming cleansers, and alcohol-based toners (with the exception of cetyl and cetearyl alcohols, which are not drying like other alcohols) will compromise the skin's hydrolipid barrier. Many of these cleansers contain solvents or detergents, such as sodium lauryl sulfate, that can cause the skin to lose water and become rough, sensitive, and prone to premature wrinkling. These products leave the skin feeling tight—which is a sign that it's been stripped. This causes it to produce more oil in a rebound effort to regulate its own moisture. But even after the sebum returns, the skin's barrier and bacterial balance remain compromised, and blemishes and other inflammatory problems are more likely to occur until the barrier is reestablished. This will require the discontinuation of soap and solvent-based degreasing cleansers.

On a purely aesthetic note, when the skin surface is dried up and deprived of its own lubrication, blemishes often stop moving through the skin and remain suspended beneath the surface for prolonged periods. Peeling often alternates with or accompanies oiliness. Blemishes spot-zapped with benzoyl peroxide become crusty, unattractive, and harder to cover. Foundation appears blotchy and unnatural. Don't destroy the beauty of your skin for the sake of temporary clarity!

How Even Moisturizers Can Dry Out Your Lipid Barrier

Finally—and this is a shocker—even natural, very emollient moistures usually leave the skin drier after several hours (after washing them off) than if you had *not applied a moisturizer at all*. This has now been verified in studies, and if you think about it, it should be no surprise. "It's a little like dish liquid," says David Pollock, a leading skin care formulator. "Dish liquid is not 'cutting grease,' it is simply emulsifying it; making oil mixable with water so it can be lifted and washed away. Emulsifiers in moisturizers unfortunately do the same

> **ANTIBACTERIAL SOAPS AND ANTIBIOTIC SKIN TREATMENTS**
>
> Most dermatologists regard antibacterial soaps as not only overkill but also potentially dangerous since they destroy beneficial bacteria and can create resistant bacteria— even in people who live with those who use them. Whether you're using over-the-counter antibacterial soaps or an antibiotic regimen from your dermatologist, you run a risk of developing resistant bacteria and the certainty that you will be more vulnerable to breakouts and other negative skin effects caused by pathogenic bacteria between uses. Oral antibiotics dramatically increase these risks throughout the body and can lead to dandruff, yeast infections, toe and nail fungus, and itchy, uncomfortable skin. They can also impair digestion and absorption of nutrients and give rise to possible lifelong sensitivities, allergies, and autoimmune issues that affect the skin and the entire body. If you're taking prescription antibiotics for a chronic skin problem, discuss topically applied options and the possibility of weaning off them completely. During the weaning process you can minimize a recurrence of infectious skin problems by incorporating natural antimicrobial topicals (see Resources)—which have not been shown to create resistant bacteria—into your skin care regimen. Also use the skin-supportive feeding and cultivating suggestions in part II, which can influence your resistance to harmful bacteria not only in the skin but also throughout the entire body.

on your skin. Once other ingredients have evaporated or been absorbed, and as the day wears on, they sit on the skin and emulsify the lipid barrier of the skin. This has been verified in some of the most expensive, richest moisturizers in the world." The answer is layering nonlotion serums, or choosing moisturizers made with new self-adjusting emulsifier technology instead of traditional creams or lotions with polysorbates or other emulsifiers.

SPARE YOUR SKIN BY UPGRADING YOUR MORNING SHOWER

What if you could dramatically improve the health and beauty of your skin and hair, reduce your allergies and your risk of cancer, and eliminate a daily source of premature aging and needless toxic exposure without altering your routine? It's as simple as installing a filter on your showerhead.

Most people are unaware of the countless ways that chlorinated shower water can undermine their efforts at beautiful skin, hair, and health. By compromising the skin's bacteria-fighting acid mantle and protective barrier and then penetrating and causing oxidative damage, chlorine represents a huge cumulative skin burden, making normal to dry skin sensitive, drier, and more vulnerable to irritation, dandruff, and fungal infections. And if the skin is already stripped, dry, or rough, your daily shower can devastate it. Chlorine also contributes to dry, brittle hair and scalp. And if you color your hair, there's the nuisance of chlorine's mild bleaching effect.

But there are even more important reasons to make this painless and inexpensive adjustment. Our pores soak chlorine directly into the bloodstream. According to research conducted jointly at Harvard University and the Medical College of Wisconsin, chlorinated water contributes to 9 percent of all bladder cancers and 18 percent of all rectal cancers in the United States.

Furthermore, the heat in your shower produces chloroform from the water, which—when inhaled—can aggravate allergies, respiratory and sinus conditions, and asthma. These issues can cause under-eye puffiness and circles.

The humble shower filter might just be the biggest beauty and health bang for your buck there is. To set yourself up with affordable yet quality filtration, look for the newer zinc-copper filter technology, which works with heat much better than the old carbon filters (see Resources).

STOP STRIPPING THE SKIN AND START PURIFYING IT

The most renowned beauty oils—among them jojoba, apricot kernel, sweet almond, squalene, and emu—are noted for their similarity to sebum, nature's perfect lubricant. The best shampoos are considered such because they "replenish" natural sheen to the hair, *which they've just stripped*. Many find it hard to grasp that it is not necessary to dissolve every trace of sebum in order to "start fresh." There are a number of effective ways to cleanse and purify the skin without stripping it. Various cleansers containing natural antimicrobial essential oils and substances can deeply purify the sebum and even help normalize its production without compromising the skin's hydrolipid barrier or causing breakouts. See the comprehensive charts in chapter 13 and the Resources section for some of the substances and products I recommend.

THE BABY WIPE TRICK, ONLY BETTER

Whenever I do makeup for the New York fashion shows, I use baby wipes. It's a popular trick for quickly cleaning makeup off models' faces. They work well, but the perfumes and other potential irritants in your average baby wipe aren't something you'd want on your face very often. Fortunately, not all baby wipes are created equal. Baby wipes available at health food stores are aloe-based and free of fragrance and propylene glycol. They are a far healthier way to wash your face than most forty-dollar fancy cleansers you could buy at the department store.

TONE DOWN YOUR TONER

If you're using a cleanser that contains a lot of petrochemicals (fragrance, colors, propylene glycol, mineral oil), which sit on or irritate the skin, it makes sense to take an extra step to make sure the residue is removed, but not if that means using a toner filled with nasty pollutants and irritants. And if you're cleansing with substances that actually purify and nourish the skin, there is little need for a toner at all. In the morning, however, when your face is essentially clean, you may want to use a nonalcohol, natural toner or my morning Teabag Trick to remove any oil or dirt it has accumulated overnight before you apply light moisturizers or serums and then makeup. Even if your skin is quite oily, fight the

MY MORNING TEA BAG TRICK

After I make my daily pot of green (or licorice or chamomile) tea using purified water, I save the tea bags in a closed glass container in the fridge and use them as little cleansing pads the next morning. They're perfect for a little exfoliation. Tea has anti-inflammatory properties and zero negatives to challenge your skin. If you have acne-prone skin that may require slightly deeper cleaning, use a washcloth moistened with tea and a dot of the right cleanser or essential oil (see chapter 13).

Save deeper cleansing for evenings, when there's makeup to remove. Mornings don't have to be scary for your skin!

urge to strip it in the morning with foaming cleansers and alcohol-based, drying toners. Go for a purifying ritual that leaves the skin's oils intact.

You can easily make a toner that keeps in the fridge for a week. Use aloe juice (healing and anti-inflammatory); a dash of apple-cider vinegar (restores optimum pH); a generous splash of strong green, chamomile, or licorice tea (anti-inflammatory and antioxidant); and a few drops of lavender essential oil (antimicrobial and calming). Add a few drops of tea tree oil, neem oil, or grapefruit seed extract for stronger antibacterial action. If you don't have time for home recipes, check out the alcohol-free toners at the health-food store. When choosing a toner, avoid potentially drying or disruptive ingredients, like fragrance, propylene glycol, sulfates, and alcohols (other than ceteryl or cetyl).

THE ONLY WAY TO REBUILD THE SKIN'S BARRIER

Letting the skin barrier recover once it's been stripped can take days to a couple of weeks, depending on the degree of damage, but we can speed the process with carefully selected topical tactics. Phospholipids derived primarily from soy and egg yolks are the only substances that possess the ability to directly rebuild the hydrolipid barrier when applied topically. They protect your skin and become a part of the skin cell membranes. They are able to form liposomes, which can nourish the skin and deliver EFAs, such as linoleic acid. Linoleic acid can rebuild the lipid barrier to prevent water loss and dry skin. At the same time, it can reduce overproduction of oil and inhibit acne. See the Resources section for products containing phospholipids and EFAs.

DON'T DEPRIVE YOUR SKIN WITH DENATURED OILS

Just as stripped foods seriously deprive the body, stripped and refined oils may seriously deprive your skin. EFAs are found in cold-pressed, skin-compatible oils, but they are lost once those oils are refined or tampered with. Mineral oil and petrolatum are highly refined petrochemical derivatives that, according to phytochemist Aubrey Hampton, PhD, can actually leave the skin and lips dryer because they block sebum's crucial functions and interfere with the skin's ability to regulate its own moisture. And both mineral oil and petrolatum have been shown to cause chemically induced acne.

THE RECOVERY AND RESTRAINT PERIOD: RESIST THE "DO SOMETHING" IMPULSE

Once you've discontinued your harsh products and incorporated the inside-out regimen upgrades in this book, you should see a marked decrease in skin sensitivity in anywhere from a few weeks to only a few days, depending on the harshness of your original regimen. You will also see an increase in skin activity, as blemishes suspended beneath the skin may move to the surface and live out their destiny over the next couple of weeks. As the skin surface recovers its integrity, makeup will go on more smoothly and last longer. Sensitivity and ruddiness will subside. Skin problems may seem worse for a few days or even a couple of weeks before they get better, but you can minimize this rebound period by immediately incorporating skin-supportive product, beverage, food, supplement, and even emotional regimens. The sum of this holistic approach will change your skin in ways your old harsh regimens never could.

TREAT YOUR HAIR LIKE YOUR SKIN

Our hair may be not be alive, but that doesn't keep us from killing it. Like fine leather, how we wash and care for our hair makes a world of difference in its quality and luster. Because hair can only be cosmetically altered once it has been harmed—although, luckily, damage grows out—it's important to cultivate resilient, strong hair via healthier scalp and hair follicles by feeding them from within and avoiding the very same stripping, irritating, and drying assaults that cause problems on the skin.

Tricks and Tweaks That Spare Your Hair

Don't overwash your hair. If you have oily hair and wash it every day, don't wash twice, and don't lather the ends. If you have dry hair, don't wash it more than twice a week, unless you use a nonfoaming radical hair-cleansing technique (see sidebar) or gentler shampoo options such as those listed in Resources. If your scalp is itchy, wash more often, but keep in mind that dandruff and itching may clear up once you install a shower filter, change your products, optimize your body's probiotic ecology, and start eating better food. You know you've achieved healthy internal ecology when your scalp stops itching, even when it's oily.

RADICAL SHAMPOO-LESS HAIR-CLEANSING TECHNIQUES

Can hair truly be cleaned without foaming cleansers or shampoo? It absolutely can. In fact, your hair can be softer and your scalp healthier than you ever imagined if you stop using or minimize your use of shampoo. The list of celebrity enthusiasts for L.A. hair pro Chaz Dean's Wen line of hair products is almost as impressive as his famous cleansing conditioner. The tea tree formula purifies the scalp and hair with essential oils. Other nonfoaming products that use essential oils and clay-based minerals include Terressentials and Logona nonfoaming hair washes. You can use these products exclusively or alternate with sulfate-free, ultra-gentle shampoos such as those listed in Resources.

Dry Your Hair Smartly

Dry your hair naturally (see the bodifying technique following) or use a super-absorbent hair chamois. Infrared or ionic blow-dryers also minimize damage by drying hair evenly, inside and out, rather than scorching the outer cuticle layer, which is frayed by conventional dryers (see Resources).

How to Get Body Without Stressing Your Hair

Wash or wet your hair in the evening. After gently squeezing (never rubbing) wet hair with a super-absorbent hair chamois, apply a touch of leave-in conditioner or moisturizer by first raking it through your hair with your hands, concentrating on the ends, and then using a wide-tooth comb to distribute. If your hair is wavy, let it dry naturally. If your hair is straight and long enough, bend over and gently comb your hair straight up, working the comb from ends to roots so as not to force it through any tangles, then twist your hair to make a loose bun on top of your head and secure with a cotton scrunchie. Sleep with your hair this way. When you let it down in the morning, you will have the body and wave you've always dreamed of. For more wave, try spraying NaPCA into your hair after using the chamois; it draws moisture into the hair without weighing it down.

Avoid a Harsh Cut

A cut should yield to your features and softly frame them, not compete with them. Cutting with a razor or a slithered or texturized scissor can create wave, lift, and movement and give you lower-maintenance hair. Let your hair change from day to day. Let it have its own life. Refrain from conquering your hair and showing it who's boss. Letting your hair do its own thing will lead you to the best cut. It can also improve your self-image.

WHAT'S GOOD FOR THE SKIN IS GOOD FOR THE HAIR

When applied sparingly, the moisturizers that are most ideal for your type of hair are often the same moisturizers and oils that work best on your skin. Some of the more expensive ingredients serve no purpose in your hair, but the basic natural moisturizers make great texturizing products. Moisturizers that penetrate the skin without leaving a greasy film are great for both oily skin and the hair type that generally comes with it. Dry hair responds wonderfully to the same textured creams and balms suited for dry skin. Distribute a dab of moisturizer on your hands by rubbing them together and apply it to hair ends only at first.

GIVE YOURSELF A PERMANENT BREAK FROM HARSH SELF-TREATMENT

We need to stop being harsh on ourselves. Stop using soaps that dry, blemish creams that irritate, lotions that sting, shampoos that strip, chemical-laden perfumes that poison, and exfoliants that leave your skin raw. As you begin to support your skin from within, you can begin to sit back and let your body deal with and heal each passing skin issue and see how a little restraint and the world of inside-out strategies can turn irritated skin into calm, glowing skin and chronic issues into transient ones that no longer cause panic.

CHAPTER 12

PURIFY YOUR POTIONS AND PAINTS

We don't need to aspire to know everything about cosmetic ingredients to set an informed criterion for what we use on our bodies, but in order to shed the true irritants and toxins that can burden your skin and your health, it is imperative to get a basic understanding of what you put on your body day in and day out. Some of it affects your skin's beauty, and some of it could be affecting your vitality and your hormonal state as well as your future. Perhaps the most realistic approach is for you to fully understand the degree of your current vulnerability. The amount of crucial information that goes unreported and undetected on labels due to the lack of testing requirements and effective regulation is astounding. Holes in your understanding could be setting you up for skin and health problems that are hard to trace. Let's close up some of those holes.

WHAT GOES ON, GOES IN

Back in beauty school, "product safety" meant not getting perm solution in your client's eyes. We learned how to pronounce and spell chemical names. We learned how they could change hair structure. We learned how to protect our hands with gloves. But we never learned about the possible proven effects of long-term exposure to some of the concoctions we slathered on our clients. At enrollment, they don't tell you that cosmetologists develop multiple myeloma—a form of bone marrow cancer—at four times the rate of the general population. This fact is more widely known to health insurers than to a budding beautician or the women on whom she applies these chemicals.

233

Skin absorption is now widely recognized as a significant way by which substances enter the body. In some cases (particularly the emerging nanotechnology trend in skin care products), it provides even more passage into the bloodstream than eating or drinking. Some scientists estimate that as much as 60 percent of typical products we apply on our skin winds up in our bloodstream. The popularity of transdermal patches to deliver synthetic drugs directly into the bloodstream is seen as one of the efficient ways to deliver chemicals into the bloodstream while bypassing the liver, but the cosmetics industry chooses whether to emphasize if a product is absorbed by the skin. In the case of vitamin C crow's-feet patches, skin absorption is boasted about, but when it comes to coal tar dyes in color cosmetics and in hair color, for example, you are unlikely to hear the claim "penetrates deep," even though they do.

There is a growing concern about the accumulation of estrogen-mimicking chemicals in the breast tissues of women and in the prostate tissues of men. Just about every day, a new industrial or cosmetic chemical is found to be a hormone-disrupting substance. Hormone disruption can cause uterine cell changes, cell proliferation, and other signs of elevated estrogen activity. More recently, hormone-disrupting substances have been linked with genetic changes believed to increase obesity risk. Estrogen dominance is becoming more prevalent in this country and contributes to breast cancer and reproductive and weight problems in both men and women. Hormone imposters are a compelling place to start with regard to cosmetic ingredients.

Phthalates, a type of chemical used in nail polish and hair spray, are confirmed estrogen mimics of growing concern to the Centers for Disease Control (CDC). The CDC has discovered forty-five times more phthalates (particularly dibutyl phthalate, found in nail polish) in women ages twenty to forty than previously estimated. More recently, phthalates have been linked with genital feminization of boys born to women who had moderately high (extremely common) levels of phthalates during pregnancy. One study found that many of the most commonly used synthetic sunscreen ingredients (which are common even in so-called "natural" sunscreen products), including benzophenone-3 and octyl-methoxycinnamates (OMC) accumulate in the breast milk and organs of rats, producing estrogenic effects, which researchers say suggests it may have the same effects in humans. The common preservatives methyl, propyl, butyl, and ethyl paraben, long thought to be safe synthetic preservatives, were found to be mildly estrogenic in a 1998 study in which researchers concluded that "given their use in a wide range of commercially available topical preparations, it is suggested that the safety in use of these chemicals should be reassessed." But this had almost no impact on paraben use in cosmetics until 2004 when a study at the University of Reading, England found high concentrations of parabens in human breast cancer tumors. By 2006, most natural products had discontinued their use of parabens, and mainstream synthetic products began to follow suit.

THE THRESHOLD PRINCIPLE

Each of us has a threshold at which we react, not just to any one irritant, but also to the number of irritants we are exposed to at a given time. And any additional exposure we encounter once we reach our saturation point could make us suddenly quite sensitive and even chronically sick. For example, formaldehyde, which can be found in all sorts of cosmetics—as well as in food, new clothes, and fumes in our homes—can build up in the body without causing acute symptoms before suddenly reaching a saturation point at which a person becomes sensitive to even minute amounts, according to Angel DeFazio, BSci, AT, president of the National Toxic Encephalopathy Foundation.

The threshold principle also applies to allergic responses. Exposure to sensitizing substances over a long period of time or too many allergens at once can cause a reaction to a substance you may never have reacted to in the past.

Remember, though, that just because a substance is natural doesn't mean it won't cause a reaction in some people. Essential oils with therapeutic effects on one person can cause an allergic reaction in another (which is why a patch test is a good idea before incorporating them into your regimens). Studies have linked talc with asbestos contamination and cancer. But unlike synthetically derived chemicals, few, if any, naturally occurring substances have been found to accumulate in the body or the environment indefinitely, or react unpredictably with other substances.

HOW REGULATION DOESN'T WORK

In a 1994 study published in the *Journal of the National Cancer Institute*, researchers examined the relationship between the use of permanent hair dyes and selected fatal cancers in 573,369 women and concluded that women who use black hair dyes over a long period of time may have an increased risk of fatal non-Hodgkin's lymphoma and multiple myeloma. Researchers urged that "the removal of carcinogens from hair dyes and appropriate labeling of hair-coloring products would help reduce this potential risk." But a prior attempt by the FDA to require a warning label on permanent hair-coloring products, after studies showed certain ingredients to be mutagenic in the late 1970s, was thwarted by a regulatory loophole that exempted these ingredients from the FDA's jurisdiction. These products remain on the shelf today, in spite of recent studies indicating that they may cause bladder cancer in humans. Many other countries, including Japan, have banned carcinogenic hair-color ingredients, the most notorious of which is phenylenediamine (PPD).

Some coal tar colors (FD&C or D&C dyes used in hair color, makeup, and skin care products) that have been tested were shown to cause cancer when injected into the skin of rodents, and yet most have never been adequately tested for safety in cosmetic use. We do know they can cause acne and allergies, but whatever else they cause is anyone's guess. This is true of most cosmetics ingredients. In fact, experts from the National Research Council and the National Academy of Science who were involved with one of the first large government studies of cosmetic ingredients back in 1984 concluded that "of the tens of thousands of commercially important chemicals, only a few have been subjected to extensive toxicity testing and most have scarcely been tested at all." In the decades since then nothing changed, until January 1, 2007, when the California Safe Cosmetics Act took effect, requiring that state's cosmetic manufacturers to report any use of known carcinogens or birth defect-causing ingredients. This does not necessarily mean that they will be removed.

Odd loopholes in regulation based on the archaic notion that cosmetics are not absorbed through the skin have literally made cosmetics a bastion for rampant use of toxic chemicals. While the government does theoretically "require" a warning label on products that have not been adequately tested, there is no congressional mandate for this, so the industry hasn't followed through. The FDA spends less than 1 percent of its budget on supervising the industry. The Cosmetic, Toiletry, and Fragrance Association (CTFA) acts as both the effective regulator as well as the special interest and key lobbying organization on the industry's behalf. The Cosmetic Ingredient Review (CIR), a small group of experts that reviews thousands of cosmetics ingredients, is largely funded by the CTFA and relies mostly on unpublished data, according to Judi Vance, publisher of *Cosmetic Health Report* and author of *Beauty to Die For*. This is just a small sample of the loopholes, delays, appeals, inactions, conflicts of interest, and exemptions that riddle cosmetic regulation and render it all but useless or worse since it provides a false sense of security. If you want more insight into the circus of cosmetic regulation, see the Resources section for suggested organizations and reading. In recent years, some great new resources have become available.

IF IT'S NOT THE CHEMICAL ITSELF, IT'S THE CONTAMINANTS, BYPRODUCTS, AND COMBINATIONS

One of the major inherent problems with synthesized cosmetic materials is that they tend to be contaminated or to form byproducts during manufacturing, storage, or while on the skin. For example, the cosmetic chemicals listed on labels as TEA, DEA, and MEA or their full names, which end in "amine," like triethanolamine, were found in 1998 by the National Toxicology Program (NTP) to form nitrosamines, which cause cancer in mice. PEG, or polyethylene glycol, a common synthetic emollient, is often contaminated with dioxane, another known hormone disruptor and a carcinogen that the Consumer Product Safety Commission has determined to be dangerous even at low-level exposure. Quaternium-15, a common cosmetic preservative, can release formaldehyde, another carcinogen, and cause skin reactions. Formaldehyde, widely known to be one of the most dangerous common chemicals, is used in nail polish and in all kinds of synthetic hair, skin, and body care products as an antimicrobial and preservative, but it is never listed on the label as "formaldehyde." It has dozens of aliases (most have the word "form" in it, like "formalin," "lysoform," and "formalith"); again, other chemicals can release formaldehyde as a byproduct, such as imidazolidinyl urea, a common preservative in shampoos.

If the formaldehyde and dibutyl phthalate don't make nail polish scary enough, there's the other key ingredient, toluene, which can cause rashes, neurological symptoms, and harm to the kidneys and liver during frequent use, according to both the EPA and the U.S. Department of Health and Human Services Agency for Toxic Substances and Disease Registry. Thankfully, professional-grade polish without the three most infamous ingredients is now available.

PERFUME OR POLLUTANT: ANOTHER MAJOR UNKNOWN

I once sat on an airplane next to a woman who got up and then returned from the restroom reeking of perfume. She sat there sniffing and messing up her perfect makeup with the tissue she used to repeatedly dab her nose and eyes. It was like looking at myself when I was twenty. Many people are sensitive to the very fragrances they use on themselves every day. In fact, fragrance is one of the top contact allergens and often contains petroleum-based chemicals identified as carcinogens and neurotoxins, according to the National Academy of Sciences.

Analysis has shown that some seriously harmful ingredients are showing up in even the finest perfumes. According to Samuel Epstein, MD, Professor of Environmental Medicine at the University of Illinois School of Public Health, Chicago, an analysis of one of the "hottest" designer perfumes in history revealed forty-one ingredients, including some known to be toxic to the skin, respiratory tract, and nervous and reproductive systems. Data about toxicity were either unavailable or inadequate on several of the ingredients. Additionally, some ingredients were determined to be volatile and sources of indoor air pollution.

Allergies to fragrance grew more prevalent in the United States from the 1980s to 1990s. In conventional skin and hair products, fragrance is impossible to avoid since it is allowed even in products labeled "fragrance free." Therefore, we can only knowingly escape from fragrance by using products with essential oil-based scents or products that are 100 percent certified organic (products labeled merely "organic" can contain up to 30 percent synthetic ingredients!). Some nonorganic products might be free of fragrance if they list only natural ingredients and no fragrance or "parfum."

WHAT'S IN A LABEL

Most of us know not to trust labels on a conscious level, and yet many of us tend to suspend our disbelief if the packaging, smell, and marketing strike our fancy. But even the term "made *with* 100 percent pure extracts" can appear on the poetic packaging of what is really a plastic, synthetic concoction. "Natural" may not actually mean natural, as it is an unregulated term. Furthermore, "hypo-allergenic" does not mean you won't react to a product; it is a phrase for which manufacturers have their own interpretations. Here's another caveat:

hypoallergenic products are also allowed to contain fragrance even if the label states "fragrance-free." And "noncomedogenic" is yet another unregulated term that tells you nothing. Mineral oil, which has been shown to be a cause of chemically induced acne, appears in some supposedly noncomedogenic products. "Dermatologist tested" can mean anything and nothing. Any dermatologist with any motive or vested interest can test a product, but the results of the test don't have to be scientific or even positive. There are no regulations setting any standard meaning for any of these terms. The term "pH-balanced" can actually indicate harmful products, according to Dr. Aubrey Hampton, who says that triethanolamine (TEA), the substance that forms cancer-causing nitrosamines, is often used in cosmetics to adjust their pH levels.

Personally, I don't spend a lot of time deciphering hard-to-pronounce ingredient lists anymore because I rarely deal with products that bear them. Even if there weren't inherent risks in synthetic chemical combinations and the serious lack of testing, I would not want to deny myself the therapeutic

---

REJECT THESE RED FLAG INGREDIENTS

I've found that rather than learn the name of every synthetic or even natural ingredient (so many are just as hard to pronounce as synthetics!), if you can avoid just a handful of ingredients, you are likely getting a product that is pretty close to natural. Here are the bare minimum ingredients to weed out first:

- Synthetic fragrance or parfum
- Synthetic emollients, such as mineral oil or petrolatum
- Synthetic preservatives such as parabens, "amines" like TEA, and imidazolidinyl urea
- Synthetic colors, such as FD&C colors (stick with iron oxide mineral pigments)
- Synthetic carriers and emulsifiers, such as glycols and polysorbates

You will be hard pressed to find even one product that is free of all five of those ingredients in typical supermarkets. I highly recommend you go to a health food store to broaden your horizons (and to do your food shopping while you're at it).

actions, purity, and life force of naturally occurring, biologically active substances. Those who are ill or chemically sensitive may choose to avoid the risks of synthesized chemicals altogether, and those who are concerned about the environment will surely take all this into account in setting their own criteria for what goes on—and in—their bodies and down their drains. Getting informed allows you to choose your potions consistently with your values.

"ORGANIC" ON LABELS: DECIPHERING THE LINGERING LOOPHOLES

The USDA's National Organic Rule (NOR) on organic standards for foods went into effect in October 2002 and was a landmark regulation that gave full credibility to the word "organic" on food labels. It assures consumers that foods labeled "100 percent organic" are completely free of pesticides, hormones, antibiotics, chemical fertilizers, irradiation, and genetically modified ingredients. As mentioned previously, though, the label "organic" only requires that 70 percent of a product be organic. This leaves a whole lot of room for synthetics, which is why I read a product's ingredients list (the only way to tell) before I consider it 100 percent natural, rather than accepting an "organic" label on the front.

Most health food stores carry a wide range of products without synthetic perfumes, colors, or mineral oil, and while it is possible to learn which ingredients are organic by reading the ingredients list, some companies count the high percentage of "organic" floral water they use (listed as "hydrosols") toward the total organic content of the product, and you could wind up using products that still contain a lot of synthetics in the remaining percentage of ingredients. The industry is working on establishing standards as I write this, but for now, one cannot trust the term "organic" on the front label of hair and skin care products—only on the ingredients list if the listing is certified. In other words, some natural products that aren't organic may be purer than some organic ones. You can learn more about the ingredients in the current brands you use, or about any ingredient, at Environmental Working Groups' (EWG) Skin Deep database, www.ewg.org (click on the Skin Deep button), where you can search ingredients or even brand name products for safety ratings. I do not do a lot of database searches on my products because I stick to the ultra-pure products like those I have listed in Resources and companies that are extremely explicit about their products, rather than those that are cryptic about them, while wowing you with clever slogans and slick graphics. Another campaign using EWG's Skin Deep database is the Campaign for Safe Cosmetics at www.safecosmetics.org. It is interesting to see which companies have and have not pledged to use known or strongly suspected carcinogens, mutagens, and birth defect-causing chemicals in their products. Ask your favorite companies if they can at least commit to that! I think America's tolerance for these things is wearing thin.

DON'T BE SEDUCED BY THE PSEUDONATURALS

Because of our desire to reconnect with the "experience" of nature, we are prone to accept pseudonatural products. From products that include token natural botanicals and fake aromatherapy candles and air fresheners that are actually toxic to inhale to flowery yet synthetic body lotions made by "green-conscious" companies that boast about their recycled packaging, to the most luxuriously packaged and ingeniously marketed "real imposters" that smell of lavender or green tea—there is no such thing as essence of green tea, by the way—we are entering a new phase of sensory exploitation. The ingredients are no different from those used in the first fruity shampoos of the 1980s, but the marketing is much more brilliant. Its success in exploiting both our senses and our sensibilities relies on one key condition: that we as individuals remain uninformed and don't look at the ingredients list.

It is exciting to remove that shiny box from that chichi little shopping bag, but your body doesn't care about the packaging. Once you've tossed out the fancy foil box, the cellophane, and the rest of the cardboard, you're probably still getting plastic *inside the bottle*. Why apply a dead and perfumed product in a beautiful package when you can use one that can give you its actual, vital life force (biologically active ingredients) in perfect harmony with your body and the environment?

There are a lot of intelligent, self-respecting women who'd be shocked to know the degree to which they've been duped into accepting cheaply made, irritating concoctions as the cutting edge in skin care. All too often a few beneficial or even patented breakthrough ingredients are carried in a soup of known irritants included primarily to benefit the manufacturer. Most drug and department store brands contain only 5 to 8 percent active ingredients, yet ads can go on and on about the effectiveness of those ingredients. And even if they do use the amount proven to have a clinical effect, the rest of what's in the bottle may be a synthetic gravy that actually weakens and interferes with the optimal functions of your skin.

The longer we immerse ourselves in fake tastes and smells, the more we lose our ability to decipher what's real. But even if you can't tell the difference between an essential oil of freshly harvested lavender and lavender-scented solvents and petrochemicals, your body knows. Just as it is offended by the denatured matter we are presented with as food, it is offended by these chemicals posing as true substance.

Nature's prohibitive cost to manufacturers, due to the care required in extracting, storing, and delivering its inimitable rewards, has kept most mainstream manufacturers from considering them in their business models. The more dirt-cheap synthetics you use and the harsher and more prevalent the preservatives, the longer your product will last in the warehouse, the cheaper it is to make, and the higher the profit; therefore, the more the manufacturer can spend on packaging, the more beautiful and prominent its ads can be, and the more exciting—yet worthless—that beautifully packaged product will be to the consumer. But this is changing as consumers wise up.

ENTER MICROBREWED COSMETICS: SUBSTANCE OVER PACKAGING

A growing number of skin companies are doing what the synthetic skin care giants claimed was impossible. These microchemists are saying no to mass production and warehousing protocol and are giving up vast profits to create biologically active skin and body care products that contain live, unadulterated ingredients. Like microbrewed beer, cosmetic products produced in small batches are likely to contain few, if any, harmful ingredients. These companies often use essential oils and citrus seed extract as preservatives, and if they use any synthetics, they are in the most minute amounts. These products are significantly more expensive to produce, and the value of the natural substances used is hard to quantify. Without as many patent profits behind them, you're unlikely to see these products advertised heavily, or at all, in your favorite magazines or on television. But among their cult following, including celebrities and fashionistas, microbrewed cosmetics are fast gaining appeal and the long-awaited acknowledgment they truly deserve. Fresh-product boutiques, beauty bars, Internet companies with no warehousing that send out fresh products as you order them, and mom-and-pop companies that mix up fresh concoctions are becoming the rage.

MY CRITERION

Choosing products is easy for me because I set my pure, potent, and proven criterion long ago. People always ask me about specific brand names. I don't enchant myself with brands as a whole (companies get bought and everything changes) or fancy marketing because they're meaningless. Look at the ingredients list; that's what counts. Some companies have amazing integrity, but not all of their products might be right for you. Don't be afraid to use a serum from one company and a cleanser from another or to alternate and evolve your products with your skin's fluctuations. It's about you, not brand loyalty. Even the individual products I recommend are based on their specific ingredients list at the time I recommended them. Be sure to check it again when you purchase it and as you continue to restock your supply. Now that you have the facts, you can set your own standards and find products that deliver the purity and potency you desire.

Purity is the new decadence.

Finally, whether you're dealing with food or with beauty and body products, always demand full disclosure. It's the very least you can do for yourself, since any product you use will become a part of you.

CHAPTER 13
STRATEGIZE A WHOLE NEW SKIN APPROACH

An inside-out approach to preventing and dealing with possible causes for skin distress will have far more impact than external care alone. Broadening your understanding of the possible issues that connect your lifestyle with your skin can save you a lifetime of wasted energy and dollars on futile treatments and save your skin the perpetual ravages of regimen overkill. The work associated with high-maintenance skin regimens seems necessary but may be in vain if the true cause of the problem is not being addressed. Getting to the cause doesn't take work; it takes information, self-knowledge, and a passion for becoming your own connoisseur. When you have truly established a cause and strategized against the cause alone (while refraining from problem-causing quick fixes), you'll be on your way to a true resolution. Best of all, addressing that cause and correcting that imbalance will make the rest of you more radiant, too.

For example, if you discover that your thyroid isn't working properly, you open a door to possibly curing your dry skin—and your weight issue. If you suffer from dandruff and itchy skin and restore the pro-beauty, good-bacteria ecology in your gut, you might save yourself a lifetime of black-sweater avoidance, dandruff shampoos, skin eruptions, and a future of more serious, compounded health problems.

A dermatologist can help you properly diagnose your skin condition, but you may need to do some work on your own or with your doctor to identify the day-to-day personal habits, treatments, and triggers behind your skin issues. Always factor in what you're putting on or into your body, any medications

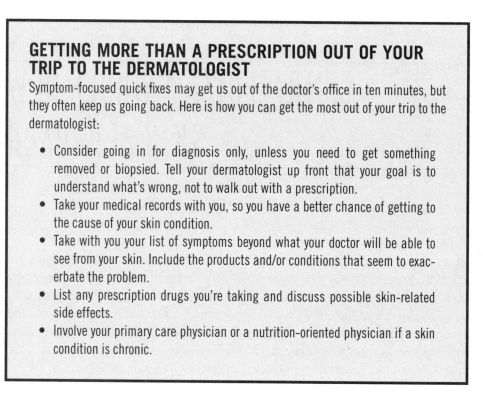

GETTING MORE THAN A PRESCRIPTION OUT OF YOUR TRIP TO THE DERMATOLOGIST

Symptom-focused quick fixes may get us out of the doctor's office in ten minutes, but they often keep us going back. Here is how you can get the most out of your trip to the dermatologist:

- Consider going in for diagnosis only, unless you need to get something removed or biopsied. Tell your dermatologist up front that your goal is to understand what's wrong, not to walk out with a prescription.
- Take your medical records with you, so you have a better chance of getting to the cause of your skin condition.
- Take with you your list of symptoms beyond what your doctor will be able to see from your skin. Include the products and/or conditions that seem to exacerbate the problem.
- List any prescription drugs you're taking and discuss possible skin-related side effects.
- Involve your primary care physician or a nutrition-oriented physician if a skin condition is chronic.

you are taking, and your emotional state. Regular health exams can help rule out or pinpoint any health issues that could affect your skin, like hormonal imbalances, autoimmune syndromes, systemic yeast, nutritional imbalances, hydration, sleep disturbances, environmental sensitivities, liver and thyroid function, stress, and prescription drug side effects.

Many chronic skin conditions can be improved and even reversed if these causes are addressed at the start rather than as a last resort, lest you pile on harsher regimens or drugs and complicate matters in an attempt to overcome issues that just can't be fixed at the surface. It's much harder to pinpoint the cause or even diagnose the real problem once it is compounded with treatments that compromise the skin's function and cause new imbalances.

The closer you are to achieving nutritional, hormonal, emotional, and digestive balance, the closer you are to healthy skin. Remember that all healthy skin is vulnerable to wild cards, like food additives, contact irritants, and prescription medications. If these issues are affecting your skin now, years of practicing the latest treatments and surface approaches won't help.

THE BRIEF HISTORY AND EXCITING FUTURE OF TRULY EFFECTIVE SKIN CARE

The detailed chart found at the end of this chapter looks at the big picture of your skin issues as they relate to possible health and lifestyle factors. But first, let's look at some new stars on the beauty scene that represent the future of skin care. These products and remedies are hot, not because they are new substances, but because they are backed by new proof for what is often ancient knowledge being relearned and technically applied by an intuition-challenged modern society.

Until the early 1990s, there was little offered by skin care technology but temporary surface-texture enhancement and protection from sun and dehydration. Vitamins and botanicals were used primarily as a marketing concept but not taken seriously by any self-respecting dermatologist. And consumers had grown desensitized to the glowing promises in skin care ads. But then came Retin A, alpha hydroxy acids, and the first science showing that vitamin C could stimulate collagen production when applied topically. From that point on, skin care—and the respect for the power of natural substances—would never be the same. Now it seems that each passing day brings a new peptide, growth factor, or extract proven to reverse past damage and change the current function of our skin simply by taking or applying it.

Special Delivery

The ongoing challenge in skin care has always been to effectively stabilize and deliver natural substances deep into the skin while retaining their potency. Between 2003 and 2006, liposomes, made from phospholipids (more on those in a moment), were the gold standard delivery system for active ingredients in effective skin care. In fact, they helped to usher in the popular term "cosmeceuticals" because of their unprecedented ability to deliver ingredients deep into the skin and effect function.

"Chiral" technology describes products formulated with the most bioactive form of a given nutrient molecule. Skin care companies that combine this technology with the best natural botanicals are at the forefront of "best-of-both-worlds" skin care. See Resources for several "Chirally correct" brands.

Nanotechnology's "Topical Injectibles": a Double-edged Sword

With the emergence of nanotechnologies applied to skin care in 2006, transdermal ingredient delivery has been taken to the "nth" degree—literally. Beyond liposomes, nanosomes (up to a million times smaller than typical liposomes), fullersomes (equally tiny substance-filled carbon "cages"), ovosomes, and the like, have arrived on the scene, and the industry, and perhaps our expectations, may never be the same.

Starting in 2006, the application of nanotechnologies took off, delivering particles so small they can enter the deep skin layers and even the cells, as no topical product ingredients have ever done before. In 2007, I attended a major beauty trade show here in New York City and was amazed to learn how nanotechnology can affect the delivery and efficacy of every topically applied preparation. Nanoparticles are so small, they can actually reach the deeper, dermal layer of the skin for the first time, sending substances like GABA (which relaxes muscles) so far into the skin that the mild, "faux-tox" effect that it has on muscles can actually be seen within minutes and last for hours. Literally, we're talking about effects that happen before your eyes from a topical product. The quantum improvements in efficacy of cellulite and hair loss preparations were equally astonishing. This is the biggest news in skin care technology in eons, but the technology also carries serious safety considerations, which many in the industry largely ignore. Delivering sometimes foreign or synthetic substances to locations and depths where they normally cannot go is a new capability that has raised some questions. Scientists specializing in nanotechnology admit that there are potential problems with substances having no way to leave the body, since these particles are smaller than atoms and literally penetrate cells. I spoke with a microbiologist at the conference who was concerned about this issue, as many formulators are. When he raised the question of what the particles of one particular product do after they bind to the receptors of the cells and if there might be any downside to that (like interfering with other functions of that receptor, or autoimmune concerns), the spokesperson giving the presentation gruffly replied "we just care that it gets there." Most of the formulators and researchers I spoke with agreed that until we know more about the actions of nanoparticles, we should avoid them or at the very least use only naturally formulated products. It's largely a matter of trust. We are simply very vulnerable to invasive nanotechnology. At a minimum, it must be very clearly labeled or even categorized as a drug. For more information about nanotechnology benefits and risks, visit the Center for Responsible Nanotechnology at http://www.crnano.org.

Here are the main categories of effective skin care ingredients and the science-backed stars of each.

Potent Antioxidants and Anti-Inflammatories

Zinc, green tea, milk thistle, curcumin, vitamin C, tocotrienols, alpha-lipoic acid, superoxide dismutase (SOD), CoQ10 (and idebinone, a synthetic variant of it), pycnogenol, and many other botanical extracts have all demonstrated both antioxidant and anti-inflammatory action in scientific studies. They scavenge the free radicals that lead to wrinkles and precancerous cell changes. Vitamin C has shown perhaps the most compelling proof as a collagen-building wrinkle-reverser. Green, black, and white teas have been found to inhibit inflammation and sun damage. Licorice and chamomile have demonstrated long-term anti-inflammatory action similar to topical steroids without the side effects. Even good old aloe is now gaining new respect for its powerful anti-inflammatory, healing, and mild collagen-building and antiseptic potential when delivered in highly potent, super-fresh formulas. It contains salicylic acid, which explains its painkilling effects when applied to sunburns.

Peptides and Other Age-Defyers

Beyond antioxidants, there's a new arsenal of potent wrinkle-reversers in this post-alpha hydroxy acid beauty world that can deliver true wrinkle reversal and stimulate collagen synthesis, skin regeneration, and other anti-aging effects without the irritation of acids, retinol products, or other peels. These include extracts of algae, soy, and yeasts; growth factors like EGF, kinetin, and TGF beta-1; peptides, like copper and marine peptides and oligopeptides, which can remodel the skin; and "faux-tox" alternatives for relaxing wrinkles, like Argireline and GABA. These substances have truly done what any self-respecting dermatologist thought was impossible not too long ago: change the functioning of the skin and reverse its aging process.

See the Resources section for products containing these ingredients. They are just the tip of the iceberg of what is to emerge over the next few years in the growing body of science-validated natural substances.

Phospholipids and Ceramides

Phospholipids and ceramides are important natural components of the skin's natural protective barrier, and when topically applied they can restore the skin's own membrane and literally become part of the skin, rebuilding its barrier function after exposure to detergents and solvents. Phospholipids also act as a humectant, while preventing water evaporation.

Cold-Pressed Oils and EFAs

According to Nicholas J. Smeh, MS, author of *Health Risks in Today's Cosmetics*, the EFA linoleic acid, present in many cold-pressed vegetable oils, walnuts, and seeds, was found to be one of the most valuable ingredients in cosmetics by German scientists, because it can help the skin retain moisture and at the same time inhibit acne. Most EFAs are anti-inflammatory. Other cold-pressed oils, such as antioxidant-rich rose hip and artic berry seed oils (including raspberry, cranberry, and sea buckthorn berry); sebumlike squalene (derived from olive oil); GLA-rich evening primrose and black currant seed oils; carrier oils, such as jojoba, sweet almond, and apricot kernel; and anti-inflammatory oils like St. John's Wort oil, are the most commonly used, truly therapeutic oils. Emu oil is worth singling out for its ability to penetrate and deliver substances deep into the skin. Heat and pressure compromise the great properties of these oils.

Essential Oils and Natural Antimicrobials

In addition to having extremely unique and powerful properties and the ability to penetrate through the skin into the bloodstream, virtually all essential oils (not to be confused with EFAs) have been shown to be antimicrobial to widely varying degrees. Unlike topical or internal antibiotics, none of these antimicrobials has been found to create antibiotic-resistant bacteria the way synthetic antimicrobials, such as trichlosan in antibacterial soaps, can. The properties of herbs and essential oils—including many biblically honored substances such as myrrh, cinnamon, and olive leaf—are proving their amazing applications in modern science. Neem, for example, is a unique oil that has been found to be antifungal and antimicrobial when applied topically or taken orally.

There are a number of other natural substances that have antibacterial benefits without the risks associated with commonly prescribed topical or oral antibiotics. Azelaic acid, for example, is a naturally occurring compound from certain grains with the antimicrobial and exfoliating properties of harsher acne treatments, only with negligible irritation or side effects. It is sometimes pre-scribed instead of topical antibiotics for acne and rosacea. It has also been proven effective in fading the dark patches of melasma, as it has an exfoliating and lightening effect. Both zinc and sulfur as supplements and topical ingredi-ents have been found to have antimicrobial action that is effective against inflamed acne.

Phototherapies

Concentrations of different light wavelengths can have amazing effects on the skin and can be viewed as another form of "nature in therapeutic doses." Also know as phototherapy, these laser, Intense Pulsed Light (IPL), Light Heat Energy (LHE), and other treatments are now successfully being used to treat sun dam-age and wrinkles, broken capillaries and redness, acne and pitted scars, and much more, often replacing harsher methods or drugs. If you have severe skin issues, such treatments make a great jump-start to your new skin and lifestyle approach but are never a replacement for regaining your health from the inside.

The following information on the ever-evolving applications of lasers, IPL, and LHE therapies, was contributed by spa consultant Gina Molinari and tech-nical consultant Thomas Paulino. Learn more at www.1800lasermd.com.

Lasers are considered the gold standard for "permanent hair reduction" (no legal claim can be made for permanent hair *removal*). They target and damage the area that causes hair growth. The wavelength of the laser used is determined by the pigmentation color and depth of the targeted skin or hair root. Longer wavelengths are safer for darker skin types due to less melanin absorption. A cautionary note: lasers in most cases cannot remove light, red, or grey hair, and the number of treatments vary per patient. Lasers can also be effective for leg veins (in combination with sclerotherapy for large ones) and tattoos.

The new generation in Erbium YAG lasers, 2940 nm (nanometer), also known as "The Whisper," is a favorite among skin professionals for pitted acne scarring, sun damage, and mild hyperpigmentation. One treatment is equivalent to 12 microdermabrasion sessions. Generally three to five treatments are recommended. Again, I recommend this as a way to reverse past damage as you start to incorporate a complete inside-out strategy to increase skin health and heal the cause of future skin problems.

Intense Pulsed Light (IPL) devices differ from lasers because they emit less concentrated, broadband, short pulses of light, reducing discomfort and damage substantially over lasers and are less expensive due to less costly equipment. Various filters are used for different effects and remove ultraviolet components that might damage the skin. Unfortunately, because most of the light energy is in the shorter wavelengths, treatment of darker skin types is less effective and more risky than with the appropriate laser.

Second generation IPL/LHE (Light Heat Energy) technology is often used to treat skin problems, such as sun damage-induced hyperpigmentation and vascular changes such as rosacea, psoriasis, broken capillaries, red spots, and pigmented birth marks, and it can kill acne-causing bacteria. This newer technology incorporates "dual mode filtering" and other advances which result in safer and more effective treatment than the older systems. Although each type of IPL/LHE equipment has its niche applications and specialties, in most cases their overall differences are negligible.

Additionally:
Deep penetrating light (DPL) therapies, such as far infrared, have been proven to reduce wrinkles, speed growth and healing of skin cells, and stimulate collagen as well.

Capacitive Radio frequency (CRF) technology, such as is used in the popular Thermage skin treatment, heats the skin's deeper layers to stimulate collagen production, which can tighten and improve tone and texture of skin, both immediately and increasingly, for several months following one treatment.

Other emerging technologies for skin rejuvenation include electrostimulation and focused ultrasound. Because treatment options are ever-expanding, always do some research before deciding on one of these treatments. The first home micro-phototherapy devices were recently cleared by the FDA, available through www.radiancy.com. But don't allow their surface results to distract you from how you treat yourself every day. Aim to glow on your own. The payoffs will far surpass any from the above treatments.

Color Cosmetics

Color cosmetics are the final frontier of nontoxic beauty products. For many years, my professional makeup kit was stocked with all kinds of synthetic concoctions that I used on photo shoots even though I was using natural makeup products on myself. While my pure moisturizers and masks usually went over big with models and celebrities, I couldn't have gotten away with using the aesthetically challenged offerings of mineral color cosmetics available then. Knowing the safety and sensitivity concerns of coal tar colors, the irritating nature of perfumes, the dangers of talc inhalation, and the pore-clogging tendencies of mineral oil, I was frustrated with the lack of sophistication and appeal when it came to natural-color cosmetics. But now I'm excited to report that the availability of high-end textures, colors, and even packaging for truly pure cosmetics has improved dramatically in recent years. Even the colors of the mineral-based foundations are now available in the wide range of global, gold-tinged shades that makeup artists seek. There are now beautiful, highly saturated, and finely textured eyeshadows, ultra-hip glosses, and smudgy pencils in must-have colors, minus the petrochemicals, perfumes, preservatives, and coal tar dyes. You can finally bring both your aesthetic desires and your desire for purity together when it comes to makeup.

Mineral Cosmetics Can Calm Irritated and Post-Treatment Skin

For those with rosacea, or allergy-prone, laser-treated, or otherwise challenged skin, or those who simply want to minimize the possible sensitizing factors and inherent toxic risks of conventional color cosmetics, micronized mineral cosmetics are the best answer. Powdered mineral foundations, blushes, and eye shadows, which are colored primarily by iron oxides, actually calm irritation, due to their anti-inflammatory properties. Because they don't contain synthetic dyes, even the lip pencils and blushes can be used in the eye area. Mineral makeup is recommended by dermatologists and plastic surgeons for use after a peel and as the first makeup usable after laser treatment. They provide broad-spectrum UVA and UVB sun protection (usually an FDA-approved SPF 17–20), which can spare sensitive facial skin the added burden and step of applying common sunscreen products. They are also water resistant but not pore-clogging. The microscopic crystals overlap, allowing the skin to breathe, but they don't crease or accentuate wrinkles as talc-based powders do. Because of the level of coverage, the loose and pressed formulas stand in for liquid foundation and powder, actually covering and calming redness all at once, without the buildup or cakiness of creme-to-powder foundations. See the Resources section for some of my favorites.

AN INSIDE OUT VIEW OF YOUR SKIN ISSUES AND SOLUTIONS

Consider the following chart an A–Z symposium of collected science and varied expert opinion on specific skin issues, from conventional to alternative and from medical to nutritional to practical. It includes what is often recommended, overlooked, proven, and observed by doctors, researchers, and experts in specific areas of concern with regard to common skin issues. From this bird's-eye perspective you can create the wisest inside-out approach.

Most of the products in the chart are available at natural-product stores. Ordering information for hard-to-find products is listed in Resources.

Note: This chart—as is all of the information in this book—is for educational purposes only. Always seek the guidance of your doctor when treating any ailment or condition. As with any therapy, use extra caution if you are pregnant.

YOUR SKIN STRATEGY MAKEOVER

Beauty-Risking Choice	Beauty-Supporting Choice	Holistic Considerations
ACNE (See also Oily Skin)		
Benzoyl peroxide: Drying and peeling regimens like benzoyl peroxide and vitamin A derivatives can destroy the beauty of the skin and compromise its protective and antiaging matrix. **Tetracycline:** Prescribed for moderate acne, this drug can cause photosensitivity, chronic yeast overgrowth, and digestive problems. **Accutane:** The drug of choice for severe acne can cause dryness of the skin, nose, mouth, lips, and vagina; itching and peeling of the palms and soles; and high cholesterol. Less common side effects include thinning hair, decreased libido, body aches, and liver damage. **Trichlosan-containing antibacterial soaps** have been found to form chloroform, a carcinogen, when mixed with chlorinated water (as in tap water).	**Phospholipids** help restore the acid balance that fights bacteria in the skin. **Azelaic Acid,** a natural compound sometimes prescribed (as Azelex) instead of topical antibiotics, has been shown to have effects comparable to topical benzoyl peroxide gel 5%, tretinoin cream 0.05%, erythromycin cream 2%, and oral tetracycline 0.5 to 1 g/day in treating mild to moderate inflammatory acne. **Tea tree oil** has an effect similar to benzoyl peroxide 5% without making the skin flaky. Tea tree oil and salicylic acid "zit sticks" are a good option for mild acne. **Essential oils** can purify and normalize skin oil. **Neem oil** is antimicrobial and antifungal. **Neroli oil** is purifying and normalizes oil production.	**Excess oil, skin-cell buildup, bacteria, and inflammation** are the issues here. Excess oil production is often hormonally induced. **High-dose pantothenic acid (B5) along with a 20 percent B5 cream or timed-release pantothenic acid** supplements on their own dramatically cleared acne in two studies. **Berberine** (from barberry) supplements inhibit the growth of the bacteria and reduced sebum production. **A combination of ayurvedic herbs,** such as guggul, turmeric, and neem, taken internally improves acne significantly. Low levels of **vitamins A, E, and the mineral zinc** have been linked with acne. **Cold-water fish, fish oil, or evening primrose** supplements have hormone-balancing and anti-inflammatory effects. **Zinc gluconate supplements** worked comparably to the antibiotic minocycline hydro-chloride against acne in one study.

Beauty-Risking Choice	Beauty-Supporting Choice	Holistic Considerations
ACNE (continued)		
	MSM, available in topical products or supplements, is a better-utilized form of sulfur that inhibits bacteria and promotes healing.

Alpha-lipoic acid topicals can help normalize oil production and shrink pore size, according to Dr. Perricone.

Phototherapy: Recent studies in the U.K. suggest isolated **red- and blue-light wavelengths** can help mild to moderate acne by killing bacteria and reducing inflammation.

The Zeno acne clearing device cleared most mild to moderate pimples in twenty-four hours in one study.

A **4 percent topical niacin product** applied twice daily significantly cleared acne in two months in one study.

See also "Phototherapies" on page 251 for dealing with acne scars. | **Contact reactions** to skin and hair products, phones, and fabrics and many **prescription drugs,** such as steroid inhalers, can contribute to acne.

Food allergies, iodine-containing foods, and **poor digestion or imbalance of intestinal flora** can contribute to acne. **Digestive enzymes** and the **probiotic** measures outlined on page 196 can increase the skin's resistance to bacteria and improve digestive issues that might otherwise aggravate acne.

Hydration is a basic defense against acne, so drink plenty of pure water.

Detox measures, such as green juices, chlorella, milk thistle, turmeric, green tea, red clover, and plant sterolins help the liver and reduce the detox burden on the skin.

The low-fiber, high-sugar, and trans fatty Western diet may be to blame for some acne. In one study, **high fiber intake** reduced inflammatory skin lesions. **Elevated levels of the androgen hormone DHT**—or sensitivity to it—are linked to some forms of treatment-resistant acne, according to the New Zealand Dermatological Society. Saw palmetto berry extract is known to block DHT. **GLA** supplements may also help. |

Beauty-Risking Choice	Beauty-Supporting Choice	Holistic Considerations
CELLULITE		
Caffeine and related chemicals, like theophylline, have limited proof and potential risk if delivered into the bloodstream via transdermal products. **Nanotechnology-based topicals** may offer the first effective topical reductions in cellulite. Use these invasive products at your own risk. **Mesotherapy** is a popular, yet controversial, procedure involving injections of various cocktails of vitamins, minerals, amino acids, and sometimes pharmaceuticals into the mesoderm (middle layers of the skin) to dissolve fat. It targets fat cells and cellulite in a way that liposuction cannot and without invasive surgery. The wild cards are that some of the substances injected may cause an allergic reaction (always do an allergy test) and some practitioners may not be experienced. Do a lot of research if you consider this therapy.	**Topically applied, concentrated seaweed extract products** can deliver minerals through the skin, helping with tissue ionization, lymph drainage, and circulation—the primary factors in cellulite. Consider any treatment or at-home routine that can improve circulation to areas with cellulite, such as **dry brush massage.** A study conducted at Vanderbilt University in Tennessee showed that fourteen to twenty treatments of **Endermologie** (a suction/massage device) caused a dramatic increase in collagen and skin smoothness.	Cellulite is exacerbated by **sluggish lymph drainage** and **circulation, inflammation,** and **hormonal imbalance.** A low-impact, organic food diet can reduce inflammation and exposure to toxins that might accumulate in the body and give you weight loss that may reduce cellulite. **Nutritional supplements** that balance hormones and reduce inflammation, such as chaste tree berry, DHEA, and blood sugar formulas and fish oil, may help.

Beauty-Risking Choice	Beauty-Supporting Choice	Holistic Considerations
DANDRUFF		
Resorcinol found in dandruff shampoos can cause discoloration and dermatitis. **Coal tar-containing shampoos** can irritate the scalp and may be toxic.	**Pyrithione Zinc** (available in shampoos) alleviated dandruff in a recent study. **Tea tree oil**-containing hair cleansers, free of SLS, can provide antifungal action without irritation. **Antifungal, antimicrobial substances** like oregano oil, grapefruit seed extract (GSE), and tea tree oil added to scalp preparations in small amounts may help. **Apple cider vinegar** normalizes scalp pH, which can help inhibit bacteria and fungus.	First rule out the simplest cause of flakes and irritation, which might be your **hair products**. See what happens if you change them. **Dry scalp** flakes may accompany dry skin and fungal or inflammatory skin and body conditions (see "Inflammatory Skin Problems" for dietary considerations). **GLA** supplements may help dry scalp and inflammation.
DARK SPOTS OR PATCHES		
Skin lighteners containing hydroquinone can cause skin discoloration and allergic reactions. Hydroquinone is made from crystalline phenol, a suspected carcinogen. **Lasers** do not perform well on melasma discolorations, according to Dr. Deborah Jaliman, a New York City dermatologist.	**Azelaic acid** is an effective and safer bleaching agent. Some data suggest that topical azelaic acid, used twice daily with a broad-spectrum sunscreen, works as well as hydroquinone 4% creams. **Kojic acid** and **arbutin** inhibit melanin. **Vitamin C**, **licorice**, and **bioflavanoids** can lighten the skin somewhat.	**Hormonal changes**, such as those associated with pregnancy or use of birth control pills, often contribute to dark spots and patches or melasma—the "mask of pregnancy." This can only be avoided by vigilantly **protecting your skin from sun exposure**. Use mineral-based sunscreens for maximum, safe protection.

Beauty-Risking Choice	Beauty-Supporting Choice	Holistic Considerations
DARK SPOTS OR PATCHES (*continued*)		
Steroid ointments are sometimes used on vitiligo. Not only are they ineffective, but they thin and compromise the immunity of the skin.	**Skin Answer** contains glycoalkaloids, which actually exfoliate raised, rough spots and patches of sun-damaged skin in four to six weeks. See also "Phototherapies" on page 251.	**Mineral makeup** gives sun protection, anti-inflammatory benefits, and aesthetic cover-age without irritation. **Antioxidants** taken internally and applied to the skin can offer added protection from sun. **Age spots faded and were prevented by both glucosamine** (often taken for arthritis) and a natural collagen drink called Toki. **Vitiligo** was markedly improved or completely reversed in almost half those who took **ginkgo biloba** in one study. **L-phenylalanine** supplements gave significant improvement (even more with UVA radiation). Vitiligo was linked with **deficiencies in copper.**
DRY LIPS		
Phenol-containing mineral oil or petrolatum-based lip balms cause skin irritation, dryness, and "lip balm addiction."	**Skin-compatible oils and lip balms** containing ingredients like shea butter, cocoa butter, coconut oil, beeswax, calendula, aloe, allantoin (comfrey root), and vitamins C and E all truly hydrate, heal, and protect the lips, not just seal them. **Oligopeptide-containing lip plumpers** can increase hydration up to 60 percent, and lip volume up to 40 percent with a month's use.	**Avoid contact with water** in the colder months. Try applying lip balm before you brush your teeth if your lips are chapped. **Avoid irritating and drying products** such as alcohol-containing mouthwashes and SLS-containing toothpastes.

Beauty-Risking Choice	Beauty-Supporting Choice	Holistic Considerations

DRY SKIN

Beauty-Risking Choice	Beauty-Supporting Choice	Holistic Considerations
Foaming and detergent cleansers, soaps, and bubble baths make dry skin worse. Dermatologist-recommended **propylene glycol–based cleansers** can still irritate and dry the skin. **Mineral oil and petrolatum-based** body moisturizers, body oil, baby oil, bath oil, and lip balms can actually leave the skin and lips dryer.	**Cleansing milks and nonstripping cleansers** free of irritants like propylene glycol and detergents help your skin recover its own protection. **Phospholipids** and **GLA-containing moisturizers and supplements** can rebuild the lipid barrier that prevents dry, rough skin. **Skin-compatible oils** such as jojoba, sweet almond oil, apricot kernel oil, primrose oil, avocado, azulene, squalane, emu oil, neem, olive oil, hemp oil, and sesame oil contain fatty acids that work in concert with sebum rather than against it or blocking it, like mineral oil.	A **humidifier** will help alleviate dryness. Increased **water intake** and decreased caffeine and alcohol intake can help. Dry skin, along with brittle hair, sparse eyebrows, or sensitivity to cold, are common symptoms of **thyroid issues**. **Chlorinated water** can contribute to dry skin. **Installing a shower filter** can make an unbelievable difference. **Injuv** is a supplement that may increase the level of hyaluronic acid in the body. Hyaluronic acid acts as a sponge, holding moisture within the skin.

Beauty-Risking Choice	Beauty-Supporting Choice	Holistic Considerations
INFLAMMATORY SKIN PROBLEMS (See also Sensitive Skin, Dry Skin, and Dandruff)		
Steroid ointments used over prolonged periods thin the skin and compromise its basic immunity, making recurrences more likely and often worse.	**Pyrithione Zinc** 0.2% sprays, lotions, and shampoos have shown remarkable efficacy for clearing up psoriasis.	**There are countless causes for dermatitis.** Rule out contact allergens first. For the best possible outcome, pay close attention to what triggers your symptoms.
Coal tar preparations can cause sun sensitivity and irritation.	**Long-term use of both licorice** (Glycyrrhiza glabra) and **German Camillosan chamomile** have been shown to be comparable in effect to long-term topical hydrocortisone treatments in inflammatory skin conditions.	**Allergies, food sensitivities, and digestive problems** are strongly linked with certain types of eczema and psoriasis. Test for food sensitivities or try an elimination diet.
Heavy petrolatum or mineral oil-based creams can ultimately inhibit the skin's healing function.	**Healing botanicals** like **aloe and allantoin** (comfrey) can speed healing.	**Compromised protein digestion and auto-immune flare-ups** may be linked with psoriasis, according to Michael T. Murray, ND, author of *Natural Alternatives to Over-the-Counter and Prescription Drugs.*
Psoriasis treatments like UVB and narrow-band UVB work on psoriasis but can raise issues of sun damage and skin cancer.	**Capsaicin** (hot pepper) cream reduced psoriasis scaling and redness significantly when using capsaicin .025 cream four times a day for six weeks.	
PUVA, which involves the use of Psoralens, a photo-sensitizing drug, plus UVA light exposure, has been found to be more effective than UVB but carries skin cancer risks.	**Climatotherapy for psoriasis** is a treatment given only at the Dead Sea clinics in Israel that includes liberal sunlight exposure and bathing in the Dead Sea. In one study, it produced a clearing of 80 to 100 percent in 88 percent of over 1,000 patients treated.	**Increased fiber intake** and **decreased sugar intake** (the antifungal diet) decreased seborrheic eczema in one study.
	High-dose topical becocalciorol (D3 analog ointment) cleared or almost cleared moderate psoriasis in a quarter of patients after eight weeks in one study.	The **probiotic** measures on page 196 may help reduce the digestive and inflammatory issues that can lead to some types of eczema and psoriasis flare-ups.

Beauty-Risking Choice	Beauty-Supporting Choice	Holistic Considerations
INFLAMMATORY SKIN PROBLEMS (*continued*)		
	Mahonia aquifolium or **Oregon grape root** improved psoriasis symptoms in sufferers over twelve weeks in a large-scale German study and has also been shown to work on eczema.	**GLA** from borage and evening primrose oil, and **EPA from fish** have been found to help inflammatory skin disorders. Four to ten grams per day were used in most studies.
	Low pH water has antimicrobial properties and may benefit inflammatory skin conditions. A small device called Charme™ delivers fresh, low pH water without the large machinery previously required.	**Anti-inflammatory supplements**, like MSM, nettle, milk thistle, green tea, and turmeric may help.
	Poison ivy, oak, or sumac rashes were prevented from breaking out or spreading with **topical preparations containing jewelweed,** a plant that grows alongside it.	**In psoriasis, esterfied fumeric acid** (should be taken under a doctor's supervision) was found in many studies to effectively reduce symptoms. **Deficiencies in vitamins A, B (including folic acid), D, and E as well as zinc** are common in psoriasis sufferers.
OILY SKIN		
Soaps and other foaming or detergent cleansers and alcohol-based astringents and products that leave the skin tight cause oily rebound and strip the skin's acid mantle protection.	**Essential oil blends** and moisturizers that include neem, ylang ylang, neroli, and lavender can purify the skin and normalize oil production.	If you have oily skin you will have fewer wrinkles as you age.
		See also **EFAs, pantothenic acid,** and **alpha-lipoic acid** under "Acne."
		GLA supplements were found to reduce enzymes that promote oily skin.

Beauty-Risking Choice	Beauty-Supporting Choice	Holistic Considerations
ROSACEA AND BROKEN CAPILLARIES (See also Inflammatory Skin Problems)		
The characteristic redness, broken capillaries, and sometimes acne associated with rosacea is commonly treated with **topical antibiotics,** which can destroy the skin's natural defenses. See **Accutane** cautions under "Acne." **Steroids** can actually cause rosacea and broken capillaries by thinning the skin and weakening capillary walls. **Conventional cosmetics** used to cover rosacea can irritate the condition by causing photosensitivity and acne. Avoid any skin products containing **solvents, alcohol, abrasives,** or **exfoliants.** Eliminate common irritants, such as perfume (see "Sensitive Skin").	**Azelaic Acid** is sometimes used or prescribed (as Azelex) instead of topical antibiotics but does not cause resistant bacteria to develop. **Vitamin K** and horse chestnut creams may strengthen weakened capillaries. **Demodicidin** is a soap that may kill both the Folliculorum and Brevis types of Demodex human associated with acne rosacea. **Strontium-containing products** have been shown to reduce sensitivity to skin products. **Blue-light therapy** may help acne rosacea. **Mineral cosmetics** achieve good coverage and sun protection while avoiding the irritation of synthetic color cosmetics and sunscreens. They also reduce inflammation. See also "Phototherapies" on page 251.	With rosacea, it's largely about **avoiding the triggers,** such as **alcohol, hot drinks,** and **spicy foods.** In *Natural Alternatives to Over-the-Counter and Prescription Drugs,* Michael T. Murray, ND, points to **hydrochloric acid (HCL) deficiency** as a possible culprit in some cases of rosacea. Early science supports this. According to Arlen Brownstein, MS, ND, and Donna Schoemaker, CN, authors of *Rosacea: Your Self-Help Guide,* **drinking liquids with meals** can dilute digestive enzymes that break down protein. **Leaky gut,** a condition in which lack of good bacteria causes increased intestinal-wall permeability, may worsen inflammatory skin issues (see also "Acne" and "Inflammatory Skin Problems" and consider the probiotic measures on page 196). **Rosacea** was significantly improved with a month of **zinc sulfate supplementation.** **Flavonoids,** found in grape seed, cocoa, citrus, and green tea strengthen fragile capillaries.

Beauty-Risking Choice	Beauty-Supporting Choice	Holistic Considerations
SCARS		
Certain lasers and IPL therapies may help but can also cause further scarring, particularly for people with medium and dark skin tones and may require downtime. Some treatments may take more than five months.	**Topical silicone gels** can reduce and flatten some raised scars over months of use. Works best with new scars. According to Dr. Perricone, **alpha-lipoic acid** can prevent and reverse scar formation. See also "Phototherapies" on page 251.	**Sunlight** on traumatized skin or even a healing pimple can leave a dark spot, particularly during hormonal fluctuations, so keep sunlight off any skin blemish. **Keeping a wound clean** is important. Picking at skin or scabs can cause scarring.
SENSITIVE SKIN (See also Inflammatory Skin Problems)		
Harsh skin products that contain solvents, fragrances, detergents, and high levels of preservatives sensitize the skin. **Foaming bath products, fragranced laundry detergent,** and **fabric softeners** can also sensitize and irritate the skin. **AHAs** and other **irritating exfoliants** can sensitize the skin by compromising its natural barrier to irritants. **Conventional color cosmetics** contain known irritants, like coal tar dyes and perfumes.	**Naturally scented and formulated products** with preservatives listed last on the ingredients list or not at all may cause less irritation. **Phospholipid**-containing moisturizers can help restore the barrier that keeps irritants from penetrating the skin. **Strontium**-containing skin products can inhibit the sensitization from cosmetic ingredients and related dermatitis. **Use mineral-based color cosmetics** and cosmetics free of perfumes, petrochemicals, and preservatives.	**Cosmetic** and **contact irritants** can sensitize and irritate the skin. **Perfume** and **nail-polish ingredients** like formaldehyde and toluene are strong sensitizers. **Formaldehyde** can also be on new clothes, sheets, or towels and can set off a reaction that can leave you sensitized for weeks. **Nickel** in fashion jewelry, car key chains, eyeglasses, and zippers can sensitize skin and cause rashes.

Beauty-Risking Choice	Beauty-Supporting Choice	Holistic Considerations
Dr. Jaliman often observes skin reactions from **nail polish**, **nail adhesives**, **hair color**, **mascara**, and eye drops containing the preservative **thimerosol**. **Soaps**, **shampoos**, **contact lens solutions** and **eye makeup removers** containing the preservative **Cat-B** can all cause redness and skin flakes.	**Kinetin (or Kinerase)** is a plant-derived substance that has been shown in some studies to effectively diminish wrinkles without irritation. **Colloidal oatmeal** and **Dead Sea salts** in the bath can bring substantial relief of irritation.	**An imbalance in body ecology** can make the skin more reactive. See "Pro-Beauty Pro-biotics" on page 195 for measures that may help. **Prescription drugs** can sensitize the skin.

VARICOSE AND SPIDER VEINS

Beauty-Risking Choice	Beauty-Supporting Choice	Holistic Considerations
Compression hose therapy for varicose veins is uncomfortable, hygienically unsmart, and doesn't address the real cause and dangers of varicose veins. **Laser procedures** can work, but they tend to be expensive and results are temporary, leaving the health issue unresolved. **Stripping of veins** has a failure rate of 30–80 percent, according to Jeffrey Miller, MD, a Detroit area vein treatment specialist.	"Large veins can be treated with **endovenous laser and microphlebectomy** with excellent cosmetic result," says Dr. Miller. "**Sclerotherapy** remains the gold standard treatment for spider veins," says Dr. Bipin Solanki, MD, FRCS, who specializes in vein procedures in New York City. "External laser has a limited role in treating spider veins in certain types of skin."	**Pycnogenol** from maritime pine bark decreased ankle swelling and varicose vein symptoms better than the drug Daflon in one study. Topical and internal pycnogenol therapies significantly speeded healing of vein ulcers in one study. **Pregnancy, sitting cross-legged**, and **constipation** are believed to contribute to varicose veins. Keeping legs elevated when possible (especially while sleeping) helps reduce swelling. Cultures with **diets low in refined foods** rarely suffer from varicose veins.

Beauty-Risking Choice	Beauty-Supporting Choice	Holistic Considerations

VARICOSE AND SPIDER VEINS (continued)

Beauty-Risking Choice	Beauty-Supporting Choice	Holistic Considerations
Spider vein treatments such as sclerotherapy will require regular tune-ups, as they often return. Spider veins are fed by reticular veins, so your physician must treat those as well, which is why some less-educated technicians will not give you satisfactory results, according to Dr. Miller.	**Address vein problems as health issues:** If you use laser, sclerotherapy, or stripping techniques, use them as a jump-start, but take steps to address the cause of the veins, which may signal trouble throughout the body. Horse chestnut seed extract, for example, strengthens the vasculature throughout the body rather than offering only a cosmetic effect. Food and beverage upgrades, supplements, and exercise may help you diminish or avoid a recurrence of the veins.	**Horse chestnut seed extract** has been shown to be comparable to compression hose therapy in decreasing ankle circumference and reducing the swelling of varicose veins in women with chronic venous insufficiency. Other natural varicose vein remedies, such as the bioflavanoid rutin, work, but horse chestnut seed extract was shown to be five hundred times more effective. **Vitamin K** is a proven coagulant that minimizes bruising and is widely used by dermatologists to minimize and strengthen broken capillaries.

WRINKLES

Beauty-Risking Choice	Beauty-Supporting Choice	Holistic Considerations
See "Dry Skin" for skin products to avoid. **Alpha hydroxy acids (AHAs):** Long-term alpha and beta hydroxy and glycolic acid use or abuse can make skin irritated, dry, tight, thin, and raw or dull. It also causes makeup to look blotchy.	**Phospholipids** can rebuild the hydrolipid barrier and prevent premature aging of the skin. Studies have proven that high-potency topically applied **vitamin C serums** can rebuild collagen.	**Smoking,** too much **sun** and **sugar**, compromised **skin barrier** due to harsh products, **fat,** or **EFA deficiency** in the diet all contribute to wrinkles. **Wrinkle alert:** If you smoke, you are two to three times more likely to have moderate to severe wrinkles at age forty or older than a nonsmoker.

Beauty-Risking Choice	Beauty-Supporting Choice	Holistic Considerations
WRINKLES (*continued*)		
Long-term effects of AHAs, BHAs, regular lasering and peels, and any other types of perpetual irritation and accelerated exfoliation are unknown. **Retin A or Renova:** Prescribed for their wrinkle- and acne-reducing peeling action that increases cell turnover, these synthetic vitamin A derivatives can be extremely irritating and leave the skin red and flaky. They also leave the skin intensely vulnerable to the sun, water loss, and offending substances that are more likely to be absorbed by the skin after treatment. **DMAE,** which can reduce sagging and visibly rejuvenate the skin, caused cultured human and rabbit cells to lose normal functions, such as division and secretions, and even caused some to die after twenty-four hours. More research is needed to assure its long-term safety in skin care.	According to Dr. Perricone, the **C-ester form of vitamin C** works without the irritation caused by the L-ascorbic acid form of vitamin C. See **Kinetin** under "Sensitive Skin." Several **peptides** have shown ability to reduce wrinkles. **Soy extracts** have been shown to have rejuvenating effects on mature skin. Topically-applied **"faux-tox" products** featuring ingredients such as **GABA and hexapeptide 3 (Argireline)** can relax deep facial furrows with continued use. **Gotu kola** has powerful skin-regenerative properties. **Seaweed extracts** can ionize and regenerate skin cells and stimulate collagen production. See also "Phototherapies" on page 251.	**GLA** supplements help to rebuild the skin's barrier from moisture evaporation and help prevent premature skin aging due to water loss. **Consuming high-glycemic foods and beverages** induces glycation and collagen cross-linking that causes wrinkles. In addition to my eating approach, **alpha-lipoic acid** and **carnosine** inhibit glycation. Topicals containing these nutrients may also offer some protection. **Wrinkle-fighting antioxidants** include: vitamins C, E (and tocotrienols), A, beta-carotene, melatonin, pycnogenol, superoxide dismutase (SOD), CoQ10 and green tea and grape seed extracts.

Beauty-Risking Choice	Beauty-Supporting Choice	Holistic Considerations

WRINKLES (*continued*)

Nanotechnologies applied to wrinkle-reducing products can give unprecedented results but are literally invasive. The safety of delivering substances into cells and cell receptors has yet to be determined, and, as of 2007, the tools for studying this have not even been developed. Consider carefully and use at your own risk.		**The supplements Biosil, by Jarrow Formulas,** as well as **Toki, by Lane Labs,** have both been proven to boost collagen levels in complementary ways with many other body-wide benefits. **Carotenoids** such as lutein, zeaxanthin, astaxanthin and lycopene, as well as flavonoids, such as those in green tea, pomegranate, and cocoa, offer added protection against wrinkling and photo-aging.

ANATOMY OF A HOLISTIC BEAUTY SPLURGE

Take a busy woman with dry skin and $125 or so to spend on her seasonal beauty splurge. Before reading this book, she might have bought the latest department-store skin regimen, with "token" botanicals or patented ingredients in a base of cheap carriers and known irritants. Now, with the same $125, she could start with a $30 vitamin C serum, buy a shower filter for $35, upgrade her current body soap to one of pure olive oil for $2, buy some fish-oil and hyaluronic acid capsules, and some health food store baby wipes to use on her face instead of a foaming cleanser. With this new regimen she may very well eliminate her dry, itchy skin and her need for heavy lotions and creams completely while improving her overall health in ways that will continue to unfold in the months and even years to come. She is now light-years beyond what any fancy dry-skin regimen will ever deliver. The degree to which our beauty splurges can truly transform us is limited only by our knowledge of the options.

WHAT REMAINS BETWEEN YOU AND YOUR BEST GLOW

Now that you've begun to consider the deeper issues behind your skin challenges, you have new clues to direct your own process of shedding and to cultivate your best glow. In the following chapters, you'll learn how to weed out and shed even more chemical and emotional wild cards that stand between you and your most radiant potential.

CHAPTER 14

YOUR BATHROOM CABINET MAKEOVER

Day-to-day discomforts quickly fixed with products that address only your symptoms will continue to impose new burdens on the body and drain the energy that could otherwise be making life—and you—beautiful. Planning and implementing your own bathroom cabinet makeover to maximize and expand your rewards while minimizing the risks are an exciting way to engage your self-respect and self-preservation instincts.

Once known only to holistic connoisseurs who did their homework, these now-proven alternatives can spare you untold assaults. As in every area of pro-beauty upgrades, each prevented assault will be beauty in the bank.

Although I've chosen to address only a small sampling of common products and safe, science-backed alternatives that you and your doctor can incorporate, I heartily encourage you to apply the same discerning principles to evaluate every single product on your shelves: read what your products contain, what side effects they may have (remember that long-term side effects aren't always listed on labels), and consider any alternatives that may serve you better.

These products can get you away
from quick fixes and don't
cause side effects.

YOUR BATHROOM CABINET MAKEOVER

Beauty-Risking Choice	Beauty-Supporting Choice	Holistic Considerations
ALLERGY AND SINUS PRODUCTS		
Most prescription **antihistamines** can cause dry mouth, dry nose, headache, and sleep problems. Most **nasal sprays** can cause swelling of nasal tissue. In addition, they are not safe for those with high blood pressure. Long-term side effects of **steroid drugs and inhalers** range from the unsightly to serious, including bone loss, "moon face," blood sugar imbalances, dowager's hump, bloated abdomen, and acne (particularly around the chin). Immunity is also compromised, leaving you more open to infections. Always consult your physician before discontinuing any kind of steroid, allergy, or asthma medication. That said, you may consider it worthwhile to look into ways to reduce your need for these kinds of medications.	**Nasalcrom, a homeopathic nasal spray,** contains cromolyn sodium, proven to both prevent and reduce nasal allergy symptoms with no side effects. **The xylitol-containing nasal spray called Xlear** has been shown to inhibit bacteria, including the bacteria that can cause ear infections, by an anti-adherence action thought to be similar to how cranberry works in the urinary tract. **Zinc-based nasal gel (Zicam)** has been proven to stop sinus infections in their tracks and reduce the duration of the common cold without side effects.	Just as **fish oil** reduces some allergic skin conditions, it also reduces allergies and asthma symptoms. Other **anti-inflammatory supplements** that help both nasal and skin allergies are stinging nettle, vitamin C, magnesium, and the bioflavanoid quercitin, which is a natural histamine suppressor. **Douching nasal passages** with salt water from your hands or a porcelain nasal cup can curtail sinus infections (if you can stand the process of snorting water through one nostril!). **Saline nasal sprays** work in a similar way without the hassle. A holistic health practitioner can help you identify **food sensitivities** and incorporate **supplements,** which may reduce **digestive issues** that can affect your allergies.

Beauty-Risking Choice	Beauty-Supporting Choice	Holistic Considerations

ANTIPERSPIRANTS AND DEODORANTS

Aluminum chlorohydrate: The man-made form of aluminum, which is contained in antiperspirants, is suspected by many scientists of accumulating in tissues, particularly when applied to broken skin. **Conventional deodorants that do not contain aluminum** tend to be highly perfumed and contain petrochemicals. Given what we are starting to learn about the accumulation of chemicals in the body, applying them over broken skin may not be a great idea.	**Natural deodorants containing antimicrobial ingredients** like tea tree oil, coriander, and GSE are getting more effective. Trial and error is the best way to find what works with your chemistry. **Lavilin** is one of the strongest natural deodorants. Caveat: it's expensive.	**Internal deodorants** containing body deodorizers like chlorophyll and activated charcoal have hit the market. All sorts of factors are responsible for our scent, so these products may or may not work for you. Detoxifying and keeping your pipes clean with **fiber, greens,** my **Beauty Detox Elixir** (see chapter 4), **liver-supportive** and **probiotic supplements,** and lots of water is the best way to usher out waste that could otherwise putrefy in the digestive tract and even affect your breath.

COLD-SORE PRODUCTS

Valtrex, Zovirax, and **Famvir** take several days to work and often fail, especially on acyclovir (Zovirax)-resistant strains of the herpes virus. **Prescription antiviral pills** may cause headache, nausea, and diarrhea.	**ViraMedx®** is the first topical treatment proven to stop the virus that causes herpes and give substantial and consistent healing in about twenty-four hours (other treatments take five to ten days). It is less expensive, and because of the nature of its mechanism of action, is effective on acyclovir-resistant strains of herpes and less likely to cause them to mutate into drug-resistant strains.	**Sun, stress,** and **illness** can bring on cold sore outbreaks, so do all you can to support your immunity and protect yourself. The amino acid **L-arginine** from any source, including nuts, can aggravate herpes, while the amino acid **L-lysine** may help prevent outbreaks.

Beauty-Risking Choice	Beauty-Supporting Choice	Holistic Considerations
COLD-SORE PRODUCTS (*continued*)		
	Tea tree oil treated cold sores comparably to acyclovir 5% in one randomized, placebo-controlled pilot study.	**Green and black tea**, even in moderate amounts, has been shown to deactivate E. coli and herpes simplex types I and II virus in the mouth. **Diamond Herpanacine** and **Herpilyn** are both supplements that inhibit herpes outbreaks.
HAIR-LOSS PRODUCTS		
Minoxidil (Rogaine): Common side effects are mainly scalp irritation or itching, though researchers at the University of Toronto found that long-term use can lead to heart changes. **Propecia (finasteride)** can throw off PSA-test results, cause loss of libido or erectile dysfunction in some men, and cannot be taken by women because of concerns over possible birth defects.	Natural **DHT-blocking hair-loss preparations** have actions similar to Propecia without the side effects. **Hair Genesis**, a nondrug formula containing the DHL-blocker saw palmetto berry and plant sterols, was shown in a recent double-blind, placebo-controlled study to be a viable, safer alternative to prescription hair-loss drugs.	**Sluggish thyroid function, trauma, surgery, stress, auto immune issues,** and **heredity** all contribute to hair loss. **Key nutrients** for healthier hair: **MSM** (sulfur), **silica, EFAs, vitamin B** (biotin, pantathenic acid, and inositol). **L-arginine's** ability to boost nitric oxide, which relaxes and dilates the hair follicle. A natural hair-loss supplement called **Viviscal** has shown significant clinical effectiveness against several types of hair loss, including alopecia areata, a type of hair loss thought to be stress- or autoimmune-related.

Beauty-Risking Choice	Beauty-Supporting Choice	Holistic Considerations
HAIR-LOSS PRODUCTS (*continued*)		
	Nitric oxide (NO) and related compounds or precursors are important to hair follicle health since they relax the hair follicle, working in a similar way to minoxidil. Dr. Peter Proctor, a noted hair-loss researcher who holds several patents for hair-loss treatments, developed hair formulas based on a nitro compound called **NANO (3-carboxylic acid pyridine-N-oxide),** which he refers to as "natural minoxidil." In one double-blind trial, an **essential oil combination of rosemary, lavender, thyme,** and **cedarwood** (a few drops each) mixed with a jojoba and grape seed oil carrier combination (20mL) sped regrowth of hair. The essential oils were thought to block the autoimmune reaction that caused stress-induced hair loss.	**Shen Min** is an herbal compound based on the Chinese medicinal herb **he shou wu,** or **fo-ti,** used traditionally to prevent hair loss and graying and aging in general. There has been no clinical proof yet regarding hair growth (though studies show it lowers cholesterol). **Circulation to the scalp** through exercise and massage is important. **Quality fats** and the **elimination of hydrogenated fats** are crucial to nourishment of the hair follicles and reducing inflammation.

Beauty-Risking Choice	Beauty-Supporting Choice	Holistic Considerations
INSECT REPELLANT		
DEET: Frequent and long-term use can cause brain deficits in vulnerable populations, especially children, according to a July 2002 Duke University Heath Note.	**Lemongrass** has been shown to be comparable in effectiveness to many commercial insect repellants in one study. **Catnip** makes DEET (and its neurological side effects) obsolete and works ten times better, according to a study done at Iowa State University.	Taking plenty of **B vitamins** makes you less appealing to mosquitos. There is a commercial insect repellant patch designed on this principle (see Resources).
MOUTH CARE PRODUCTS		
Toothpastes that contain SLS are proven skin and mouth irritants. They are also known to cause canker sores. **Conventional mouthwashes** with an alcohol content of 25 percent have been shown to increase the risk of oral cancers by more than 90 percent. They also dry the mouth, which can cause tooth decay. **Professional teeth whiteners** and home whitening programs are expensive and can contain irritants that make teeth more porous and prone to staining.	**Herbal toothpastes and mouthwashes** without SLS and alcohol can spare you irritation and canker sores and provide a spectrum of proven oral healers with ingredients like aloe, echinacea, goldenseal, neem, CoQ10, Xylitol, pomegranate extract, and clove to keep your mouth clean and teeth and gums healthy. **Hydrogen peroxide** (the basis of most expensive teeth-whitening products) made into a paste with baking soda whitens teeth very well and can reverse some gum problems that might otherwise require surgery, according to many dentists.	**Avoiding mouth infections** is important to maintaining fresh breath and also affects your overall health. Supplements like **CoQ10** and **grape seed extract** have been shown to improve gum health. **Oolong tea** reduces plaque deposits on teeth. **Green and black tea,** even in moderate amounts, have recently been shown in preliminary studies to inhibit the bacteria that causes tooth decay and even deactivated E. coli and herpes simplex types I and II in the mouth.

Beauty-Risking Choice	Beauty-Supporting Choice	Holistic Considerations
MOUTH CARE PRODUCTS (*continued*)		
	Sonic toothbrushes can disinfect the mouth below the gumline and whiten teeth while stopping some gum infections and canker sores in their tracks. **Xylitol-containing gum and oral care products** can protect teeth from bacteria, including streptococci, and aids in the remineralization of tooth enamel.	
NAIL PRODUCTS		
Nail fungus drugs: The prescription antifungals **Sporanox** and **Lamisil** are associated with liver toxicity. **Typical nail polishes and strengtheners** only coat the nail to thicken it, which protects the nail from breakage while actually drying out the nail and burdening the nail bed (and your system) with harmful chemicals like **formaldehyde, toluene,** and **dibutylpthalate.** These ingredients can also cause severe skin rashes.	A double-blind study compared **TTOs** (tea tree oils) effectiveness against nail fungus to its prescription counterpart, clotrimazole, and showed TTO to be just as effective. To eliminate nail fungus, Dr. Julian Whitaker, editor of the newsletter *Health and Healing*, recommends rubbing the oil onto the nail and adjacent skin twice daily. It may take eight to ten months before the infection is gone. **Myrrh** is a substance that is known to substantially penetrate and strengthen the nails. The product Vivinal features myrrh.	**Nail fungus** can signal systemic yeast overgrowth problems in the digestive tract. **Staying away from sugar and flour** and taking **probiotics** can reduce symptoms and help treatments work better. **Skin, hair, and nail supplements** contain connective tissue-supporting nutrients like sulfur (or its more bio-available form, MSM), silica, B vitamins, and EFAs to create resilient, healthier nails (and hair and skin) in a few months. Biosil is the premier silica product.

Beauty-Risking Choice	Beauty-Supporting Choice	Holistic Considerations
STEROID OINTMENT		
Using **steroid ointments** regularly thins the skin and compromises its immune function.	In one study, **poison ivy, oak,** or **sumac rashes** were prevented from either breaking out or spreading with **topical preparations containing jewelweed,** a plant that interestingly grows alongside poison ivy.	See also "Inflammatory Skin Problems" in Your Skin Strategy Makeover chart for safer ways to address specific conditions.
SUNSCREEN		
These common chemical sunscreen ingredients rarely block most UVA (aging rays), they have also been found in animal studies to accumulate in breast milk and to influence hormonal systems: 4-Methyl-Benzylidencamphor (4-MBC), Oxybenzone, Benzophenone-3, Octyl-methoxy-cinnamates (OMC), Octyl-Dimethyl-Para-Amino-Benzoic Acid (OD-PABA), and Homosalate (HMS). There is unprecedented skepticism regarding the strong marketing of sunscreen use in light of the fact that it rarely does not protect from the most fatal skin cancers, and also the fact that vitamin D deficiency—made even worse by vigilant sunscreen use—could be causing far more cancer deaths.	**Micronized zinc oxide (Z-cote) and titanium dioxide-based sunscreens:** Titanium dioxide can block both UVA and UVB rays with no known toxicity if used externally. Avoid micronized titanium dioxide, which showed some negative health effects. Zinc oxide complements titanium dioxide. The new sprays go on easily and lightly and don't make you white. **Antioxidant ingredients** like vitamins C and E and green tea have been proven to make sunscreens more effective.	**Antioxidant supplements** such as **green tea, alpha-lipoic acid, carotenoids** like **beta carotene** and **astaxanthins,** and **vitamins C** and **E** have been shown to inhibit sun damage and reduce inflammation. More and more studies have shown a connection between **the quality of fat we eat** and our skin's ability to withstand the sun. **EFAs** have been shown to offer some natural sun protection when taken for a few months in doses of up to 10 grams per day.

Beauty-Risking Choice	Beauty-Supporting Choice	Holistic Considerations
TALC OR BABY POWDER		
Talc has been linked with ovarian cancer. One study showed ovarian cancer risk to be 3.28 times higher in women who used talc in the genital area than for those who didn't. Talc has been discovered in ovarian tumors and in lungs.	**Cornstarch or silk-based powders** are a safer choice, especially for babies!	Whether it's you or your baby you're taking care of, you can avoid myriad confirmed irritants and toxins by using **natural baby products** instead of standard powders, mineral oil, and baby wipes.

HULDA: CHRONIC DERMATITIS CLEARED UNEXPECTEDLY

Until she attended my seven-day cruise program in November 2000, Hulda had been plagued by hives for a few years. She would get welts over her entire body, especially under her arms and breasts. She had been to several doctors, was given different diagnoses, including shingles, for which she was given Valtrex, and contact dermatitis of unknown origin, for which she was given antihistamines, and finally psoriasis, for which she was prescribed steroid ointments. These prescriptions gave only minimal and temporary relief. She was desperately seeking a solution.

After one of my sessions on cosmetics ingredients, Hulda counted her antiperspirant/deodorant roll-on, which was labeled as hypoallergenic, among one of the products she would phase out of her personal care routine. She wanted to use a product that would keep her fresh without blocking her normal perspiration. To her complete surprise, she experienced a marked reversal of her hives only a few days after discontinuing the product, and in about two weeks her skin had cleared completely. She now uses a calendula-based deodorant and has never had a recurrence of her problem.

THE BIG GUNS: NEW BATHROOM CABINET STAPLES TO STOCK

The following is a short list of particularly powerful, natural antimicrobials and immune boosters you should know about for occasional times of need. Available through health and vitamin stores, these substances can be used in a wide variety of applications, and with your doctor's supervision, you may even use them to avoid resorting to antibiotics and the cascade of syndromes and skindromes that come with them.

THE BIG GUNS	
Echinacea/goldenseal tincture	Echinacea and goldenseal tincture can enhance your resistance when you're under the weather. Echinacea has proven immune-boosting effects, and goldenseal has proven antimicrobial effects.
Grapefruit seed extract (GSE)	Grapefruit seed extract (GSE), not to be confused with grape seed extract, has demonstrated strong antibacterial action against a wide range of nasty bacteria. Ask your doctor if you can try it before resorting to harsher drugs. Available in capsules, liquid, sprays for the skin and feet, foot powders, deodorant, and other products.
Oregano oil	Oregano oil has been shown to destroy Candida albicans yeast both in vitro and in vivo, as well as strep, pneumonia, staphylococcus, and E. coli bacteria in vitro (test tube studies). The oil is strong and can be blended in small amounts into topical preparations. Do not apply to delicate skin. A few drops can be added to water and taken internally. And it's fantastic in cooking!
Tea tree oil (TTO)	The essential oil of *Melaleuca alternifolia* (tea tree), or TTO, has broad-spectrum antimicrobial activity and fights nail fungus, cold sores, and Candida yeast. TTO nasal ointment and body wash has worked against antibiotic-resistant strains of staphylococcus aureus better than conventional antibacterial nasal ointment and antibacterial (trichlosan-containing) soaps. Used in minute amounts, it can be added to scalp, foot, and skin preparations and used in mouth products.
Cranberry capsules	Cranberry helps prevent urinary tract infections.
Xylitol	Xylitol is an amazing natural sugar found in birch. It can prevent and halt sinus and middle-ear infections and inhibit bacteria by an anti-adherence action. Xylitol-containing gum inhibits tooth and gum infections.

Several other "Big Gun" immune boosters are available at your health food store.

KAREN GETS OFF THE ANTIBIOTIC MERRY-GO-ROUND WITH GSE

After making the connection between her frequent antibiotic use and her chronic digestive problems, Karen decided to try GSE for her yeast infection. With her gynecologist's blessing, she decided to fight her impulse to use antibiotics in the early stages of her infection. She took one GSE capsule three times a day. After only a few days, the infection cleared up. Karen is now a convert and grateful to be saving herself the antibiotic aftermath.

CHAPTER 15

MINIMIZE YOUR BEAUTY WILD CARDS

Beauty wild cards are the factors that can come up in our lives that we can't always control, even when we play our other cards wisely. Wild cards such as the growing risks of standard healthcare, prescription drug side effects, environmental and household chemicals, and our increasingly stressed-out world can jeopardize our precious vitality. Even our mother's choices when we were in the womb were wild cards we could not control that are affecting us today. Here are some steps you can take—recapping some previous discussion—to protect the future of your beauty and quality of life.

STEP 1: HELP YOUR DOCTOR GIVE YOU BETTER CARE

In today's awkward transitional period, at the dawn of the most major medical upheaval in history, we need to be armed with our own working knowledge of both our issues and our options so as not to fall victim to the current power struggle between the past and future of healthcare.

The average doctor's appointment is down to less than seven and a half minutes. It's no wonder we're so often discouraged from getting to the cause of our health complaints. If we merely control low-grade complaints with the help of over-the-counter symptom-mufflers, we're far more likely to progress to a full-blown disease state.

Consider these statistics when you consider standard guidelines or treatments:
- Life expectancy of Americans is ranked forty-second in the world, while we are number one in health spending, according to the World Health

Organization. Health in several countries that spend up to 75 percent less on healthcare is significantly greater.

- At least 65 percent of Americans are overweight or obese (that figure is projected to hit 75 percent by 2015).
- A 1999 Institute of Medicine report concluded that medical errors contribute to over one million injuries and up to ninety-eight thousand deaths annually. A 2002 study published in the *Archives of Internal Medicine* noted that errors occurred in nearly one in five doses in a typical three-hundred-bed hospital, which translates to about two errors per patient daily.
- Properly prescribed and used prescription drugs cause over 106,000 deaths each year, making it the fourth leading cause of death (more than AIDS and gun fatalities combined), according to the *Journal of the American Medical Association (JAMA)*.
- More drugs have been recalled in the last fifteen years than in all of history.

If healthcare goes universal, there's no telling where these stats might head. Obviously the issue isn't not having *enough* healthcare. It is the lack of effectiveness of standard care. When you seek medical intervention for each issue that comes up without trying lifestyle changes first, you play Russian roulette with your health. Upgrade any health practitioner who urges you—at the first sign of trouble—to forego the possibility of function-restoring health approaches in favor of costly, risky "fixes." Trying health-building, natural approaches before symptom-blocking drugs that allow the original problem to progress is a basic principle of vitality preservation. And when drugs or surgery are required, studies consistently show that they have better results when combined with nutritional and alternative therapies.

Protect Yourself with an Informed Grasp of Your Options

Keeping up on your health issues and on the variety of options that exist for addressing them is your first defense against the wild cards. Regardless of what you've heard, some of the best information you can get is available on the Internet. A quick search of some of my favorite databases (see Resources) will show you a world of clinically proven integrative health options for your whole family that will actually improve your overall health rather than endanger it. Where issues of surgery or starting a controversial drug seem like the only choice, be sure to get a second opinion. The second opinion of a nutrition-oriented specialist or naturopath who is also an MD is the best of both worlds, and provides a rare perspective that is not limited by major blind spots in training and knowledge. Remember, if published research is rejected without discussion, find another doctor who is informed about, or at least open to, nondrug approaches.

Get a Real Checkup

Integrative or complementary physicians combine the diagnostic technology of conventional doctors with extensive nutritional and alternative perspectives and, where truly necessary, drugs or surgery. Dr. Ron Rosedale of Advanced Metabolic Labs contributed to this checklist:

CHECKUP CHECKLIST

- Bring/get copies of all recent or past abnormal blood work and X-rays.
- Keep a list of all drugs you're taking if you have multiple doctors.
- Write down all symptoms and discuss them at your appointment.
- Get a full analysis of your blood, urine, and hair (if possible).
- If you're over thirty-five, Dr. Rosedale suggests having your "free" hormones (especially testosterone) tested as well as a urine test for certain proteins to indicate bone health more accurately than a bone density test.
- Get colon cancer screening if you are at risk or over fifty.
- If you suspect food or environmental allergies, arrange to be screened.
- Ask to have your homocysteine and C-reactive protein (CRP) levels checked as well as your LDL (important: ask for LDL particle size test or LDL "fractionation" test) and HDL cholesterol levels and triglycerides.
- If you're a male over forty or a post-menopausal female, get ferretin (stored iron) checked. If you are concerned with weight or onset of disease or premature aging, a fasting insulin test is in order.
- Bring any studies you have come across regarding safer alternatives proven to help your condition.

DR. ROSEDALE EXPLAINS SOME OF THE CAVEATS OF CONVENTIONAL TESTS

"Bone density testing does not determine bone *strength*. A better way to do that is to monitor bone breakdown by measuring certain proteins in the urine. These tests are performed by the same labs that do hair analysis, such as Great Smokies Laboratories. The blood ferritin (stored iron) test is important for older men and post-menopausal women because high ferritin will literally 'rust' you from the inside out and is a pro-oxidant—the opposite of what you want happening in your body. Conventional measures say that up to 225 is normal, while I recommend ferritin be kept between 40 and 60. I also recommend leptin testing for pre-diabetics and diabetics, as well as overweight and obese people. The problem is, most physicians will not know the right thing to do once an abnormal level is discovered. Same with insulin. It comes down to the same dietary principle Kat James and I suggest, which allows insulin and leptin sensitivity to return. As far as most hormone testing goes, it is the same problem: if imbalances are discovered, the conventional treatment is unsatisfactory. Since doctors who prescribe risky synthetic estrogens rarely even monitor free estrogen once they've prescribed it, one can avoid much unnecessary risk by working with a physician or naturopath who is experienced in proper testing and comprehensive natural and bio-identical hormone treatments."

STEP 2. GET A HANDLE ON YOUR HORMONE ISSUES AND OPTIONS

Your state of hormonal balance is one of the most consequential factors impacting your beauty and quality of life at every stage. The extent of the influence of hormone-mimicking chemicals in our products or our environment—or even while we are in the womb—has only begun to become clear in recent research. We accept hormonal problems throughout life as normal occurrences, but the fact is, more and more clues tell us that much of our suffering might be aggravated by environmental and nutritional issues. In our youth, we experience acne or menstrual discomforts. By our thirties, tens of millions experience thyroid hormone imbalances. Soon thereafter (particularly as a result of stress and lack of sleep) come the decline in DHEA, the youthfulness and libido hormone I spoke about earlier, as well as human growth hormone (hGH) secretion. And then there are menopause and andropause with health risks all their own.

Until 2002, the odds were that your doctor was unlikely to know about natural, plant-based, or bio-identical hormone replacement therapies (HRT) or hormone-balancing supplements. In the fall of 2002, the National Institutes of Health's Women's Health Initiative study on synthetic estrogen and progestin-based HRT drugs was halted after showing higher breast cancer, heart attack, and blood-clot risk in women taking them for five years. Spokespeople for the drugs emphasized that no effective alternatives existed. In the meantime, GlaxoSmithKline sent out thousands of its salespeople with samples and literature about its black cohosh–based herbal supplement, Remifemin. Black cohosh was proven in placebo-controlled clinical trials in the eighties and nineties to offer similar—and in some ways superior—effects to synthetic HRT in relieving hot flashes, mood symptoms, and vaginal dryness. Since then, two studies have revealed that the rates of breast cancer decreased between 2003 and 2004 in direct correlation with the decrease in

HEDGING THE HYSTERECTOMY WILD CARD

Hysterectomy—despite published research in 2005 that confirmed it is unnecessary in nine out of ten cases—is the most common major surgery for women in the U.S. Researchers at the University of California, Los Angeles, concluded that unless it's in response to a high cancer risk, the outcome of hysterectomy is that it actually increases overall health risks. Translation: over 540,000 women are subjected to the devastating loss of quality of life and sexual health only to be left sicker (more heart disease and bone loss for starters) and poorer. This is all the more tragic since well-known, effective alternatives, such as myomectomy (removal only of the fibroids), arterial embolization, and endometrial ablation are often not presented to hysterectomy candidates. Even less likely to be mentioned are the battery of natural approaches that can actually reverse the estrogen dominance that causes most of the issues that lead to hysterectomy. Again, the antidote is information.

synthetic HRT use. Some analysts suggested that this was because mammograms had also been decreased, but this was disproven by the second study, which was published in the summer of 2007 in the *Journal of the National Cancer Institute*, which confirmed that mammography screening rates had remained stable.

Those with mild hormonal imbalances and PMS often experience marked to complete relief after making the food and beverage upgrades in this book and taking proven hormone-modulating herbs such as lignan concentrates (Brevail), black cohosh, dong quai, gamma oryzanol, DIM, and chaste tree berry (vitex). These herbs can also play a role in balancing the "estrogen dominance," which causes fibroids and fibrocystic breasts, heavy periods, endometriosis, and an exaggerated pear shape in hips and thighs. I experienced astounding benefits firsthand by taking several of the above as my own exaggerated pear shape, which was my "God-given" trademark for the first half of my life, was re-proportioned in a way I never imagined possible. I was a textbook case of estrogen dominance, and my weight problem itself contributed to it, as fat itself is now known to produce estrogen.

Plant-based or bio-identical estrogen and progesterone therapies, including prescribed sprays, creams, and transdermal patches, offer relief of menopausal and andropausal symptoms without the risks inherent to synthetic HRT. Bio-identical hormones used in the right balance act identically to the hormones naturally found in the body. Most naturopathic doctors (NDs) are versed in their use and proper monitoring. Before you make any decisions with your doctor about bio-identical HRT, I advise you to read a good book on the subject. Dr. John Lee pioneered the successful use of natural progesterone creams, and his books are widely respected and followed by holistic and integrated practitioners. *The Sexy Years* by Suzanne Somers presents the differing views of several prominent physicians regarding bio-identical hormone replacement therapies. Dr. Eugene Shippen's book, *The Testosterone Solution*, presents ample research to dispel common myths about testosterone therapy, which deserves a whole lot more attention, given its ability to dramatically improve health and quality of life for both men and women.

While natural hormone replacement can do incredible things for one's skin, shape, virility, and outlook, its true importance is in the documented improvements in heart, metabolic, immunological, mental, sexual, and many other health issues that are behind those rejuvenating benefits that are seen and felt.

Mind Your Thyroid: The Limitations of Blood Tests

Thyroid problems are major beauty and quality-of-life issues that often go undetected, and yet affect up to one in four women. If you're cold all the time, can't lose weight, are tired, or have droopy lids, sparse eyebrows, brittle hair, or dry skin, get your thyroid hormone levels checked. Thyroid problems can arise from stress, exposure to fluoride and mercury, autoimmune issues, pregnancy, heredity, exposure to radiation, and more. Be aware that conventional thyroid hormone tests are notorious for missing real thyroid issues since blood levels of the hormone don't always reflect thyroid function. The Broda O. Barnes, MD Foundation is a nonprofit organization considered to be the premiere educational organization on thyroid issues (see Resources). The Barnes Basal Body Temperature home self-test is widely considered to be the most reliable indicator of thyroid function.

THE BARNES BASAL BODY TEMPERATURE SELF-TEST

Basal temperatures are taken first thing in the morning before you get out of bed and when your body is completely at rest. Menstruating women must take this test on the second, third, and fourth days of their periods only. Nonmenstruating women, women who have had hysterectomies, and men can take their temperature at any time.

The night before you take the test, do not drink any alcohol. Shake a glass mercury thermometer down and leave it by your bed. In the morning, before getting out of bed and with as little movement as possible, place the thermometer under your arm and leave it there for ten minutes.

The normal temperature range is 97.8–98.2. A lower temperature means you might be a candidate for thyroid hormone therapy. If your thyroid function is borderline-sluggish, a nutrition-oriented doctor may recommend supplements such as kelp and L-tyrosine, thyroid glandulars, and incorporating virgin coconut oil into your diet to stimulate thyroid function.

If your temperature is below normal range, most doctors prescribe synthetic thyroid hormone (levothyroxine, which contains only the T4 hormone). However, a natural dessicated bovine thyroid used for nearly a century called Armour Thyroid may have advantages due to a broader spectrum of hormones (both T4 and T3), according to a letter by Dr. Alan Gaby to the *Journal of the American Medical Association*. In addition, a 1999 study published in the *New England Journal of Medicine* showed that patients had greater improvements in mood and fewer negative symptoms when treated with Armour Thyroid as opposed to synthetic T4 drugs. One synthetic levothyroxine product manufacturer in particular has encountered legal trouble for suppressing information on competing thyroid drugs, including generics. Its generous contributions to endocrinologists and the American Thyroid Association (whose opinions doctors, and even publications such as *Worst Pills, Best Pills*, often accept as truth), call the merits of the widespread bias against Armour Thyroid into even greater question. Because most people on synthetic thyroid hormones do not have satisfactory results, I suggest that you look into these issues closely before you make such a quality-of-life-impacting choice.

STEP 3. STRATEGIZE CREATIVELY AGAINST STRESS, SLEEP, AND MOOD ISSUES

Another hormone that wreaks havoc is cortisol. Stress and a lack of deep sleep can lead to elevated levels of cortisol, which can in turn cause a cascade of immune and inflammatory issues, like skin eruptions, tissue and muscle breakdown, fat accumulation, water retention, thyroid imbalances, and bone loss. In his book *Caffeine Blues*, Stephen Cherniske, MS, notes that overworked women may have higher than normal cortisone levels. As mentioned in chapter 4, caffeine—like stress—causes the release of stress hormones and raises cortisol. A study at the National Institutes of Mental Health comparing bone mineral density in women with both normal and elevated cortisol found that those with elevated stress hormones had bone density similar to that of seventy-year-olds!

Relieve Your Stress Creatively
- Express yourself—speak up!
- Pursue your passion.

EXERCISE: THE ULTIMATE STRESS- AND BLUES-BUSTER

Exercise—in both strenuous (though not prolonged), and less intense forms, such as yoga and tai chi—can effectively reduce stress and cortisol levels while improving your overall health. A team of Duke University Medical Center researchers demonstrated in late 1999 that thirty minutes either riding a stationary bike, walking, or jogging three times a week was just as effective after sixteen weeks as Zoloft in treating major depression in the middle-aged and elderly. Keep in mind that more than half an hour of nonstop aerobic activity will bring you diminishing returns, cause cortisol to kick in and actually signal the body to hoard—rather than burn—fat for hours after your workout. The cortisol issue is a problem for long-distance runners, who are likely increasing their inflammation issues via chronically elevated cortisol. Recent research has shown that repeated short bursts of activity for approximately 12 to 20 minutes with rest breaks in between (called interval training) are more beneficial than prolonged aerobic activity. This means that doing rigorous household chores, taking a few flights of stairs, and taking breaks to wrestle or toss a frisbee with your kids throughout the day may be more effective than forty minutes on a stair climber after a day at the computer.

- If you feel trapped, set new boundaries.
- Choose physical activities you find uplifting (such as dancing, playing with your kids, walking with a friend, or meditative movement such as yoga or tai chi) to relieve stress and lift your moods.
- Use alone time to tune in to yourself (i.e., music, journaling, creative pursuits), not tune out (i.e., TV, food).
- Keep a journal.
- Get or spend time with a pet.
- Read books that address your emotional issues.
- Spend time with people who expect great things of you.
- Support yourself nutritionally with stress adaptogens, like ginseng and plant sterolins, and the previously discussed brain function-supportive supplements, if needed.

- If you suspect you're depressed, seek help. But also remember to listen to how depression sometimes leads us to reevaluate our lives.

Take Your Beauty Sleep Seriously

Getting your beauty sleep goes way beyond the avoidance of under-eye circles. It can greatly affect your health and even your weight. It is during "deep-wave" sleep that hormone activities—like the release of human growth hormone (hGH) and regulation of cortisol—really kick in, protecting us from inflammation, the cumulative aging effects of stress, and other cortisol-related effects such as weight gain in the belly and immune problems. HGH is the body's fountain of youth, keeping skin thick and supple and the body lean and muscular. It also helps keep every other system in the body energized and in working order.

- Getting some sun early in the day and using a sleep mask at night will help your body produce more melatonin, which helps you sleep. Melatonin supplements can help.
- Nose strips, antisnore sprays, and pillows that support the neck can reduce or stop snoring, which interferes with deep sleep.
- Upgrade coffee or alcohol to herbal nightcaps such as Teeccino or tulsi tea for deeper sleep.
- Herbs such as valerian and 5Htp work in different ways to help you sleep. Look into them.
- Hypoallergenic and dust-mite-proof bedding can vastly improve your mornings and your under-eye circles if you deal with allergies (see Resources).
- Some MSM-based antisnore throat sprays actually work by reducing inflammation of the soft throat tissue and increasing airflow.

STEP 4. AVOID THE REMAINING WILD CARDS

From the fluoride, chloroform, and drug residues in your tap water (which we're told is safe) to the cosmetic and household chemicals and sun that could either give us cancer or save us from it and the newly confirmed dangers of electromagnetic fields (EMFs) from our Wi-Fi gadgets, what once seemed like paranoid concerns have emerged as real ones we need to keep on top of. I urge you to explore these issues even if you spend only an hour on the

Internet. You have a good head on your shoulders, and I know you'll find your way past the hype to what has been substantiated.

If you are a parent, you have even more reasons to be vigilant. Even our unborn babies deal with the wild card choices we make which can affect their appearance and quality of life decades from now. In a recent animal study at Duke University, a chemical from plastic, BPA, was introduced to pregnant mice in much smaller amounts than were thought safe, and was shown to cause their babies to be born with dramatically altered coloration and size and a predisposition to obesity, diabetes, and cancer. But when folic acid and genestein—a component of soy—were given to pregnant mice, they were both independently shown to interfere with the negative genetic expressions induced by BPA, sparing the newborn mice from the physical alterations and genetic response to the chemical. Dozens of additional studies have shown

THE DENTAL WILD CARDS

When we think of following the advice of dentists and doctors as kids, we think of what it means to be "good." And while not even a dentist would dispute the fact that mercury is a potent toxin, accumulating evidence points to a danger that lurks literally right under our nose. Some studies have now found that the amount of mercury found in various organs such as the brain and kidneys was proportionate to the number of fillings the test subjects had, and that gum chewing could increase mercury vapors in the mouth, and accumulation in the body. German, Italian, and Australian researchers have voiced concerns, and in fact Canada as well as several European governments have recently called for discontinuation of amalgam fillings for pregnant women. The FDA has recommended further research. In the meantime, it's easy (and important) enough to do your own.

I applaud the American Dental Association's decisive new warnings against using fluoridated water to mix with infant formulas for newborns. It's stated concern is with the possibility of dental fluorosis (mottling of the teeth and enamel). Recent research has also linked fluoride with child brain development problems and possible bone cancer in boys. Most of Western Europe no longer fluoridates.

how a mother's nutrient intake—and avoidance of chemicals—can affect the entire life of their unborn child. So this is the wild card only you can protect your unborn child from.

Luckily, we live in an information-empowered age when it is no longer necessary to accept unquestioningly that any drinking water additive is harmless, or that anything we are told to slather onto our bodies every day to avoid cancer is truly protecting us. And if we are informed, we needn't sign up as test subjects for experiments. We need only stop rushing to "be the first" to try the latest nanocreams or injections, and rethink our "innocent until proven guilty" attitude toward untested chemicals and procedures and put that notion in reverse. Finally, we must embrace the real means to quality of life and beauty healing, such as whole foods and supplements (which alone could save us an estimated $24 billion in national healthcare costs). So much great information and so many great companies are countering the wild cards. Play your cards right and you just might live better than ever.

CHAPTER 16

MAKE LIFE AN AUTHENTIC
BEAUTY RITUAL

Throughout the course of this book I've applied the three tools—the magic motivation of health, complete information, and access to the best resources—to each area of our dawn-to-dusk lives. With these powerful new tools and the Resources to follow, you now have everything you need to become your own passionate connoisseur. After you finish reading this book, return to your notebook and choose your first cycle of strategic, pro-beauty upgrades. As each cycle of shedding and upgrades becomes second nature and propels itself into the next, you'll release more burdens and sidestep countless new challenges. You'll soon be adept at tapping the transformative power that lies dormant in every choice until no choice remains mundane in your evolving recipe for self-creation. You'll gain an exhilarating new sense of freedom and awareness that will empower and uplift you in unimagined ways, and you'll continually reset your own criteria for what goes on in your body and how you live. As you cultivate yourself with growing clarity and the ever-expanding options that enable you to have it all, your concept of the good life, the nature of your beauty splurges, your spirit, and the person staring back at you from your mirror will never be the same. And here's the most amazing part: once your tastes, your concept of decadence, and your desires have evolved to become one and the same with your body's innate desires, you will be home free. You will have achieved a state I affectionately call "beauty nirvana," an effortless, joyful state that lifts you in an upward spiral toward nature's intention: an ageless beauty that is never static.

SHEDDING FREES US UP FOR MORE PURPOSEFUL PURSUITS

The beautiful thing about the process of shedding is that it frees up so much energy that was once tied up in the old merry-go-round. Each of us has gifts we've either cultivated or neglected. Now is the time to focus your newfound energy into that greater purpose. Vitality is the point where our physical manifestation connects with our inner spirit, and when all is said and done, what comes from that spirit is what really counts. Vitality and radiance are simply joyful mediums for the expression of our truest gifts from the heart.

CULTIVATE YOUR INTRINSIC BEAUTY

When we are disconnected from our unique essence, there is a hole in our foundation for self-creation. Discounting the inner wisdom we are born with is like asking the painter Gauguin, "Which artists have influenced you?" and then shaming him for daring to say his work came from his own soul. We have so much inside that we've been shamed out of tapping in to and expressing by parents, siblings, coworkers, spouses, and others whose approval we seek or who are threatened by the part of us they can't understand or control. I have worked with women whose gurus, hairstyles, designer clothes, facialists, bikini waxers, and Pilates instructors are the same as their mother's or their friends'. These women fear that they might fall out of favor if they were to go in their own direction or make some of those choices privately. A different situation has been described by many of my website readers who have shared their battles with husbands or family members who unwittingly contribute to their struggles with food by interfering with their attempts to break their own patterns or establish needed boundaries. It takes vigilance to establish and defend our own boundaries. By giving others the space and unconditional support that fosters and encourages their own self-creation, you set the stage for granting yourself that same nonjudgmental room to explore, fail, and grow as you cultivate the path to your own truest purpose.

Vitality is the point where our physical manifestation connects with our inner spirit.

Perhaps the real key to developing our independent spirit is not in finding the time or the right group with which to pursue a spiritual path but finding ways to avoid having our own innate spirit trampled or imposed upon. We need to give our own inner wisdom its platform within our hearts. Evolve your self through self-knowledge and truth and what they lead you to. Draw on the wisdom of others, but don't accept that your own unique collection of beliefs and instincts is inferior in any way to any other belief systems.

USING OUR MOST BEAUTIFUL GIFTS

What's even more important than the gifts we possess is how we channel and use them. There are so many passionate and bright people whose gifts fail to manifest their much-needed good in the world. This quiz was forwarded to me by e-mail (author unknown). It is a beautiful testament to the nature of our truest gifts:

1. Name the five wealthiest people in the world.
2. Name the last five Heisman Trophy winners.
3. Name the last five winners of the Miss America contest.
4. Name ten people who have won the Nobel or Pulitzer Prize.
5. Name the last half-dozen Academy Award winners for Best Actor and Best Actress.
6. Name the last decade's World Series winners.

How did you do?

The point is that none of us remembers yesterday's headliners. They're the best in their fields, but the applause dies, awards tarnish, achievements are forgotten, and accolades and certificates are buried with their owners.

Now here's another quiz. See how you do on this one:

1. List a few teachers who aided your journey through school.
2. Name three friends who helped you through a difficult time.
3. Name five people who taught you something worthwhile.
4. Think of a few people who make you feel appreciated and special.
5. Think of five people you enjoy spending time with.
6. Name a half-dozen heroes whose stories have inspired you.

Easier? The lesson: the people who make a difference in your life aren't the ones with the most credentials, the most money, or the most awards. They're the ones who care.

LET YOUR BEAUTY RIPPLE OUTWARD

Another potential gift each of us can give to the world is a passion for the stories and the values behind the products we buy. My own passionate pursuit of high-quality products and meaningful services and support for pro-beauty living has led me to some of the most amazing and passionate people I've ever encountered. One couple who knew nothing about organic farming developed one of the most profitable organic-produce companies in the world out of a strong desire to do something for the environment and for people. A maker of some of the purest body care products I've found healed herself of non-Hodgkin's lymphoma by detoxifying her life and using homegrown herbs in her microbatch body delicacies. The creator of one of the most cutting-edge supplement lines transformed himself from diseased and emaciated to healthy and robust. These are people and companies after my own heart. We share a creative spirit that has come out of transforming our own lives and the need to share what we have learned and created with others. There are no spokespeople or number-crunchers fronting or vouching for or compromising the quality of their products. These products and companies are as rare, real, and precious as the most beautiful endangered butterfly. If we want the hope of a more beautiful future, we have to seek out companies that reflect what we want to see more of in the world, before they are gone or sold to entities with other agendas. Capture this beauty and make these companies a part of your life. Many of them are listed in the Resources section.

Doing Better for Your Self Is Doing Better for the Planet

You can see how these simple, "green" choices are examples of how improving your own beauty and health does the same for our planet:

- Upgrade bottled water to filtered water. Spare the landfills while doing better for your body.
- Upgrade factory-farmed "organic" foods to local organic food.
- Upgrade synthetic cosmetics to petrochemical-free personal care.
- Upgrade conventional animal products to grass-fed meat and dairy.

- Upgrade synthetic, perfumed cosmetics to pure ones.
- Upgrade driving to walking, biking, or public transport.
- Upgrade to eco-smart home, lawn, and pest-control products.
- Upgrade processed, "dead" foods to live, unprocessed, whole foods.

GUARD YOUR BEAUTY WITH YOUR LIFE

As cultivators of our own lives, we need uninterrupted access to true sustenance and untainted raw materials. If we want to have continued access to food that still has nutrients and life force in it; water that doesn't harm us more than it helps us; clean, quality seafood; pure body care products; quality supplements; and innovative, accountable healthcare, we need to express these demands through our choices and recognize their true value by being willing to pay—and maybe even fight—for them. We mustn't take these precious needs for granted. Beauty has no real future without them.

STAY AWARE, STAY BEAUTIFUL

It has never been more important for each of us to understand the issues that occasionally threaten the future of our beauty and quality of life. Fortunately, it has never been easier to get hooked in to the resources that can elevate our quality of life and to the complete, unfiltered, and unpackaged information we need to stay ahead of the game and steer clear of beauty wild cards.

PRO-BEAUTY HEALTH CHOICE ISSUES

Since 1989, industries have contributed more than $68 million to political candidates who support laws that allow them to release untold chemicals into the environment. Laws sweeping through Europe threaten our future freedom to improve our health and quality of life with supplements. And the agricultural biotechnology, seen by many scientists as an uncontrollable threat to the world's food supply, is running neck and neck with the emerging hope of sustainable agriculture and the unstoppable passion of consumers.

On top of all of this lies the inarguable fact that globalization gives corporations unprecedented protection from any accountability for our health, our environment, and our quality of life. Fortunately, this disturbing reality is still somewhat vulnerable to the power of your choice. But more and more, that choice is being threatened. Hundreds of millions of people in this country are actively seeking deeper meaning in their choices, purchases, and lives, and this passion is felt and quantified with fascination by economists and market analysts. We are in an age of great upheaval. The medical guard is changing, and many current practices will soon be relegated to the archives of a medical Dark Age. Agriculture is changing. Environmental frivolity is becoming intolerable, even to the mainstream. Fat-free is over. Consumers' blind faith is over. For the uninformed, life will continue to get worse before it gets better, but for the informed, it can be better than ever right now.

STAND UP FOR YOUR BEAUTY AND YOUR QUALITY OF LIFE

Though it may seem daunting to be up against polluters and soulless corporations that don't want consumers to be informed, consumers have begun to make a huge difference with their dollars and with their computers. Perhaps the most exciting contribution that computers have made to society is their ability to connect and mobilize huge numbers of people in support of important issues. One of the most encouraging examples of this new kind of grassroots power was demonstrated in the late 1990s, when efforts by over fifty organizations informed and mobilized an unprecedented 275,603 Americans to e-mail comments and successfully defeat the USDA's attempt to degrade the definition of organic-food standards to include GMO foods and other potential health hazards. Several important organizations representing the crucial issues that can make or break our quality of life have made the act of raising our voices as easy as a couple of mouse clicks. You can certainly make a difference without a computer as well. See Resources for a list of organizations that will inform and inspire you to make a difference.

SAVE YOUR OWN BEAUTY AND YOU HELP SAVE THE WORLD

It used to be nearly impossible or at least inconvenient to reconcile your desire for high-end results and appeal with your desire to do no harm to yourself or the planet in the process. But for the first time in history, you no longer need to compromise any of those desires. It is now easy, pleasant, and more rewarding than ever to live in harmony with the values so many of us have suppressed within ourselves for far too long. Corporations that make mediocre, harmful, and polluting products are now at your mercy like never before. Start with your choices on a personal level to turn the tide. Let your own beauty ripple outward and you can begin to save the world.

TAKE YOUR TOOLS ALONG FOR THE JOURNEY

No one can or should tell you how to proceed from here. Part of the power of shedding is the joyful spirit of discovery and creativity that feeds your own unique process. All you need to take with you from here are your new tools. Keep them honed and by your side, and they will surely take you where you want to go. Shedding is forever. Enjoy the process.

THE LIVING BEAUTY RESOURCE GUIDE

Stocking up on superior product upgrades is the surest way to get yourself on track for serious self-transformation—minus the suffering. This process will ultimately simplify your life as it enables you to leave behind the merry-go-round of problem-causing choices most people are dependent on. The following is a special, annually updated collection of exceptional products I have continually honed over several years that lets you experience the good life wherever you live. Many products mentioned here are available from natural food stores or online. I've limited this collection to one-of-a-kind or hard-to-find products, so not all products mentioned in previous chapters are mentioned here if they are widely available. New products will be launched, and others may be discontinued, but better products are being created every day for you, the informed consumer. For additional products, information, and recipes between official updates of this book's resource guide, I invite you to subscribe to my free quarterly newsletter at www.InformedBeauty.com. I also welcome your suggestions for standout products that meet the specific ingredient criteria laid forth here, for consideration in future listings for either this book or InformedBeauty.com.

Finally, I've also included some of the most reliable resources for staying on top of new science and quality-of-life issues in your areas of interest. Welcome to a world where science and companies serve you, where substance counts and so does the impact of your choice. Everyone should live this well!

FOODS AND BEVERAGES

These are the hard-to-find items featured on my Total Transformation® Programs because of their low-glycemic status, superior taste, and healthfulness. They have taken me years to compile. Many are one of a kind. It's important to stock up on the low-impact versions of foods you normally crave until your body's "sugar pendulum" comes to a halt. I've gathered some of the best foods and beverages (many award and taste test winners) while avoiding sugar, high-impact flours, synthetic sweeteners, and genetically modified ingredients.

Beverages

Cranberry Juice, Unsweetened, by Lakewood and R. K. Knudsen

Because of its low sugar content, unsweetened cranberry juice is the only juice besides aloe, tomato, noni, or goji (in small quantities) that I recommend. It is both tart and highly concentrated, so use only a splash of it in water or seltzer and add a low-glycemic sweetener to taste. Proven effective against bladder infections and loaded with vitamin C, it makes an elegant spritzer that won't spike blood sugar levels. I serve these with lime in tall-stemmed glasses on my programs instead of wine. Stay away from the sweetened or blended varieties if you want to avoid blood sugar spikes.

Ito En Teas' Tea Bottled Artisan Teas

718-250-4000 • *www.itoen.com*

Teas' Tea is the only widely available bottled artisan's true tea without sugar, so it is the one bottled tea I serve on my programs. The Jasmine is my favorite (like drinking flowers!). Ito En's elegant teashop in New York City was rated number one by *Zagat Guide* in 2006.

Loose Tea, Mail Order, from In Pursuit of Tea, Special Teas, and Teance

www.truetea.com • *www.specialteas.com* • *www.teance.com*

In Pursuit of Tea offers the highest-end traditional teas, including Yinzhen Silver Needle (the finest white tea) and potent Japanese matcha (powdered tea that is whisked to a froth in bowls). I use the matcha for heavenly, homemade green tea ice cream (simply freeze half-and-half ice cubes with matcha and xylitol, then process in a Vita-Mix). SpecialTeas carries exotic and nontraditional blends, including Osmanthus green, a fruity, peachy blend that will please former sugary fruit tea addicts. Earl Grey rooibos, rooibos with bourbon-vanilla pieces, and Berry Lapacho with black currant are both caffeine-free options that taste sweet without sugar. Teance has a wide selection of the highest-end traditional teas. Bauchong Oolong has an unusual, almost buttery taste, making it a favorite on my programs.

Numi Artisan Teas

One of the only full-leaf teas sold in teabags, Numi uses no "natural flavors" or added flavor oils, unlike the oxidized and flavored "tea dust" featured in most teabag brands. The Monkey King (Jasmine) is my favorite.

Steaz Diet Green Tea Sodas, Diet Black Cherry flavor

800-295-1388 • *www.steazsoda.com*

Sugary soft drinks are linked with mental problems and obesity in kids. Steaz diet (but not their regular) soda is the only stevia-sweetened soda with no synthetic sweeteners. It does contains a low 5 grams of sugar (compared to the 30+ grams in regular soda), so I still dilute the Diet Black Cherry flavor with plain selzer, which makes it last twice as long, and it still has an amazing flavor that will fool even your kids.

Teeccino Mediterranean and Maya Lines of Herbal Coffees

800-498-3434 • *www.teeccino.com*

This is the number one-selling—and best-tasting—herbal coffee alternative I've found. It gives you the same aroma and brewing experience as coffee, and it also makes espresso. The newer Maya line (Maya Chai, Maya Caffe, and Maya Chocolate) is the most coffeelike and features potassium-rich ramon nut, a Maya traditional food as a main ingredient.

Tisana Traditional Tuscan Herbal Infusions

212-255-7773 • *www.spatechnologies.com*

More potent than most herb teas, these "liquid dietary supplements" are produced by one of Italy's leading herbalists. These herbal infusions are based on centuries-old European formulas for issues such as digestion, stress, cellulite, and sluggish circulation. Grown from prized volcanic soil in Tuscany, Tisana is featured at European medical spas and increasingly in the U.S.

FOODS AND BEVERAGES

Tulsi Teas by Organic India

www.omorganics.com

These are the finest Holy basil teas I have found, and the only ones that are 100 percent organic. Tulsi (Holy basil) has been used for centuries to reduce stress, support strength and stamina, promote immunity, and enhance calm and clarity. It has a naturally uplifting tangy mint flavor and aroma, and this company features sophisticated Tulsi blends with chai masala, lemon ginger, pomegranate green tea, sweet rose, and more.

Breads, Cereals, Crackers, Chips, and Pastas

Cereals, Low-Glycemic by Flax Z Snax and Uncle Sam

www.low-carb.com • *www.carbsmart.com*

Flax Z Snax may be the only natural hot cereal that won't spike your blood sugar (your oatmeal will if you are the average American). Uncle Sam (original) is a one-of-a-kind, low-glycemic, whole wheat and flaxseed cold cereal that has been around since 1919. Find it in regular and health food stores. Its glycemic content is the lowest when sprinkled over full-fat yogurt or with nuts and organic cream (organic berries puts it over the top).

French Meadow Bakery's Healthy Hemp Bread, Bagels, and Tortillas

These rare, naturally low-glycemic products found in your health food store freezer are the only sprouted bread products I serve on my programs because they meet my standards for taste and have the lowest impact on blood sugar. The bread is great toasted with butter, egg salad, grilled cheese, or even as French toast (skip the syrup and top with warm mashed berries spiked with maple flavoring). Keep frozen. The better the bread, the quicker it spoils.

The Kitchen Table Bakers Cheese Wafer Crisps

800-486-4582 • *www.kitchentablebakers.com*

These flourless, savory gourmet crisps have been featured in the *New York Times* and other respected culinary reviews for their rare, melt-in-your-mouth delectability. They scratch both the cheese-y and the crispy cracker "itch" but are very low-glycemic.

La Tortilla Factory Tortillas, Low Carb Variety

www.latortillafactory.com

These are the low-glycemic tortillas that are most like regular tortillas. I love the green onion flavor and use these in breakfast burritos, quesadillas, wraps, and pizzas. Unlike some low-carb foods, they contain no unhealthy fillers or trans fats.

Lydia's Organics Grainless Herb Crackers

www.lydiasorganics.com

I feature these mouthwatering, no-flour, no-grain, organic, raw, herb-loaded crackers on my programs because they appeal even to health food-phobics who might reject other flax crackers. They're uncommonly tasty because of the ingenious use of herbs (the curry flavor is my favorite) and the zingy Himalayan salt. Find them in the raw foods section.

Flax Crackers by Glutino Cracker Flax and Yaya's Raw Rah

www.carbsmart.com • www.yayasrawrah.com

Flax crackers are unique in that they can scratch your crunch "itch" or make perfect dipping snacks without the carb, grain, or gluten consequences. Check the raw foods section of your health food store as some great brands come and go. Glutino Cracker Flax tomato onion flavor is widely available and wonderful with avocado or hummus. The award-winning Spicy Flax Crackers by Yaya's Raw Rah are wonderful and far more exotic in their use of herbs.

Pasta: Dreamfield's and Shirataki Noodles

www.lowcarbdiner.com • www.carbsmart.com • www.low-carb.com

Beware of "reduced carb" and whole-wheat pastas if you are trying to dismantle a carb addiction. It's not something you can go halfway with. Dreamfield's is the only truly low digestible carb pasta made from durum semolina. It tastes like fine Italian pasta but with twice the fiber. Shirataki noodles are great for Asian dishes. The Tofu Shirataki Noodles are basically fettuccini-shaped tofu. They are also thicker and more full-bodied than the traditional Shirataki noodles, which are like super-thin cellophane noodles. The latter is made of konjac root flour (ultra low-glycemic because it's just soluble fiber). I use both to make my "Pad Thai without the Padded Thighs" dish.

Pizza Crust Mixes, Low-Glycemic

www.carbsmart.com • www.lowcarbdiner.com • www.low-carb.com

Believe it or not, you will lose your cravings for things like pizza once you're weaned off blood sugar-spiking foods, but it's good to have low-glycemic (as in low-carb) pizza crust mixes in the cupboard for nostalgic indulgences. Pizza truly becomes non-fattening health food with these mixes and fresh ingredients to top them.

Soy and Flaxseed Corn Tortilla Chips by R.W. Garcia

www.rwgarcia.com

This is the only tortilla chip I serve on my program because it is organic and naturally very low-glycemic (the spicy flavor is my favorite). The best part is that it doesn't taste anything like the tough, tasteless low-carb chips of yesteryear. It is great with guacamole and more filling than conventional chips because of the protein and flax.

Chocolate, Candies, Cookies, and Sweet Snacks

Betty Lou's Nut Balls, Coconut Macadamia flavor

www.bettylousinc.com

This chewy and delicious creation is the only xylitol-sweetened, all-natural nut butter ball I know of, and it comes from the nut ball queen (she's been making them for decades).

Jennies Coconut Macaroons, Unsweetened

888-294-1164 • *www.zerocarbsjenniesmacaroons.com*

With zero sugar or flour and available in coconut, chocolate, and carob, this amazingly tasty macaroon will scratch that chewy-sweet cookie "itch" without the blood sugar spike, gluten, sulfites, or trans fats in other macaroons. They are sweetened with maltitol, which is natural to the body (unlike Splenda/sucrolose) but can be a laxative if you eat too much.

Dagoba Organic Dark Chocolate

www.dagobachocolate.com

Among the finest dark, organic chocolates I have tasted. Once you've eliminated blood sugar spikes from your life, you will train your taste buds for the adventures of their Eclipse 87 percent and maybe even their daring 100 percent cacao Prima Materia bar (take a nibble first thing in the morning, when taste buds are most sensitive, to really understand the depth of this exceptional unsweetened chocolate), as well as their amazing Apothecary collection of herb-packed bars—this is what scratching the dark chocolate "itch" is all about. Avoid any bar under 87 percent if you're still weaning off sugar.

Nature's Sweet Life Dark Chocolate Bars from Nature's Sunshine Products

734-233-5303 • *www.mynsp.com/gerette*

One of the only chocolate bars I know of sweetened with xylitol (my favorite natural sweetener that actually prevents tooth decay). Comes in two varieties—Cardio Raspberry Dark Chocolate and Calcium Crunch Dark Chocolate.

Ross Chocolates No Sugar Added Dark Chocolate

www.carbsmart.com

These maltitol-sweetened (which I prefer over synthetic sweeteners any day), Belgian dark chocolate bars are for discerning chocolate eaters. I love Ross's green tea dark chocolate bar, which contains organic green tea.

Snack bars by Living Fuel, Designs for Health, Think, and BioGenesis Nutraceuticals

www.livingfuel.com • *www.totaltransformation.com*

These very low-glycemic bars are rare because they contain no synthetic sweeteners or fillers. Coco chia (original flavor) bars from Living Fuel are a chocolaty blend of organic coconut and chia seeds, sweetened with TheraSweet (a natural blend of xylitol, tagatose, and probiotics). PaleoBars (I like the chocolate-covered one) are whey and almond butter-based and contain phosphatidyl choline, omega-3s, and glutamine. Think offers many natural, low-impact bars. Ultra Low Carb Bars from BioGenesis are also whey and nut butter-based and full of vitamins and minerals, including chromium. All scratch the chocolaty-chewy "itch" perfectly.

Tearrow Organic Green Tea Chewing Gum

866.4U2.CHEW • *www.tearrowgum.com*

This is the only natural, sugar-free organic green tea gum in the world. In green, black, oolong, jasmine, mint, osmanthus, and lemon-black tea varieties infused with cavity-fighting natural xylitol as a sweetener.

Theo Chocolate

www.theochocolate.com

This new artisan chocolatier is the only American roaster of organic cocoa beans. Its 84 percent cacao Ghana bar is transporting and fair trade-certified. Remember though: if you're just getting off sugar, start with a sugar-free bar, such as Ross's or Nature's Sweet Life.

FOODS AND BEVERAGES

Cooking and Baking Supplies
Coconut Flour and Coconut Fiber from Simply Coconut
www.simplycoconut.com

This is the amazing low-glycemic flour I now do all my baking with at my programs. Your brownies and piecrusts can be made with 100 percent coconut flour. Coconut four and coconut fiber have a high fiber content and have far lower glycemic levels than whole grain flours, and they are much better tasting and lighter than soy or nut flours. Coconut fiber, a sister product, offers a far more pleasant alternative to psyllium fiber (and it's antifungal). Find these and the *Cooking with Coconut Flour* cookbook by Dr. Bruce Fife at the above website.

Decadent Desserts Bake Mixes
www.carbsmart.com • *www.lowcarbdiner.com*

These exceptional low-carb brownies, almond cookies, and cheesecake mixes are sweetened with xylitol, while most others use synthetic sucrolose. Almond flour stands in for wheat flour, giving you great taste without the normal baked goods consequences.

Essential Oils, Food Grade, by Young Living Essential Oils
https://www.youngliving.org/bluesummit

Cooking with essential oils has added an amazingly tasty and healthy new dimension to my culinary creations, both at home and at my programs. My favorite essential oil "spice rack" staples include lemon, nutmeg, peppermint, rosemary, sage, tarragon, fennel, lime, tangerine, clove, and basil essential oils. Add one or two drops of these incredibly powerful oils (don't subject them to high heat) to dressings, sauces, homemade sugar-free ice cream (the peppermint is amazing for that), eggs (tarragon transforms them), and even pumpkin pie. The well-being benefits are a wonderful side effect. You can get these from any YLEO distributor or at the above link.

Flavorings and Extracts by Flavorganics and Frontier Natural Flavors
www.flavorganics.com • *www.frontiercoop.com*

Natural flavorings and extracts like cherry, almond, vanilla, maple, rum, and coconut are some of the best ingredients to use to create tasty sugar-free desserts, beverages, and toppings. I use the maple flavor to make sugar-free (xylitol-sweetened), mashed berry syrup for my low-glycemic French toast, the almond to pump up macaroons, the cherry flavor in seltzer and homemade ice cream, and the rum flavor in healthy eggnog.

Hempola Hemp Seed Flour

www.hempola.com

This is a revolutionary, nutty-tasting, super high in protein (41 percent), gluten-free flour for baking low-impact foods. Blend with other flours (like coconut) for best results.

Mushroom and Truffle-based Sauces and Condiments from FungusAmongUs

www.fungusamongus.com

This line of exotic, wild-crafted mushroom and truffle products includes dried mushrooms, sauces, marinade rubs, soup mixes, and seasonings. Its award-winning Truffle Gatherer's Sauce features hand-picked black truffles from Tuscany, Champignon mushrooms, black olives, capers, yeast extract, olive oil, anchovies, and aroma of truffle. It's magic in my raw hemp seed "risotto."

Nut Flours and Guar Gum by Bob's Red Mill and Now Foods

Available at health food stores, low-glycemic nut flours, such as almond and hazelnut flour, can be used in baking tasty pie crusts, as crumb toppings, or as a coating for fish or chicken. Guar gum is a low-impact alternative to cornstarch for thickening sauces.

Real Salt by Redmond Trading Company

800-367-7258 • *www.realsalt.com*

The American Culinary Institute awarded this natural, untainted, true sea salt its 2004 Best Taste award. From ancient sea bed mines in Utah, Real Salt is a perfectly balanced source of over 50 trace minerals (including iodine), and—because it doesn't cause a sodium-potassium imbalance like typical white salt—it's not been found to raise blood pressure or cause water retention. But beware: other so-called "sea salts" are often still stripped and bleached.

Sauce mixes by Organic Gourmet

800-400-7772 • *www.organic-gourmet.com*

Organic Gourmet's sauce mixes include old-fashioned sauce and gravy mixes, mushroom and miso stocks, and vegetable bouillon cubes without additives like MSG and hydrolyzed vegetable oil. It also carries organic peppercorns and other spice rack staples.

Spices and Seasoning packets by Simply Organic

This company offers organic versions of every spice in your spice rack, all-natural versions of seasoning mixes, like taco and tabouli mix (use shelled hemp seed instead of the bulgar wheat for a low-glycemic version), and even mulling spices (use unsweetened, diluted cranberry juice and stevia for a much healthier "cider"). I almost cried when I found its no-MSG, nonhydrolyzed sloppy joe mix!

See also:"Sweeteners."

Meat, Poultry, Fish, and Dairy

Canned Gourmet Wild Fish by Dave's Gourmet Albacore and G'Day Gourmet

www.davesalbacore.com • www.g-daygourmet.com

Dave's Gourmet Albacore's Santa Cruz, CA-based fishing, canning, and retail operation ships its premium and eco-friendly canned and fresh wild fish from the North Pacific to anywhere in the U.S. Its canned tuna is top-rated by the *New York Times* and, unlike other canned fish, is pressure cooked in the can, preserving much more of the juices and omega-3 fats. G'Day Gourmet's use of herbs and seasonings is what makes its wild-caught, canned skipjack (low-mercury) tuna from Australia unique. Comes in single servings, and there is no refrigeration needed, so it's perfect travel food yet elegant enough for hors d'oeuvres.

Shelton's Free Range Ground Turkey

Find this in natural food stores' freezer sections. I use it in sloppy joes, chili, and my fennel seed tomato sauce (fennel gives it a sweet sausage taste). Shelton's free-range holiday birds (order directly from the company) and turkey jerky are also terrific.

Total Classic Greek Yogurt by Fage

www.fageusa.com

This traditional, strained yogurt is a staple in Greece, and a thick, creamy treat to be enjoyed often on its own or in any sweet or savory dish. I put a dollop on soups and atop spicy meat dishes, or I use it on coconut flour pancakes or to make a parfait with berries and chocolate. As long as you avoid all B.S. foods, this will not put weight on you (skip the reduced-fat ones). Produced without antibiotics or hormones.

U.S. Wellness Meats

877-383-0051 • *www.grasslandbeef.com*

This mail-order source for grass-fed beef, lamb, bison, and organic dairy was sin-gled out two years in a row by the *New York Times* for the superior taste of its steaks. Grass-fed is a completely different meat and cheese experience for your body, providing an omega-3 essential fatty acid profile similar to fish and twice the beta-carotene of grain-fed beef.

Vital Choice Seafood

800-608-4825 • *www.vitalchoice.com*

This is the premier online mail-order source for what is regarded as the highest-quality wild Alaskan salmon and other wild fish. It is a great gift resource, especially if you want to send salmon or lox that is naturally red in color and high in omega fats, as opposed to most farmed salmon that is full of red dyes and devoid of healthy fats.

Nut and Seed Products

Almond and Nut Butters by Maranatha, Once Again, and Futters

Nut butters won't spike your blood sugar. Buy raw when you can for the greatest health benefit. The above are all widely available except Futters (find them at www.futtersnutbutters.com), whose rare varieties include pistacio, walnut, macadamia, and cherry. Its Chocolate-Cherry Almond Haze (as in hazelnut) is obscenely tasty.

Hemp Seed and Hemp Shakes by Nutiva

www.nutiva.com

Amazing, sustainable hemp foods were legalized in the U.S. in 2004 (they never contained THC after all . . .). Hemp seed is unusual because it is grainlike, yet is high in protein, low-glycemic, high in omega fats (3, 6, and 9), and requires no cooking! I use it in pilafs, stuffed peppers, soups and chili, to replace bread crumbs in meatloaf, and even in desserts. It is crucial for vegan and raw diets. Nutiva's award-winning Amazon Acai Hemp Shake combines super-healthy hemp protein and acai fruit in a low-glycemic, very tasty shake. Hemp milk is a new craze, and while it is loads healthier than soy milk, be sure to avoid high sugar content. Remember not to drink down more than about five grams of sugar (always in a creamy drink) at a time.

Nuts, Organic and Germinated, by Living Nutz

www.livingnutz.com

Your health food store will have a good bulk nut section, but if you want to experience germinated nuts (more digestible and nutritious), visit this website and your mouth will water at the descriptions of Italian Herb Almonds, Pesto Walnuts, and Spicy Onion Garlic Pistachios.

Raw Nuts and Seeds by Nature's First Law

www.rawfood.com

Find the best and most affordable selection of truly raw nuts, seeds, and much more here. Information on the raw food lifestyle is also available. Remember, it's easy to spike our blood sugar while eating a lot of typical raw foods, with all the high-impact sweeteners, juices, and dried fruits. Use my principles and you can't go wrong.

Salba

www.totaltransformationstore.com

This chia-related, white seed possesses the highest omega-3 content of any known food, is raw, gluten-free, GMO-free, low-carb, and as versatile as hemp seed, and has many times more of most minerals and vitamins you can think of than the foods that are famous for being highest in those nutrients. I'll warn you about the price, but the serving size is two tablespoons, and you can store this food at room temperature for up to five years. Sprinkle on or in anything, as it will take on the taste of the dish and add a great texture. Thicken or bake with it. Make protein balls with it. The possibilities (and benefits) are endless!

See also: "Nut Flours" under "Cooking and Baking Supplies."

Oils, Organic and Gourmet

Biodynamic Tuscan Olive Oil Imported by Scarangello Company, Inc.

800-871-4741, ext. 00 • *www.etruscanelixirs.com*

This aromatic, spicy olive oil comes from the region known to produce the world's best olive oils. My program participants and I enjoyed a tour and tasting at this producer's pristine orchards during my program in Tuscany.

LaTourangelle Artisan Oils

www.latourangelle.com

This company's award-winning walnut oil (a personal favorite) was voted "Best Food Product" by the *San Francisco Chronicle* in 2005. Its grape seed oil withstands high cooking temperatures while it benefits cholesterol ratios. Its roasted almond, sesame (great in Asian dishes), pecan, pistachio, or hazelnut oils are all great in pesto or on my Decadent Meal Salad (see recipe in chapter 6, page 128).

Mac Nut Oil

This is another versatile, high-temperature cooking oil with a very adaptable, nutty flavor and heart health benefits. Available at health food stores.

Organic and Virgin Coconut Oils from Nutiva, Simply Coconut, and Tropical Traditions

www.nutiva.com • www.tropicaltraditions.com • www.simplycoconut.com

These companies sell the freshest organic virgin coconut oils I've found. Unlike olive and other more delicate oils, coconut oil does not degrade during high-temperature cooking and also offers slimming and energizing MCTs (medium-chain triglycerides) and antifungal and antimicrobial actions in the body. Nutiva also sells high-GLA hemp seed oil.

Pumpkin Seed Oil from North American Herb and Spice

800-243-5242

This oil is so therapeutic that it is sometimes taken as a supplement, but the taste is unbelievable and will make any risotto, salad, or appetizer amazing.

Spectrum Organic Mayonnaise and Shortening

www.spectrumorganics.com

Spectrum's organic olive oil mayonnaise is the only egg-based (as in real) mayo that is not loaded with nonorganic (usually genetically modified) canola oil. Other so-called "health" mayo is soy-based, which is not great for everyone. Spectrum's organic shortening is rare because it's nonhydrogenated. A must-have for health-savvy bakers.

Produce, Organic

Acai Fruit Unsweetened Purée from Sambazon

www.sambazon.com

The trendy acai fruit, or Brazilian palm berry, not only tastes like slightly chocolaty berries, but it also has ten to thirty times the anthocyanidin antioxidants of red wine. The unsweetened purée (avoid the sweetened one) comes frozen and ready to put in your favorite smoothies and sweetener. Recent studies suggest skin and digestive benefits.

Black Soybeans from Eden Organic

Canned soybeans are the only very low-glycemic beans. I prefer the black soybeans in chili, soups, salads, or mashed with garlic and olive oil in place of refried beans.

Goji Berries from White Dragon

707.823.4932 • *www.gojiberryintl.com*

These certified Mongolian goji berries, one of the most nutritious foods in the world, are of the highest quality. I prefer to eat them in creamy foods to keep their impact on blood sugar extremely low. They turn a smoothie or my home-made ice cream into the most gorgeous, colorful treat. Avoid other dried fruits, which are too sweet.

Local or Mail-order Organic Produce at Local Harvest and Diamond Organics

www.localharvest.com • *www.diamondorganics.com*

Farmers markets and local co-ops are the freshest, most environmentally conscious ways to buy organic produce. Local Harvest is an online resource for locating the farmers markets and co-ops nearest you. It is also a clearinghouse of online sources for organic product delivery. Diamond Organics also delivers a vast array of organic produce and products to most areas of the U.S. overnight.

Salad Greens, Organic Packaged, by Grateful Harvest and Earthbound Farm

Convenient, ready-to-eat organic greens in resealable bags found in the produce department can spell the difference between good intentions and follow-through. They make easy work of my Decadent Meal Salad recipe in chapter 6.

Sweeteners, Natural and Low-Glycemic
Erythritol, Powdered, by Now Foods

Powdered erythritol tastes like sugar but has 70 percent of the sweetness, is harmless to the teeth, is easily digested, and safe for diabetics. For those who still obsess about calories (as in those who still battle cravings, which will diminish by using this sweetener), erythritol has zero calories in a teaspoon. Best of all, it has been a part of the human diet for thousands of years.

Sweet Fiber

www.sweetfiber.net

Naturally sweet inulin fiber (from chicory) blended with luo han guo fruit extract makes this a not-too-sweet powder. Three packets provide the same amount of soluble fiber as a serving of oatmeal or a slice of whole wheat bread (without the spike), so it is great for cooking and baking healthier foods.

NuStevia No Carbs Blend and Vanilla Stevia by NuNaturals

800-753-HERB • *www.nunaturals.com*

NuStevia is the best tasting stevia I've tried. Its liquid Vanilla Stevia is made with its artisan Singing Dog vanilla extract from New Guinea rather than the artificial flavors some other vanilla stevia products use. It's fantastic in yogurt and smoothies.

Xylitol by Emerald Forest, NuNaturals, Now Foods, and The Ultimate Life

Xylitol is an amazing, natural, low-glycemic sweetener because of its array of potential health benefits, from inhibiting tooth decay and ear infections to building bones, from stimulating collagen synthesis to inhibiting stress-related tissue breakdown in the body. Use measure for measure like sugar. Not recommended in drinks or large quantities due to its natural laxative effect. The Ultimate Life brand is the birch source for those who prefer that over corn or unknown sources that may be genetically modified.

ZSweet

866-227-9338 • *www.zsweet.com*

This is a nearly perfect, nonglycemic, zero-calorie (for those who are counting), very sugarlike (in both taste and its baking and browning actions), natural sweetener derived from non-GMO corn that won't disrupt your digestion. What more could you want?

SUPPLEMENTS

The most potent beauty supplements in the world rarely bear the word "beauty" on the label or reach the status of the "beauty pills" with cult followings that are sold next to over-priced synthetic skin care products. But make no mistake: a well-chosen beauty supplement regimen based on the support *you* need specifically can transform you like no beauty pill ever could.

SUPPLEMENTS

I learned in a powerful, amazing way how supplements can make all the difference, even once you've done all you can with diet and exercise. Knowing your own needs and going at your own transformation from every angle possible is your ticket to an "extreme makeover" with far greater transforming power and without the disappointment of external or shortsighted extreme measures.

While these are by no means the only great supplements in their categories, the following are undisputed standouts (in many cases one of a kind) and available in fine vitamin stores. The amazing "side effect" you'll experience from transforming yourself physically with these supplements will be improvement to many health issues you might never have otherwise been compelled to address. Please note: the listings and information below are not intended to diagnose or treat disease. Always read the labels for dosages and precautions during pregnancy and enlist your doctor's supervision when addressing health complaints or illness.

Advanced Multi-Nutrient Regimens by Ola Loa, Garden of Life, and New Chapter

www.drinkyourvitamins.com • *www.gardenoflifeusa.com* • *www.new-chapter.com*

Ola Loa's powdered vitamin drink is the most advanced powder multi, for those who can't swallow pills, featuring methylation-enhancing nutrients rarely found in a multi. Garden of Life and New Chapter offer state-of-the-art, fermented, multivitamin, mineral, and herbal formulas with whole-food concentrates, enzymes, and ionic minerals. New Chapter's Every Woman and Every Man are the first organic, whole-food-based multivitamin introduced to the public.

Appetite Suppressants by Health Direct, Gencor Pacific, Inc., Millennium Health, and Kemin Foods

www.healthdirectusa.com • *www.swansonvitamins.com* • *www.hoodiahoodia.com*

Each of the following contains ingredients proven in clinical studies to effectively reduce appetite. I like the oral spray (instantly absorbed) delivery of Health Direct's popular Binge Buster product, which changes taste and aroma responses to foods with hoodia and blood sugar stabilizers. Gencor Pacific's Slimaluma (caralluma fimbriata) extract is powerful, as is Millennium Health's Hoodia—the same

100 percent-pure South African hoodia gordonii featured on CBS News. Kemin's Slendesta is a potato-derived extract that enhances CCK, a satiety compound in the body. If I still had my eating disorder, I'd try all of these for damage control while upgrading to all low-impact foods and taking measures to rebalance every biochemical challenge naturally. The goal is to not need them.

Antiacne Supplements from Clear5 and Skinutrients

www.skinutrients.com • www.acne-vitamins.com

Accunatural Acne Control Factors by Skinutients features Berberine (from barberry), which was found to inhibit the growth of bacteria and reduce sebum production in published research. Clear5 is based on preliminary research into timed-release vitamin B5, which caused remarkable remissions in most cases of acne in a Singapore study.

Antiaging Supplements from Life Extension and PhytoPharmica

www.lef.org • www.phytopharmica.com

Mitochondrial Energizer with SODzyme is one of the most advanced antiaging formulas available. It helps prevent one of the key contributors to aging: mitochondrial decay. Contains the super-antioxidant R-lipoic acid (far more potent than common lipoic acid) and energizing acetyl L-carnitine-arginate (more potent than common carnitine). It also contains carnosine, the glycation-inhibiting di-peptide that reversed various aging markers in animal studies. Ubiquinol CoQ10 is the first highly absorbable, and thus more affordable, form of CoQ10, achieving the same blood level of conventional CoQ10 with one-eighth the dosage. This product caused stunning decreases in typical aging markers in mice in one study. Resveratrol-Forte by PhytoPharmica features the red grape skin component resveratrol, which showed remarkable antiaging effects in animal studies, mimicking the effects of calorie restriction, including blood sugar control. Two capsules equal the resveratrol content of 42 bottles of red wine.

See also:"Antioxidant Catalyst Supplements."

Anticandida Yeast Supplements from Forest Herbs Research

www.kolorex.com

Kolorex by Forest Herbs Research was proven more effective against yeast infections than even oregano oil or olive leaf extracts (both are extremely powerful in their own rights). Kolorex contains Horopito, a botanical from New Zealand.

Anti-Inflammatory Skin Supplements by Himalaya Herbal Healthcare

www.himalayausa.com

DermaCare (internationally known as Vegecort) has been clinically proven to improve a broad range of inflammatory skin problems by supporting the underlying mechanisms behind skin health, including liver and immune health and structural integrity. A complex combination of first-rate Ayurvedic herbs is incorporated.

Anti-Inflammatory Supplements by New Chapter

Zyflammend is one of the most celebrated anti-inflammation supplements, having demonstrated strong anticancer, COX-2-inhibiting, and antioxidant actions in preliminary published research. Because of its state-of-the-art formulation of several of the most powerful anti-inflammatory and antioxidant substances (such as turmeric, ginger, and rosemary), it is one of the most popular supplements among informed supplement users. I am a personal devotee.

Antioxidant Catalyst Supplements by LifeVantage Corporation

www.protandim.com

Beyond ORAC-rated antioxidants, Protandim is a next-generation antioxidant "catalyst" (a proprietary blend of botanicals and extracts) proven to trigger a dramatic increase in SOD and CAT enzymes, thus offering thousands of times the protection of conventional ingested antioxidants.

Antioxidant Skin-Protective Supplements from AstaVita

www.astavita.com

Skin Defense System from AstaVita contains AstaReal, the most industry-respected form of the super-antioxidant astaxanthin that has been found to protect the cells from free radical damage. It also contains other carotenoids, including lutein (recently proven to protect the skin from the effects of the sun) and tocotrienols, a powerful form of vitamin E.

Antiviral Skin Supplements from Diamond Herpanicine

www.diamondformulas.com

This supplement addresses the viral and immune function that affects outbreaks of cold sores and other skin problems. Contains Lysine and immune-strengthening astragalus and echinacea, among other effective herbs.

Antiwrinkle Supplements by Ferrosan, Injuv, CosmedeX

www.imedeen.us • *www.dermasilk.org*

Imedeen's Time Perfection and Prime Renewal supplements by Ferrosan are clinically proven to improve structure, density, and moisture levels while diminishing fine lines and wrinkles, unwanted pigmentation, and dilated capillaries, and it features its Biomarine Complex from deep sea fish protein, as well as a proprietary grape seed extract and lycopene blends. Prime Renewal increased skin density an average of 20.9 percent in post-menopausal women after six months of use. Injuv hyalouronic acid supplements may actually build up the skin's inner "moisture sponge"—and do the same for joints. The ingredients in DermaSilk Anti-Wrinkle by CosmedeX were shown to promote skin firmness and elasticity and increase collagen production via SOD, algae extract, tocotrienols, collagen, carnosine, and benfotiamine.

Beauty Supplements (Specialty) by Santica Beauty Recipes and Lane Labs

www.nutritionwholesalers.com • *www.compassionet.com*

The Santica Beauty Recipes Line is a truly impressive, Italian-researched array of cutting-edge supplements (and some topicals) for acne, wrinkles, and even cellulite and couperose. The acne formula, for example, addresses DHT (a form of testosterone found to play a part in treatment-resistant acne). The blueberry bioflavanoids and horse chestnut in the couperose formula work to desensitize capillaries. Each is backed by solid research. Clinical research shows that Toki from Lane Labs, a lemon-flavored "skin" drink, increases collagen levels in the blood and significant reduction of lines and age spots. Also, anecdotal evidence is compelling for its effects in plumping up the skin. Takes approximately forty-five days to show effects. Toki Color from Lane Labs has been shown to support melanocyte production, which is responsible for forming pigment in the hair color.

Beauty Injectibles and Homeopathics by GUNA Biotherapeutics

www.gunainc.com

A leading homeopathic company in Italy, Guna expanded its cutting-edge offerings in both homeopathy and mesotherapy into the United States in 2000, with the latter soon to be offered through doctors and medical spas. These treatments target beauty- and antiaging-specific conditions, chronic and acute. Learn more at its website.

SUPPLEMENTS

SUPPLEMENTS

Berry and Green Tea Concentrates (liquid) by Pure Inventions and Chi Tea
www.pureinventions.com

These travel-friendly, concentrated liquid blends, such as Pomegranate with Acai Berry, can be added to bottled water for an upgrade to sweet bottled juices. Both lines offer several green tea-based, caffeine-free, needs-targeted blends.

Blood Sugar Formulas by AML, Himalaya Herbal Healthcare, and NuNaturals
www.advancedmetaboliclabs.com • *www.himalayausa.com* • *www.nunaturals.com*

Advanced AML Select is a state-of-the-art, blood sugar-therapeutic, multi-nutrient line created by metabolic pioneer Dr. Ron Rosedale. GlucoCare (known internationally as Glucosim) by Himalaya is a clinically proven Ayurvedic herbal formula shown to stabilize blood sugar, cholesterol, and triglyceride levels, and it even did so in diabetics and those with high cholesterol. LevelRight by NuNaturals is a comprehensive mix of proven blood sugar normalizers, including gymnema, cinnamon bark, and banaba leaf extracts, two forms of chromium, and alpha lipoic acid.

Breast Health Supplements by Brevail, Nature's Way, and Schiff

Brevail is the first breast health supplement based on lignans, which is shown to decrease breast cancer risk by docking into estrogen receptors and providing weaker estrogenic messages, while blocking harmful, stronger ones. DIM-plus, from Nature's Way, contains diindolylmethane, a phytonutrient found in cruciferous vegetables that has been shown to increase the level of favorable estrogens while reducing levels of less favorable ones. Breast Health by Schiff contains detoxifying D-Glucarate, shown to offer some protection against breast cancer.

Bone Support Supplements by Lane Labs and Jarrow Formulas
800-510-2010 • *www.compassionet.com*

Advacal from Lane Labs is the only calcium supplement proven at this writing to increase bone density in the critical spine. Jarrow Formulas' BioSil was clinically shown to have superior benefit over other types of silica sources, such as horsetail and colloidal silica, and was proven to stimulate collagen synthesis and bone-building cells (osteoblasts).

Carb- and Fat-Blocking Supplements by Natrol and Swanson Ultra
www.swansonvitamins.com
Supplements containing the carb-blocking ingredient Phase 2 (many brands feature it) are key transitional tools for anyone seeking assistance with blood sugar metabolism or recovery from carb addiction, though you won't need them once your cravings are gone. Phase 2 products (by many names, such as Carb Intercept, Carb Blocker, etc.) block the enzyme that converts starches to sugar, so they are largely passed through the body. Ultra Carb Control C-120X (available through Swanson) is by far the strongest carb-blocking product. As far as the need for fat blockers goes, when one eats the way I recommend, gaining weight from fat ceases to be an issue. But during the first week or so of transition to becoming a fat-burner, chitosan products (by Swanson and others) really help. They do what the first over-the-counter (formerly prescription-only) pharmaceutical fat-blocking drug did, only naturally. Chitosan is shellfish derived, so steer clear if you're allergic.

Female Hormonal Support by Dr. Susan Lark, Futurebiotics, and StopFlash USA
www.drlark.com • www.totaltransformation.com • www.stopflash-usa.com
Dr. Lark's Daily Balance PMS, Hot Flash, and Menorrhagia (heavy menstruation) supplements are cutting edge. Progest E, a natural progesterone in a spray, is also available. Futurebiotics' EstroComfort menopausal balancing complex is one of the only comprehensive formulas incorporating the most researched hormone balancers, along with the L-theanine, and the powerful anti-hot flash substance, gamma oryzanol. StopFlash is an instantly absorbed spray incorporating proven anti-hot flash ingredients and essential oils.

Fiber Products by Genesis Today and Simply Coconut
www.genesistoday.com • www.simplycoconut.com
4Fiber by Genesis Today provides powerfully effective nutritive fiber and probiotic and antifungal support with zero harshness. Coconut fiber is a new fiber that is similarly effective to psyllium, but has a better taste and blends better with food, as well as having the additional antifungal characteristics of coconut.

Fish and Cod Liver Oils and Skin Health Supplements from Nordic Naturals
800-662-2544 • *www.nordicnaturals.com*
Nordic Naturals is the highest-grade and best-tasting overall fish oil product that I've found. Nordic won the "Best Choice" award from Environmental Defense, an

environmental organization, as well as a "Best Taste" award for its cod liver oil from the American Culinary Institute. In addition to the head-to-toe benefits of fish oil, Nordic's Skin Synergy supplement and GLA-containing fish oils successfully target a wide range of skin issues.

Green Foods from Garden of Life, New Chapter, Herbs, Etc., and SGN Nutrition
www.vitaminshoppe.com

Unless you're getting dark greens twice a day, green supplements are smart insurance. Perfect Food by Garden of Life contains among the highest amounts of superfoods and antioxidant complexes, while Berry Greens by New Chapter leads the way in non-grass sources of organic greens and the most nutrient-dense berries, all fermented in probiotics for superior digestability. ChlorOxygen from Herbs, Etc., is the most concentrated liquid chlorophyll (oxygenating and blood-building) on the market. Emerald Balance blends traditional green foods along with hair, skin, and nail nutrients like silica.

Hair Growth Formulas by Alphactif, Hair Genesis, Viviscal, and BioMed Health
www.alphactif.com • www.hairgenesis.net • www.viviforyou.com • www.biomed-health.com

The Alphactif Nutritif supplement from France was clinically proven to dramatically reduce hair loss, increase growth, and strengthen hair more than 300 percent after three months. Hair Genesis, a DHT-inhibiting supplement, worked as well as prescription hair-loss drugs without the side effects in a double-blind, placebo-controlled study. Viviscal showed effectiveness against alopecia areata as well as androgenic hair loss in several published studies via a marine concentrate which changes the tissues surrounding the hair follicle, re-establishing the passage of key nutrients required for hair growth. Bao Shi Restorative Hair Nutrients is a comprehensive formula of both Chinese as well as Ayurvedic herbs used traditionally for hair growth and color restoration. See also "Hair Loss Topicals" in the following section.

Hair, Skin, and Nail Supplements (General Support) from BioSil and Megafood
www.megafood.com • www.jarrow.com

BioSil is the most bio-available form of silicon, which not only has body-wide connective tissue benefits, but also increases collagen content in the skin, strengthens nails, and strengthens the hair by improving keratin integrity. Skin,

Nails, and Hair DailyFoods by MegaFood provides 100 percent whole food forms of key nutrients such as silica, sulfur, licorice, and GLA for superior absorption.

Liver Support from Himalaya Herbal Healthcare

LiverCare (internationally known as Liv.52) from Himalaya, with 182 clinical studies proving efficacy, is the number one-selling liver formula in the world. Proven to buffer the liver from a variety of challenges and shown to outperform milk thistle in at least one study; had I known about it when I was having my liver crisis I might have even recovered from it sooner.

Mood Support from CraniYums, FTH, New Chapter, and Next Pharmaceuticals

www.craniyums.com • www.fth-inc.com • www.vitaminshoppe.com
CraniYums offers "feel-good" brain chemical support lozenges, as do the pharmaceutical-grade L-tryptophan, L-theanine, L-tyrosine (precursor to dopamine), and other amino acid supplements from FTH. New Chapter's "supercritical extract" of Holy basil is the most potent form on the market. Both Holy basil and Relora, from Next Pharmaceuticals (though marketed under many brands), reduce cortisol and anxiety by different mechanisms and can be used together. If you are seeking solutions to depression and anxiety, ask your doctor about these options.

Weight Loss Support from NSP, Enzymatic Therapy, and Garden of Life

www.mynsp.com/gerette • www.pharmaca.com
Nature's Cortisol Formula is a phenomenal combination for weight loss, antiaging, and stress reduction. This product not only combats stress with top ingredients Holy basil, I-theanine, and Relora, but it also contains top blood sugar-stabilizing ingredients such as banaba leaf, chromium, vanadium, and DHEA. Naturalean with 7-Keto (a form of DHEA) by Enzymatic Therapy contains thyroid-supportive nutrients, which demonstrated profound weight loss in placebo-controlled studies. FucoTHIN by Garden of Life is the first nonstimulant supplement to be shown effective at increasing thermogenisis (fat burning) in human clinical trials.

NKO Neptune Krill Oil from Jarrow Formulas and Source Naturals

Neptune Krill Oil has been shown to promote cellular integrity and cardiovascular function. It supports nerve, brain, and joint function, healthy skin, and even helps with PMS issues.

Probiotics by Ganeden, Essential Formulas, and Jarrow Formulas

These probiotic products are recognized leaders. Ganeden's Sustenex and Digestive Advantage feature superior ability to maintain potency throughout the digestive process, and there is clinical proof showing benefits for IBS and more. Dr. Ohhira's Probiotics 12 Plus, by Essential Formulas, is the only probiotic containing the E. faecalis TH 10 strain of lactic acid bacteria, shown to be 6.25 times stronger than any other known bacteria. Fermented for five years, it requires no refrigeration. Jarrow's Jarro-Dophilus+EPS is room temperature stable and features 8 different strains of bacteria, while its Fem Dophilus is the only oral probiotic clinically documented to restore healthy vaginal flora and support a healthy urogenital tract.

Seaweed and Algae Supplements from Sun Wellness, Spa Technologies, and E3Live

www.vitaminshoppe.com • www.spatechnologies.com • www.E3Live.com

These detoxifying supplements contain high amounts of chlorophyll, minerals, protein, vitamin B12, and other nutrients lacking in most (particularly vegetarian) diets. Sun Wellness' chlorella is the highest in chlorophyll. It, along with seaweed supplements, such as those from Spa Technologies, is known to remove heavy metals from the body. Seaweed, offered by Spa Technologies, also has strong detoxifying and remineralizing properties that can be absorbed from pure micronized external products and baths. E3Live is the only raw, very potent liquid algae (from Klamath Lake in Oregon).

Thyroid Support from MegaFood Nutritional Therapeutix and World Organic

www.megafood.com • www.vitaminshoppe.com

Thyroid Strength from MegaFood is the most comprehensive, quality thyroid support I've come across, from a company that pioneered food-based supplements. It contains not only the tyrosine and iodine-rich, food-form herbs, but also ashwagandha extract and other metabolic boosters. Liquid Kelp from World Organic is a valuable tool for anyone with a challenged thyroid. Work with your doctor to try natural tools first.

Varicose Vein Support from Futurebiotics, Nutrica, and Planetary Formulas

www.totaltransformationstore.com • www.venarin.com

VeinFactors by Futurebiotics incorporates citrus rinds, gotu kola, and horse chestnut to provide clinically proven support for normal vein function. Horse chestnut seed extract has been proven to reduce varicose veins and ankle circumference in those with chronic venous insufficiency (varicose veins). It also includes diosmin, which has been shown to help maintain blood vessel tone and support healthy circulation. Venarin by Nutrica features the most studied botanicals for vein health, including Japonese pagoda tree extract, horse chestnut, vitamin K, butcher's broom, and grape seed extract to strengthen vein walls, normalize their permeability, and improve microcirculation. A corresponding topical product is recommended. Full Spectrum Horse Chestnut by Planetary Formulas is the most potent horse chestnut product I've found. Pycnogenol, available from many brands at most health food stores, reduced the swelling associated with chronic venous insufficiency (varicose veins) better than the drug Daflon in a controlled Italian study.

Whey Powders (Raw Milk) from Mercola.com and Mt. Capra Products

www.mercola.com • www.beyondprobiotics.net
Whey protein is one of the best and lowest-impact ways to start your day, either in a smoothie or stirred into plain organic yogurt with berries. It has proven satiety, detoxification, blood sugar-stabilizing, and breast cancer-fighting effects. Dr. Joseph Mercola's preferred Whey Healthier Protein Meal raw milk whey product is from untreated cows, making it rare in its range of nutritional and immune-boosting benefits. Bonus: it's sweetened with xylitol. Mt. Capra Mineral Whey is another raw milk whey but from goat milk, and it is regarded as one of the best whey products for its easy digestibility and super high mineral content.

SKIN CARE

The endless array of new, high-performance, natural (or nearly-natural) skin and personal care products is both exciting and overwhelming for professionals and laymen alike. The following standout products correspond with my tough criteria for purity and potency and include the hard-to-find ingredients in my charts and guidelines throughout this book. I've attempted to hit a broad price range for most categories and have chosen to feature only the most active-strength delivery of the most effective ingredients in the purest formulas available. Feel free to mix, match, and (for best results) layer these products to take advantage of the complementary actions of different natural compounds. Most are free of mineral oil, perfumes, stripping detergents,

SKIN CARE

synthetic colors, and synthetic preservatives (which is why you usually don't see the most famous brands listed). Products containing nanoparticles don't require label disclosure at this writing, so I've done my best to avoid them here until they are better researched and understood, but some companies are keeping them secret. The best policy is to ask the manufacturer if they are used. There is DMAE in a few of these products. While the more recent study showing cell damage is not conclusive, you can make that call yourself. Review all product ingredients yourself before investing in skin care. I can't list all ingredients here. When straying from this list, keep in mind that some organic products may not be as clean as a product where each ingredient listed is natural. A certified organic product is only required to be 70 percent organic, and the remainder can be synthetic. And remember that if companies get sold, their ingredients often change, so keep reading the labels closely!

Acne and Oily-Skin Products

Acne Soothing Lotion, Neem Oil, and Kapha Essential Oil by Pratima Skincare

www.pratimaskincare.com

Dr. Pratima Raichur's Ayurvedic Acne Soothing Lotion contains essential oils to heal infections and skin irritations. Neem oil has unique antimicrobial properties. Kapha Essential Oil blend is designed to balance the Kapha skin type, which is often oily and blemish prone. Learn more at her website or from her book listed in Suggested Reading.

Acne Spot Treatment by Osea

www.oseaskin.com

Osea Essential Corrective Complex, a super-potent, 30 percent essential-oil blend of tea tree, rosemary, grapefruit, lavender, white thyme, and juniper, is 100 percent natural and creates a calming, antibacterial, nondrying acne treatment. Cypress may help heal broken capillaries. Vitamin E promotes healing of scarred and damaged skin. It also relieves cold sores and insect bites.

Balancing Elixir by Zia Natural Cosmetics

800-334-7546 • *www.zianatural.com*

Tea tree, lavender, and clary sage essential oils in a rosemary hydrosol help balance and treat excess oil production. MSM speeds the skin's natural detoxification.

Blemish Remover and Cleansing Gel by Naturopathica

800-669-7618 • *www.naturopathica.com*

Moss Mask Blemish Remover purifies blemishes and eliminates redness without destroying the beauty of the skin, using potent antibacterial extracts of comfrey, sage, rosemary, chamomile, and moss. Its Aloe Cleansing Gel purifies oily skin without stripping its lipid barrier.

Clear Skin Serum with Azelaic Acid by MyChelle Dermaceuticals

800-447-2076 • *www.mychelleusa.com*

Azelaic acid (one of the best tolerated, yet most powerful acne treatments), niacinamide, totorol (a lesser known but super effective acne fighter), retinol, d-biotin, and hydrolyzed yeast protein make up just a part of this comprehensive, A-list acne treatment.

Grapefruit Complexion Mist by Burt's Bees

Essential oils of lemon, lime, and grapefruit help balance overactive oil glands, while rosemary helps clear trouble spots. Contains only lime oil, lemon oil, rosemary oil, and grapefruit oil.

Happy Skin Light Box by Verilux

800-786-6850 • *www.verilux.net*

Recent studies in the United Kingdom suggest that isolated red- and blue-light wavelengths help mild to moderate acne by killing bacteria and reducing inflammation. Verilux guarantees results in twelve weeks.

Lotion for Problem Skin with Tea Tree Oil by Arboretum

877-767-9367 • *www.arboretum-skincare.com*

This lotion contains conifer-needle extract, tea tree oil, and Sea Buckthorn oil. It has been shown to have anti-inflammatory and antimicrobial effects, reduce pore size, and regulate sebum while improving the acid-mantle supportive barrier function of the skin with phospholipids.

Naturally Clear All-Natural Acne-Fighting System

888-24-CLEAR • *www.naturallyclear.com*

This impressive, research-based, inside-out system uses a multivitamin emphasizing zinc, chromium, and selenium, while its topical products include a unique, nonstripping cleanser, spray, and blemish stick with niacinamide, l-lysine, aloe,

SKIN CARE

and PCA. Topical 4 percent niacinamide (Vitamin B3) was shown to reduce certain types of acne in a 4 percent gel.

Normalizing Day Oil by Dr. Hauschka

www.pharmaca.com • *www.drhauschka.com*

This sebum-balancing oil blend includes St. John's wort and neem to calm irritation, slow oil production, and refine pores.

Skin Healing Gel by Youthful Essentials

877-916-1212 • *www.youthfulessentials.com*

Combines carnosine, detoxifying MSM, and vitamin D to speed the healing of skin lesions, acne, burns, and cold sores and to reduce large pores.

See also:"Inflammatory Skin Problems."

All Skin Type Products

Basic (Great) Moisturizers by Jason and Kiss My Face

www.vitaminshoppe.com • *www.dermstore.com*

Tea Time from Jason Natural Cosmetics is one of my favorite photo shoot moisturizers because everyone loves how it feels on their skin and no one ever reacts with it. With green tea, algae, aloe, squalene, polyphenols, and the super antioxidant SOD, it's quite therapeutic. My other photo shoot moisturizer is Kiss My Face's Under Age Ultra Hydrating Moisturizer from its Obsessively Organic line. It smells unbelievable because of the honeysuckle extract and rose oil. GLA-rich borage oil calms and protects skin from water loss.

Body Polishes by Trillium Herbal Company and Zia Natural Cosmetics

www.trilliumherbal.com • *www.zianatural.com*

Brown Sugar Body Buff by Zia incorporates brown sugar and sea salt, with organic clover honey, sea kelp, and algae extracts that soften and nourish the skin. Trillium's Body Polishes are made with Pacific sea salt and phospholipid liposomes to hydrate and maintain the skin's lipid barrier, and cold-pressed olive and essential oils, such as cedar leaf and rosemary, give you amazingly soft skin.

Foot Care Products from Gilden Tree and Betty K

www.gildentree.com • *www.vitaminlife.com*

Gilden Tree knows feet, and knows the spa experience. Its luxurious shea butter-based foot creams and beautiful terra-cotta foot scrubbers are topnotch (the latter also supports children of Pakistan through the women who make the scrubbers). Its blow-up foot baths and reflexology marble dry foot "bath," along with its luxurious organic cotton velour and waffle robes, have been staples at my own programs and top spas for years. Betty K's New Feet is a fantastic lecithin- and papaya-based foot "tenderizer" that softens calluses and corns for gradual removal with daily use.

Masks by Reviva Labs, Astara, Eminence, and Spa Technologies

www.revivalabs.com • *www.dermstore.com* • *www.spatechnologies.com*
Another great, green papaya-based mask that exfoliates with enzymes from green papaya, rather than irritating acids, is the Hydrogen Peroxide Instant Oxygen Mask with Green Papaya by Reviva Labs. It is terrific for drier or lifeless skin. Astara is famous for its super-natural mask, "dynasty." Its green papaya, activated sea mineral, and nourishing vitamin mask (with phosophlipids) are my favorites. Eminence Organics of Hungary has an unbelievable, nearly edible but deceptively powerful array of fresh, concentrated, specifically targeted plant-based masks with no synthetics. Finally, if you want to understand what a real seaweed mask is all about, try any of the 100 percent pure and potent masks from Spa Technologies.

Massage and Bath Oils by Nature's Formulary, Erbaviva, and Young Living

www.naturesformulary.com • *www.erbaviva.com*
www.youngliving.org/bluesummit
Because essential oils should be enjoyed often via massage, baths, skin care, and even in cooking (food-grade oils only) and cleaning, affordable products of high quality are key. Nature's Formulary offers affordable authentic Ayurvedic massage and bath oil blends (and much more), such as its popular Calming oil, with sandalwood, jasmine, frankincense, and more, in a sesame, jojoba, and wheat germ base (recommended for all skin types). Erbaviva's products are a bit pricier, but are the most elegantly prepared bath oil, mother-to-be, and spa gifts you can buy. Young Living Essential Oils are widely considered the purest essential oils in the world and offer myriad uses for blending yourself. Ranging widely in price, most oils are so powerful they go a very long way and need to be dispersed in a carrier oil (such as sesame), though some, such as lavender, can be sprinkled directly into the bath or used on the skin full strength.

SKIN CARE

SKIN CARE

Petroleum Jelly Upgrades by Alba and Jing Jang

www.totaltransformationstore.com • *www.jing-jang.com*

Un-petroleum Jelly by Alba Botanicals is a petroleum jelly alternative made from plant oils, with none of the skin function-inhibiting and pore-blocking consequences of petroleum jelly. Jing-Jang Crème is a higher grade and moister healing balm to use anywhere to calm, soothe, and protect the skin.

Seaweed Balancing and Detoxifying Treatments from Spa Technologies

800-998-8728 • *www.spatechnologies.com*

The Women's Balancing Formula features calcium- and magnesium-rich seaweeds in both supplements and an amazingly pure (no fillers or perfumes) bath that is literally an ionic mineral supplement for the body, and it's scented only with essential oils. Completing the program is the Drainage Oil with hormone-balancing sage and juniper for bloating. The Seaweed Vital Energy program steps up lymph drainage with fuccoidan and laminaria capsules (high in iodine, removes heavy metals, and supports breast health), Firming Cream with bio-fermented algae targets cellulite, and Anti-fluid gel helps with lower leg swelling.

Shaving Products by Total Shaving Solution and The Art of Shaving

www.totalshavingsolution.com • *www.theartofshaving.com*

Total Shaving Solution is the best unisex shaving product I've found. Carefully formulated carrier and essential oils soften hair or beard, soothe skin, and are super-economical because you use only a drop in water. Reduces irritation and bumps. Great all-purpose travel oil. The Art of Shaving's Ingrown Hair Night Cream releases ingrown hairs, soothes skin, and smoothes razor bumps overnight with gentle exfoliation and anti-inflammatory white willow bark and other ingredients while essential oils keep bacteria in check. It's the natural upgrade from yucky, mineral oil-based ingrown hair lotions.

Soap-Free Facial Cleansing Products by Aubrey Organics and Wonder Cloth

www.aubrey-organics.com • *www.wondercloth.com*

Unless you have acne, a facial cleanser is one thing you should never spend a lot of money on. Fancy antiaging cleansers are a waste of money since they are a wash-off product. The trick is in finding a product that doesn't destroy your skin's natural balance. A nonfoaming cleanser from Aubrey Organics, such as its Seaware and Rosa Mosqueta or Green Tea cleansing products, will do the trick perfectly.

The Wonder Cloth is an unusual plant fiber and cotton cloth alternative to microfiber cloths that you can use with or without cleanser to thoroughly clean your face. It exfoliates gently, removes makeup without remover, and—here's the miracle—rinses stain-free with only water.

Makeup Remover by Reviva Labs

www.revivalabs.com

Aromatherapy Eye and Lip Makeup Remover by Reviva Labs is carrot oil in a base of sweet-almond and wheat-germ oil—an effective and nourishing makeup removal that won't disrupt the lipid barrier of the delicate eye area.

Soaps and Body Washes by Kiss My Face, Terressentials, and Earthlight Organics

www.kissmyface.com • *www.terressentials.com* • *www.earthlightorganics.com*

Classic Olive Oil Soap by Kiss My Face is a 150-year-old formula containing 86 percent olive oil. Switching to this super-affordable soap from typical soaps makes a huge difference in skin health and comfort. Avoid the scented variety. Cool Mint Body Wash by Terressentials is the most herbally decadent and potent real mint wash I've found. Zero synthetics, yet far more affordable than fake, bath boutique-chic, perfume-laden "natural" products that actually cause problems. Great summer coolant for body and for tired, burning feet. "Rubb It In" soaps from Earthlight Organics are the most luxurious (and expensive, but worth it) soaps I've found. Wrapped in elegant foil, they bear a "nutrition panel." What's inside is even more impressive: the purest, most prized cold-processed, "live" organic oils, like cranberry, carrot seed, black seed, and blueberry seed, infused with an incredible array of essential oils or even Kombucha. They're wonderful for dry or troubled skin and for shaving.

Baby Products

Amikole's Baby Butter

877-576-2825 • *www.sheabutter.net*

Amikole's beautifully packaged blend contains blue chamomile, lavender, melissa, and geranium for a barrier protector, a calming skin effect, and scent.

Desert Essence Baby Talc-Free Powder

800-439-5506 • *www.desertessence.com*

Contains blue cypress to calm irritated skin.

SKIN CARE

Erbaviva Baby, Pregnancy, and Personal Care Products

877-372-2848 • *www.erbaviva.com*

The most elegant line I have seen for new babies and their mothers, or anyone who loves amazing oils, body and room sprays, and sensitive-skin bath products. Gift sets for mothers-to-be and lavender and oatmeal washing sachets for baby are as beautiful as they are healthful.

Seventh Generation Baby Wipes

Cleanse with pure aloe instead of propylene glycol and synthetic fragrance. Better for removing makeup and cleansing the entire face than 95 percent of the cleansers out there.

Color Cosmetics, High-End Mineral-Based

The following cosmetics do not contain coal-tar colors, petrochemicals, or perfumes in their products. All powder mineral makeup has SPF of 18 to 20, is anti-inflammatory, and won't clog the pores. Every color can be worn anywhere on the face. Many "me-too" mineral lines are popping up. These are some pioneers.

Annemarie Borlind

800-447-7024 • *www.borlind.com*

Better foundations and mascaras in beautiful colors like Laguna (a gorgeous turquoise) and gold-tinged, creamy concealers that I use on photo shoots.

Bare Escentuals

800-227-3990 • *www.bareescentuals.com*

This is the widest selection of loose mineral eye shadows, both matte and shimmery. Any color you could want.

Dr. Hauschka

www.pharmaca.com • *www.drhauschka.com*

These cosmetics are biodynamically produced (the highest form of sustainable agriculture) and elegantly packaged. They offer some great colors and skin formulas. I particularly like the golden peachy blush. Julia Roberts is a Hauschka fan.

Ecco Bella

www.eccobella.com

Beautiful shadow and blush colors. An excellent, newer bronzer, Sunflower, is exactly like a tan and could work for men. All the lipsticks contain organic chamomile, calendula, and jojoba. Flower wax is what makes these products luxurious. They also have very good concealer that gets the shades right.

Gabriel and ZuZu Luxe Cosmetics by Gabriel

800-439-5506 • *www.mothernature.com*

The glosses, such as Diva, are the perfect nude colors that don't leave you looking washed out. And the gloss really lasts—an impressive feat, especially with no synthetics.

Hemp Organics

877-524-4367 • *www.colorganics.net*

I love the new 97 percent organic Karma Gloss line from this company, particularly the Nirvana and Calm shades. Paradise is a vivid plumish-magenta that, when dotted on the center of an otherwise neutral lip, can really enliven the face. The hemp and castor oil-based lipsticks and lip pencils come in great, wearable colors. Crimson is an amazing blackberry-tinged, juicy burgundy lipstick that has made an impression with models.

Jane Iredale

www.janeiredaledirect.com

This is the highest-end, most color- and texture-savvy, truly full line of mineral makeup I've found out there. Recommended by plastic surgeons and makeup artists alike. The pressed and loose mineral powder foundations come in the global, golden tones makeup artists like myself prefer. The taupe eye pencil, terracotta lip pencil, and Ripe Plum mascara and liquid liners are must-haves. The Circle Delete #1 concealer duo has the perfect fair shades and creamy texture. The Brush Me Bronze delivers sparkle-free, authentic looking tan from a high-end automatic brush that simultaneously shields skin from UVA and UVB rays. The lip gloss in Melon is a "shot of optimism" I've used for the runway and on photo shoots. Jane's men's line, H/E, offers bronzers that also give coverage, so men can cover skin flaws and get SPF protection without feeling girlie!

SKIN CARE

Lavera

877-528-3727 • *www.lavera-usa.com*

Its award-winning organic lip glosses contain berry extracts, and its beautiful blue-toned pencils look great on blue eyes.

Sevi Cosmetics

www.sevicosmetics.com

Sevi has got some fresh innovations with mineral-based, vegan makeup. My favorite is her "Coffee with an Attitude" eyeshadow solids that can be used for brows, or lining and shadowing the eyes in rich warm (Java) and bitter (Mocha) brown shades.

Dark Spots and Patches

Pigment Correction Products by Sircuit Skin and CamoCare

www.sircuitskin.com

Brilliance serum by Sircuit Skin comes just in time for the removal of most hydroquinone products from the market. This skin-lightening serum provides a safe alternative, with 4 percent l-arbutin and 2 percent lactic acid. It's also fortified with neem leaf extract (a newly discovered brightener) and lemon peel extract.

Raised Sun Spot Smoother by Lane Labs

800-526-3005 • *www.lanelabs.com*

SunSpot, ES is the only product I know that can eliminate raised, rough sun-damaged spots while leaving healthy skin alone. Requires four to six weeks' daily compliance, and skin will feel irritated—but only the unhealthy tissue—before it is sloughed off. Always have spots checked and supervised by your dermatologist.

See also: BIOSKINCARE under "Scars and Stretchmarks."

Dry Skin Products

Dry Skin Creams by Aubrey Organics, Weleda, and Jurlique

www.vitaminshoppe.com • *www.jurlique.com*

Lumessence moisturizer and eye cream from Aubrey Organics (available at most health food stores) contain dry skin delicacies like phospholipids, liposomes, hyaluronic acid, seaweed, rosa mosqueta rose hip seed oil, and proline at a price similar to creams that are all packaging and no substance. Skin Food by Weleda is a pure, biodynamically produced cream for super-dry areas that can be applied to body, face, or lips. Contains pansy extract, chamomile, calendula, and the finest rich oils. Jurlique Day Care Face Cream is an extremely decadent, hydrating infusion full of dozens of first-rate extracts and regenerators.

Nondrying Cleansers from Aubrey Organics and Burt's Bees

www.aubrey-organics.com • www.burtsbees.com

Spending a lot on cleansers will get you into trouble with dry skin, as most expensive cleansers (and drug store brands) are full of synthetic emollients and irritants that ultimately dry the skin. Aubrey's Seaware and Rosa Mosqueta cleansing cream is extremely luxurious for the price, with fine rose hip oil, seaweed, and non-GMO soy protein, and zero irritating synthetics. Orange Essence Facial Cleanser from Burt's Bees is an award-winning, heavenly smelling, olive oil-based cleanser that really works.

Skin Barrier-Rebuilding Serums from Arbonne International and Zia

Bio-Hydria Naturesomes by Arbonne International is a phospholipid serum that is applied under moisturizer. Zia Natural Cosmetics Replenishing Elixir contains phospholipids, MSM aids repair of damaged skin, and neroli hydrosol hydrates.

See also: Petroleum Jelly Upgrades and Masks under "All Skin Type Products."

See also: "Wrinkle Products."

Anti-Inflammatory Skin Products

Aloe Vera Skin Gels by AloeLife and Aubrey Organics

www.aloelife.com • www.aubrey-organics.com

Skin Gel Ultimate Skin Treatment by AloeLife is the quintessential, powered-up aloe gel product for sunburns, skin flare-ups, shaving, and skin renewal. Features the highest-quality whole-leaf aloe concentrate, as well as vitamins A, E, C, and extracts of chamomile and comfrey. Not your grandma's aloe! Aubrey Organics also has a good, pure, organic product available at most health food stores. Keep it in the fridge.

Antibacterial Topicals from Nutribiotic, Manu Nutraceuticals, and Aidance

www.vitaminshoppe.com • www.manuka-skincare.com • www.tetrasil.com

These products can spare you the risks of using synthetic antibacterials, since natural antibacterials have not been found to give rise to resistant bacteria strains.

SKIN CARE

Skin Ointment by Nutribiotic contains powerfully antibacterial grapefruit seed extract and tea tree oil, along with healing l-lysine, echinacea, bee propolis, honey, cajeput oil, calendula, and goldenseal in a natural base. Manu Nutraceuticals' Active Manuka UMF® Honey and East Cape manuka oil from the New Zealand manuka plant offer powerful antibacterial and antifungal properties for a wide range of uses, including acne, rosacea, eczema, athlete's foot, scalp conditions, and more. Tetrasil, by Aidance, skin and feminine care creams feature a proprietary silver oxide compound shown to have broad-spectrum antimicrobial effects. All of these are bathroom cabinet staple-worthy.

Cortisone Cream Alternatives by Boericke & Tafel, Herbalab, and CamoCare

www.vitaminshoppe.com • *www.herbalab.com* • *www.camocare.com*

Herbacort by Herbalab Products has been formulated to achieve powerful anti-inflammatory effects without steroids. Called a cortisone alternative by the manufacturer, Florasone and Psoriaflora creams by Boericke & Tafel Homeopathics are clinically proven to significantly reduce the itching and flaking of rashes, allergies, and psoriasis. Consistent use of CamoCare Soothing Cream may result in the clearing of your rash. The German camillosan chamomile featured in CamoCare products has been shown to be a powerful anti-inflammatory.

Climatotherapy for Psoriasis

To learn more about the proven Dead Sea psoriasis-treatment programs, contact the Dead Sea Research Center (*www.deadsea-health.org*) and the Dead Sea Psoriasis and Arthritis Treatment Foundation (*www.psoriasis-dead-sea.org*).

Dead Sea and Moor Mineral Muds and Glacial Clays by Ahava and Torf

www.ahavaus.com • *www.torfspa.com*

Ahava's Dead Sea Mineral Mud is the real thing: pure, mineral-rich, and antimicrobial. Recommended for acne, psoriasis, and other inflammatory or fungal conditions. Relieved swelling in arthritic hands in one study. Saprox Glacial Clay and Moor Mud Products by Torf are both antifungal and high in sulphur, trace minerals, and humic acid, which fight bacterial skin infections, fungus, and rashes.

Naturopathic Skin Therapies and Infusions by Sunshine Botanicals

www.sunshinebotanicals.com

Developed by master herbalist and naturopath Dr. Philip Fritchey, ND, these are as fresh (literally) and innovative as any products I've seen. Their skin infusions, such as their Firming and Repairing infusions, offer concentrated, very specific therapies for acne, rosacea, scars, and more. Always ahead of the curve, it's been among the first to use ingredients like cajeput oil (strong antifungal), Oregon grape root, and shepherd's purse (great rash fighter).

Neem Products from Neem Aura Naturals

877-633-6287 • *www.neemaura.com*

The ultimate multitasking herb for irritated skin or acne. This company pioneered concentrated pure neem products in the U.S. The cream is a phenomenal pain- and itch-calming, antimicrobial blend of neem, arnica, white willow bark, barberry, and many other herbs. The oil is nothing but pure neem oil. No preservatives needed.

Oregon Grape Root (Mahonia aquifolium) Cream by Vital Botanicals

800-609-4326 • *www.vitalbotanicals.com*

Ecz-cream by Vital Botanicals contains Oregon grape root, which is proven to reduce the symptoms of eczema and other inflammatory skin problems. For even better results, take Vital Botanicals' Oregon grape root tincture simultaneously.

Zinc Pyrithione Products from ThiOne International, Inc.

www.thione.com

ThioSkin products contain Zinc pyrithione, long recognized for its antifungal and antiseborrheic effects. More recent studies reconfirmed its power against dandruff. Available in sprays, lotions, and shampoos.

Lip Balms and Plumpers

Lip Balms by All Terrain and Jurlique

www.allterrainco.com • *www.jurlique.com*

Lip Armore by All Terrain featurs unrivaled Z-cote sun protection, shea butter, and high-EFA hemp oil moisture. Lip Care Balm by Jurlique really fixes dryness. A great protective balm for any skin area for winter.

Lip Plumpers by MyChelle and SircuitSkin

www.mychelleusa.com • *www.sircuitskin.com*

Both Lip Plumping Treatment by MyChelle and Suggah Anti-Aging Lip Plump- ing Treatment by SircuitSkin utilize oligopeptide technology to hydrate the lips immediately and give you plumper lips in 30–45 days. MyChelle's product includes a bevy of antioxidants, lysine, and sun block. SircuitSkin's features shea butter.

Tinted Lip Moisturizers by Juice Beauty

www.dermstore.com

Lip Trio: SPF 15 Tinted Lip Moisturizers by Juice Beauty are what I'd call "tropical ambrosia" for the lips. These decadent balms feature coconut oil and shea butter infused with guava and peach essences spiked with honey and algae, vitamins, aloe, and more. Mineral pigments give them their gorgeous anyone-can-wear-them colors, as well as their SPF protection.

See also:"Cold Sore Products."

Perfumes and Essential Oil Fragrances, Natural

Each of these precious blends and essences will spare you the forty to two hundred or more petrochemical pollutants and neurotoxins commonly found in any one synthetic perfume. Averaging around $20, they also spare your pocketbook.

Aftelier Natural Perfumes

www.aftelier.com

Celebrated master perfumer Mandy Aftel has been formulating these custom solid and liquid natural perfumes for decades, and they are unequaled. The fig and Cacao scents are the only real (and amazing) ones I know of. They'll also customize one for you.

Eau by Jules and Jane

www.julesandjane.com

An androgynously clean, Ayurvedic elixir of prized Holy basil, peel of lime, and East Indian sandalwood. No petrochemicals.

Essential Oils by Young Living Essential Oils

www.youngliving.org/bluesummit

These food-grade essential oils are widely regarded as the purest in the world. The only thing more amazing than the aromas is accumulating scientific evidence of their amazing effects on the body. Get your hands on the Essential Oils Desk Reference to learn more.

Florin and Freesia Parfums by Jurlique

800-854-1110 • *www.jurlique.com*

Both of these perfumes are developed from twenty to thirty organic essential oils and resins designed to celebrate purity and beauty.

Men's Stock, Aftershave, Balms, and Colognes by Aubrey Organics

www.aubrey-organics.com

Well-formulated, sophisticated, 100 percent natural scents and shave products for men. I particularly like the City Rhythms scent, which blends real sandalwood, ylang ylang, and patchouli essential oils. The shave products are terrific skin formulas as well.

Perfume with a Purpose by Trillium Herbal Company

www.aromafusion.com

These synergistic roll-on aromatherapy blends feature essences found to have specific effects on mood and mental focus. Love, Work, Play, and Rest blends smell wonderful.

Rosacea and Broken Capillaries

Demodicidin Soap and Chang Sheng Soap

800-669-0987 • *www.shoplifestyle.com*

Demodicidin soap may kill the bacteria associated with acne rosacea.

Firming Infusion by Sunshine Botanicals

866-907-9546 • *www.sunshinebotanicals.com*

Pure and powerful, this infusion contains only extracts of horse chestnut, shepherd's purse, alum root, and yarrow flowers to strengthen blood vessels and reduce redness and broken capillaries in rosacea and chronically flushed skin. Tightens skin tissues.

Herbal Celandine Cream by Arboretum Natural Cosmetics

877-767-9367 • *www.arboretum-skincare.com*

An organic, freshly made cream containing celandine and horse chestnut extracts, potentiated by liposomes to minimize redness and tone and strengthen broken capillaries.

SKIN CARE

Redness Reducing Serum from Derma E

800.521.3342 • *www.dermae.net*

Pycnogenol, the main ingredient in this product, has been shown to stabilize the capillary system. With the addition of arnica, calendula, and proprietary type of willow herb, this serum helps reduce blotchiness and skin reactivity.

Rosacea-Targeted Moisturizers, Serums, and Calming Lotion by Rosacea Care

800-696-9791 • *www.rosaceacare.com*

These offer a therapeutic concentration of skin calmers and rebuilders like phospholipids, willowherb, green tea, vitamin K, glutathione, selenium, and grape seed. Calming Lotion contains the breakthrough COSMEDERM-7™, a strontium compound proven to block irritation-producing nerve endings (type C nociceptors) that cause itching, burning, and stinging. The lotion diminishes skin reactivity over time.

See also:"Inflammatory Skin Products" and Sunshine Botanicals and Happy Skin Light Box under "Acne and Oily Skin Products."

Scars and Stretchmarks

Alpha-Lipoic Acid Products by N.V. Perricone, MD and Pure Skin - PSF

www.clinicalcreations.com • *www.essentialdayspa.com*

Dr. Perricone recommends alpha-lipoic acid for scar reduction. His Advanced Face Firming Activator is his latest, higher-potency, alpha-lipoic acid product. ALA Complex by Pure Skin - PSF is a very concentrated, all-natural, squalene-based complex with high-potency R-ALA (a superior form of alpha lipoic acid). Both water and fat soluble, it can penetrate both water and fat barriers of skin cells.

Rosa Mosqueta Rose Hip Seed Oil from Aubrey Organics

www.aubrey-organics.com

Rose hip seed oil, and particularly Chilean rosa mosqueta rose hip seed oil, has been shown in some Chilean studies to reduce scarring.

Scar-Dissolving Products by BioCutis

www.abateit.com

Definitely not for vegans, BIOSKINCARE from BioCutis is—believe it or not—a snail-secretion-based, revolutionary, almost-natural line of scar-dissolving, skin-restoring products backed by impressive preliminary research showing its main ingredient's ability to normalize the cascade of immune and skin regeneration events that determine the formation of scars. Via enzymatic hydrolysis, scars are dissolved and fibroblast and collagen activity are enhanced. If I had scar issues, I would consider this product line in spite of its few synthetics. BIOSKINEXFOL targets raised, old scars, BIO STRETCH MARK CREAM helps prevention and treat stretch marks, while BIO SKIN CLEAR targets acne and acne scars. This line is also a breakthrough for wrinkles and pigmentation issues.

Silicone Scar-Reducers by Dermatix, KeloCote, Mederma, and Others
www.spabeauty.com • *www.skinstore.com*
The silicone gels and sheeting products sometimes soften and flatten raised scars. See also Sunshine Living under "Inflammatory Skin Products."

Sensitive Skin Products
Chamomile Cleansing Cream by Naturopathica
www.naturopathica.com
This therapeutic nonfoaming cleanser contains linden flower, ginseng, and German chamomile, all of which are known for their soothing properties.

Supercritially-extracted Skincare by PlanteSystem from Arkopharma
www.plantesystem.com
This is the first skin care line composed of CO_2 supercritical extracts, meaning there are no traces of solvents and no potential allergy-causing proteins common to most natural ingredients, making it naturally hypoallergenic and suited to sensitive skin. These formulations target specific challenges such as redness, overreactivity, scaliness, wrinkles, oiliness, and more.

E3 Light Creme by Vision, Inc.
888-800-7070 • *www.e3live.com*
This is a particularly calming cream with healing MSM, evening primrose oil (good source of GLA to rebuild lipid barrier and inhibit inflammation), CoQ10, aloe, chamomile, grape seed and carrot oils, and Aslan formula GH-3.

See also:"Inflammatory Skin Products."

Sun Products

In seeking to avoid potential harm from sunscreens, one must not only be conscious of chemicals shown to collect in tissues and have estrogenic effects, such as octylmetoxycinnimate or benzophenone (which also generates free radicals), but also be aware of the fact that many of these chemicals do not protect from all UVA (skin aging) rays, only burning (UVB) rays, and may even contribute to skin damage. There are also new questions arising regarding the safety of nano-sized titanium dioxide (TiO_2). Normally a very safe mineral pigment, micronized TiO_2 (similar to that used widely in nonwhite sunscreens) has shown some harm in animal studies. No problems have been found with micronized zinc, which appears to offer slightly broader protection as well. The good news is that this new knowledge, plus studies confirming the benefits of antioxidants as sunscreen-boosting ingredients, has inspired some great new products.

Sunscreens by Aubrey Organics, UV Naturals, Benedetta, and Marie-Véronique Skin

www.uvnaturalusa.com • *www.organicskintherapy.com*

Aubrey Organics (available at most health food stores) has a wide range of affordable, safe, non-nano TiO_2-based, nonchemical sunscreens with antioxidants like green tea, for the whole family. UV Naturals offers micronized zinc-based (Z-Cote) protection that doesn't go on white, with added extracts of green tea and grape seed. Its sports and golfers' lines aren't greasy or prone to migrate into your eyes while sweating. Benedetta's ingenious Ombra Del Sole is the first antioxidant-only sun protection product without minerals. On its own, it is great for mild sun exposure, and in strong, prolonged sun, it adds another type of protection on top of what mineral blocks can. In terms of the first intelligent sunscreen to combine high-end treatment, Marie-Véronique's Crème de Jour TiO_2-free SPF 15 and Sun Serum from her Serumdipity line take sunscreen to the next level with cranberry seed, sea buckthorn, emu oils, and glucosamine.

Sircuit Soleil Firming Mineral Self-Bronzer

www.sircuitskin.com

As natural as self-tanners get, with firming and enhancing features like horse chestnut extract for strengthening capillaries and a patented French botanical complex for tightening and improved elasticity. Most notably, iron oxides (mineral pigments) provide an instant bronze tone to help with even application.

Under-Eye Circles

Under-eye circles are caused mainly by thin skin revealing weak, leaking capillaries, puffiness (from inflammation, allergies, and edema) that casts a shadow, or, less frequently, hereditary pigmentation.

Under-Eye Circle Serums by Mainely Naturals and MyChelle Dermaceuticals

www.mainelynaturals.com • www.mychelleusa.com

The main component in both of these serums is now the gold standard ingredient for reducing dark circles: Haloxyl, from the herb chrysin, which helps heal capillary blood leakage that creates most dark circles. The Mainely Naturals formula also has high potencies of skin-thickening peptides and cucumber extract to diminish puffiness. Fresh Eyes from MyChelle also incorporates the pigment-inhibitor kojic, the compound called EYELISS, which has been proven to reduce puffiness and increase drainage while strengthening skin and capillaries. Kojic acid, a pigmentation reducer, rounds out MyChelle's hard-to-beat formula.

Antiwrinkle Products

These are advanced natural, or nearly natural, products based on cutting-edge antiaging technologies. The synthetic-sounding chemicals and peptides upon which these products are based (such as the hexapeptides or oligopeptides) are actually natural or nature-identical. Most natural products at this level will sneak in a synthetic preservative here or a silicone or glycol there. Many of these are the only such products that do not include those things. Since these products can be expensive, I recommend that you try to get samples and double-check ingredients before you buy, as many of these more natural formulators change their ingredients frequently.

Antioxidant Serums from Jason, Lluvia, PCA Skin, PSF, and Youthful Essentials

www.amazonherb.net • www.essentialdayspa.com
www.youthfulessentials.com

Hyper C Serum by Jason Natural Products (available at most health food stores) is an affordable, nearly natural, high-potency 10 percent vitamin C serum that made a big difference in my skin. Lluvia Camu C Serum from Amazon Herbs (amazing company) combines camu camu berry, the most concentrated source of natural vitamin C, and sagre de drago, an Amazonian tree sap composed of up to 90 percent super-potent proanthocyandin (OPC) antioxidants, as well as stevia (surprisingly), a

SKIN CARE

humectant that is three times as effective as glycerin. PCA Skin pHaze 15+ C-Quench features vitamin C, polysaccharides, proline, squalene, black currant seed oil, resveratrol, glutathione, and more. PSF Berry Beneficial Antioxidant Serum is not ony packed with super-antioxidants like extracts of wild harvested acai, grape seed, green tea, pomegranate and blueberry, but also with amazing spin trap, which captures free radicals before they do damage, then redirects them to support tissue respiration. Youthful Essentials Wrinkle Serum is the only 100 percent natural C ester serum I've found, and the only one with a high potency of carnosine, the remarkable antiglycation dipeptide.

Eye Wrinkle Treatments by Hydron, Benedetta, and Sundari

www.hydron.com • www.essentialdayspa.com

Hydron Organics Eye Cream is the first and only eye cream at this writing to use the new self-adjusting emulsifying technology to promote homeostasis of the skin. Clinically proven to reduce wrinkles by 14 percent in one hour and up to 50 percent in one week. Contains oxypeptides for oxygenation, hyaluronic acid, sodium PCA, and soy protein for hydration, phospholipids, sphingolipids to rebuild the lipid barrier, and more. Benedetta's The Eye Creme is a 100 percent natural and organic melding of organic alfalfa, green tea, and amalaki fruits extracts, with organic rose and immortelle essential oils in a base of organic pumpkin seed and borage oil. Sundari's Gotu Kola and Boswellia Eye Serum de-puffs with Ayurvedic traditional herbs, while layering the antiwrinkle, skin rejuvenating effects of a state-of-the-art multipeptide complex.

"Faux-tox" Wrinkle Relaxers by DermaE and PSF

www.dermae.net • www.essentialdayspa.com

Peptides Plus Double Action Wrinkle Reverse Crème by Derma E is an affordable, almost all-natural, wrinkle-fighting combination of two proven wrinkle-diminishing peptides: palmitoyl pentapeptide for collagen building and "faux-tox" ingredient acetyl hexapeptide to relax deeper, expression-caused wrinkles. PSF Brow-tox Wrinkle Relaxer gets its relaxing effects from acetyl hexapeptide-3 (Argireline), which inhibits the neuro-receptors where applied, gradually reducing muscle constriction, and thus, wrinkle depth. Amazonian curare extract (which also has a muscle-relaxing effect) is also included, along with hyaluronic acid and galangal root for hydration and firming.

Growth Factor Products by Reviva, MyChelle, Sircuit Skin, and Solange

www.revivalabs.com • www.mychelleusa.com • www.sircuitskin.com • www.wellnesstrader.com

TGF beta-1 by Reviva is a growth factor shown to play a key role in skin cell nourishment uptake and construction. Use over serums and under moisturizers. Soy Rejuvenating Serum, also by Reviva, is one of the most effective of the affordable products in the natural (almost natural) arena. Soy extracellular matrix is a proven firming and fibroblast-stabilizing stimulator for younger functioning skin. Deep Repair by MyChelle contains Epidermal Growth Factor (EGF) to accelerate skin regeneration, algae to detoxify cells, and D-beta fructan to strengthen skin immunity. Dream Weaver Night Time Skin Repair by Sircuit Skin also has EGF, and incorporates spin trap (to convert free radicals before they get radical), aminoguanidine (antiglycation agent) and skin-strengthening D-beta glucosamine. DNA Skin Repair Complex by Solange Skincare revives dry, depleted skin, tightens pores, and promotes scar healing with a potent, concentrated blend of seaweed, gotu kola, horsetail, RNA, and DNA extracts in a pure essential oil base.

Peptide Wrinkle Serums by Annemarie Borlind, MyChelle, and PCA Skin

www.borlind.com • www.mychelleusa.com • www.dermstore.com

Annemari Borlind's NatuRoyale Series features wrinkle-reducing peptides, plankton extract for collagen stimulation, hyaluronic acid, cold-pressed sea buckthorn and macadamia nut oils, rhizobiam gum, and chitosan lactate to bind moisture, lift, and smooth skin both immediately and long-term. MyChelle Dermaceuticals' Supreme Polypeptide Cream is an advanced, natural, "chirally-correct" (as in truly bio-available) combination of highest-potency peptides with many extras, including resveratrol, sodium hyaluronate (the best-utilized form of hyaluronic acid), astaxanthin, d-beta-glucosamine, and much more. It is still more affordable than many synthetic-laden products with fewer actives. PCA pHaze 25 ExLinea Peptide Smoothing Serum (quite a mouthful!) is one of the highest-end formulas—natural or otherwise—with acetyl hexapeptide (Argireline), cassia leaf extract, sodium hyaluronate phospholipids and ceramides (skin barrier builders), MSM (an anti-inflammatory form of healing sulfur), vitamin C, EGCG (a super-antioxidant from green tea), rose hip seed oil, tocotrienols (a superior form of vitamin E), sandalwood, and more.

Seaweed-based Serums by Aubrey Organics, Seaflora, and Spa Technologies

www.aubrey-organics.com • www.spatechnologies.com • www.sea-flora.com
Seaweed extracts are unbeatable to regenerate and detoxify the skin—if you can find a serum of high enough concentration. Aubrey Organics' Vegecell is a very good product packed with algae, aloe, and over two dozen herbs at a great price. Seaflora reigns in the area of whole seaweed serums and body wraps (not extracts) freshly harvested from ultra-pure Canadian Pacific seaweeds. Bio-Active Marine Complex by Spa Technologies is perhaps the most potent seaweed serum on the market—made with 100 percent pure marine algae extracts that truly penetrate and ionize tissue to stimulate cell regeneration, along with phospholipids, proline, yeast extracts, and essential oils. Spa Technologies' other premier product, Oxygenated Renewal Complex, adds dissolved liquid oxygen.

HAIR PRODUCTS

Cleansers and Conditioners, Nonstripping

These shampoos contain no sulfates and are packed with the world's most amazing substances.

Clarifying Shampoo by Avalon Organic Botanicals

Avalon's Lemon Verbena Clarifying Shampoo is something to use every other week to remove product residue. It's also great for detoxing your hair before starting to use non-foaming cleansers and periodically thereafter.

Leave-on Moisturizing Treatment and Hair Growth Formula by Sea Chi Organics

www.seachi.com
This unusually luxurious product is formulated to stimulate circulation, which is a key for hair health. Contains kombucha, seaweed extract, and biodynamic essential oils.

Nonfoaming Hair Cleansers by Wen, Terressentials, and Logona

www.chazdeanstudio.com
Wen Conditioning Cleanser, created by celebrated hair stylist Chaz Dean, doesn't lather up, softens the hair on contact, and rinses out completely. People with dry, coarse hair that gets big after washing will love this product. Clay-based hair washes

by Terressentials and Logona are nonfoaming aromatic washes that are better suited to oily hair, with organic shavegrass, natural clay minerals, nettle, and other scalp-clarifying extracts; they absorb oil and get rid of buildup without stripping.

Shampoos and Conditioners by John Masters, Giovanni, and Max Green Alchemy

www.johnmasters.com • *www.giovannicosmetics.com*
www.maxgreenalchemy.com

John Masters Organics is the highest-end, purest organic hair care line available. With regular clients like Sarah Jessica Parker and Winona Ryder, it has to perform. Evening Primrose Shampoo is one of the only shampoos for dry hair that actually moisturizes the hair. Citrus and Neroli Detangler conditions weightlessly. Herbal Cider Hair Rinse and Clarifier removes buildup and restores proper pH to hair and scalp. Lavender and Avocado Intensive Conditioner quenches the driest hair. Giovanni is a salon-quality, nearly natural line that has a super-wide array of high-end yet affordable custom cleansing and styling products. Scalp Rescue Shampoo and Conditioner by Max Green Alchemy are 100 percent pure and uncommonly great for dry hair. Therapeutic for troubled scalps.

Dandruff Shampoos by John Masters Organics and ThioSkin

www.johnmasters.com • *www.thione.com*

Zinc and Sage Shampoo with Conditioner by John Masters Organics is a great alternative to synthetic dandruff shampoos. This will help diminish itching and flaking. ThioSkin Shampoo, though not entirely natural, contains powerful zinc pyrithione for proven antidandruff effects, along with a less synthetic, more therapeutic formula than standard dandruff shampoos.

Hair Color

Logona Herbal Semi-Permanent Hair Color Creams

www.logona.com • *www.budcosmetics.com*

All permanent hair colors (even so-called natural ones) contain PPD, a carcinogenic ingredient. Henna is safe but hard to work with. This is the first ready-to-apply cream color that blends henna with other coloring herbs. Not everyone will find their color, but the three colors blend with your own and blend gray: Copper Blonde, Indian Summer (medium reddish brown), or Tizian (deep red-tinged brown). Always do strand tests first.

HAIR PRODUCTS

Hair Loss Topical Formulas

By taking an inside out, comprehensive approach, incorporating topicals such as these, along with the supplements in the previous section, and with consistency and patience, hair regrowth without drugs is possible for many (though not all) people. If the best products will work for you, the process takes at least three months to merely stop hair loss, another few months to show regrowth, and up to nine months to fully restore the hair. It's about inhibiting DHT (a type of testosterone responsible for hair loss) and, more importantly, the hair follicles' autoimmune and free-radical response to it. Increasing circulation to the follicles is also important. Some products use nanotechnology, which has not yet undergone long-term safety studies and, therefore, are not included here.

Hair Loss Topical Formulas by Dr. Proctor, Shen Min, and John Masters

www.lef.org • www.shenmin.net • www.johnmasters.com

Hair Regrowth Formulas by Dr. Peter Proctor are based on a compound called NANO (3-carboxylic acid pyridine-N-oxide), which Dr. Proctor, one of the most published hair loss researchers, refers to as "natural" minoxidil. He claims an 80 percent success rate in hair regrowth and holds several patents. In addition to DHT-inhibiting saw palmetto, Nu Hair by Shen Min contains fo-ti, also known as he shou wu, which is prescribed widely in Chinese traditional medicine to combat premature aging and graying hair. John Masters Organics Deep Scalp Follicle Treatment & Volumizer For Thinning Hair is a unique combination of organic herbs and essential oils that works to improve nutrient intake, stimulate circulation, balance sebum production, and neutralize free radicals while providing volume and shine.

See also:"Hair Loss Supplements."

Styling and Texturizing Products

Ionic Far-Infrared and Low EMF Hair Dryers by Wigo

www.americanprohaircare.com

Ionic and infrared blow-dryers dry hair in half the time with far less damage because they use a different kind of heat that evenly penetrates and does not scorch the hair. A must if you blow-dry often. Wigo takes smart blow-drying a step further by offering low-EMF (electromagnetic field) models to meet that legitimate health concern. Other popular professional and even drug store brands will surely follow suit as our wi-fi society wakes up to the dangers of EMF exposure.

Jason Fresh Botanicals Hairspray

Contains no PVP (a common ingredient in hairsprays that causes buildup, drying out the hair as well as flaking). Amino acids, soy, and wheat proteins give body as glycerin, yarrow, cherry bark, and natural gums give a hydrated, flexible hold. I like to spray it on my fingers and rake them through the hair for texture that looks wild but stays.

Primrose Tangle-Go Conditioner, Lusterizer, and Styling Spray by Aubrey Organics

www.aubrey-organics.com

A really great lusterizer for styling or moisturizing the hair at home or at the beach.

Texturizing Product by John Masters Organics and Sante

www.johnmasters.com • www.budcosmetics.com

John Masters' Bourbon Vanilla and Tangerine Hair Texturizer is a versatile styling delicacy for the hair and the senses. His Dry Hair Nourishment and Defrizzer offers light control without impeding the therapeutic action of sebum as silicone serums can (they actually dry the hair). Sea Mist contains sea salt and lavender to give you day-at-the-beach hair texture. His Hair Pomade with organic mango butter and babassu oil controls and shapes short styles and frizzy hair and makes a great elbow, heel, and cuticle balm. Sante Natural Hair Wax is particularly great for giving texture to short or thick hair (guys will love this). Tames dry ends and gives a piece-y texture with coconut oil, jojoba, lecithin, and beeswax. No synthetics.

NAIL PRODUCTS

Nail Products by Acquarella, Firoze, and Earthly Delights

www.acquarellapolish.com • www.firoze.com
www.totaltransformationstore.com

Acquarella is the first and only water-based nail polish you can apply on a plane or in the back of a taxi without offending anyone near you. It also lasts unlike any other water-based polish I've tried. Firoze nail polish is professional performance polish that, while not necessarily natural, lacks the three worst nail polish ingredients: toluene, formaldehyde, and dibutyl pthalate. Naked Nails polish remover by Earthly Delights has no chemical smell and removes even glitter polish.

Antifungal Treatment Products by NonyX Nail Gel and Aidance Skincare

www.swansonvitamins.com • www.aidanceproducts.com

This nontoxic gel containing naturally derived ethanoic acid can clear nail fungus and restore normal nail growth in about twelve months, even if you've had fungus all your life. It's a great alternative to dangerous antifungal drugs. Pedi-Cure Footcare and Nail Restoration by Aidance Skincare ointment is formulated to restore the nails and feet to health with multi-patented tetraSILVER® silver oxide and antimicrobial and essential oils.

BATHROOM CABINET PRODUCTS

Allergy and Sinus Products by NasalCrom and Xlear

www.nasalcrom.com • www.xlear.com

These products have been proven to prevent and relieve nasal allergic symptoms without side effects. Available at most drug stores. Xlear Nasal Wash has been shown to inhibit bacteria adherence and reduce or halt sinus infections.

Cold Sore Treatment by ViraMedx

800-224-4024 • *www.totaltransformationstore.com*

ViraMedx Releev 1-Day Cold Sore Treatment is the only cold sore medication—natural or otherwise—shown in published studies to give substantial, consistent healing in twenty-four hours against drug-resistant outbreaks.

See also: Diamand Herpanicine under "Supplements," page 320.

Deodorants by Benedetta, Weleda, Lavilin, and Dr. Mist

When switching from the world of function-inhibiting, dangerous conventional antiperspirants to a natural deodorant that still lets you sweat, the difference can be discouraging. But if you experiment you'll find a natural deodorant that works for you. Benedetta's "The Best Deodorant" (that's actually what it's called!) is a truly effective deodorant made of a proprietary blend of certified essential oils. Weleda Sage has been a favorite of mine, and it smells incredible. Lavilin is one of the strongest natural deodorants, but it's expensive and a little awkward to apply. Dr. Mist Body Hygiene Flotation Fluid Spray is an international award-winning, multipurpose, all-natural odor-fighting antibacterial spray containing only minerals and specially-treated water. Based on Dead Sea principles, it is not yet widely available in the U.S., so I have not tried it personally but would be remiss not to mention it as it is purported to fight odor for up to three days (used widely in hospitals) without synthetic chemicals. Keep an eye out for it!

Hand Sanitizer, Natural and Trichlosan-Free, by Sensibility Soaps

www.sensibilitysoaps.com

Iced Mint and Vanilla Waterless Hand Sanitizer is a must-have in this ecologically-challenged hand-sanitizer society! With no synthetic antiseptic chemicals to give rise to resistant bacteria (*natural* antimicrobials are too complex for bugs to adapt to), this effective aloe and tea tree oil-based product is a great carry-along wherever kids and other concerns call for cleanup.

Insect Repellants from Mosquito Solutions and OmeZone

www.mosquitosolutions.com • *www.defendpatchfla.com*

This is news: catnip makes DEET (and its neurological side effects) obsolete, and works ten times better, according to a study done at Iowa State University. Catnip Oil Insect Shield from Mosquito Solutions is the answer! A subscriber at my website, www.informedbeauty.com, gave me the lead on this product. Thanks, Karla! OmeZone Defend Insect Repellent Patch is based on research showing that thiamine (vitamin B1), when applied topically, actually helps repel insects like mosquitoes and flies. Works for thirty-six hours.

Jewelweed Poison Ivy Remedies by Ivy Block and Alternative Nature

www.ivyblock.com • *www.altnature.com*

Jewelweed, which grows alongside poison ivy, is clinically proven to prevent poison ivy, oak, and sumac rashes before they take hold. It also gives almost instant relief. These lines include a variety of lotions, cleansers, and salves.

Mouth Care Products by BlanX, Jason, and Young Living Essential Oils

www.blanxusa.com • *www.youngliving.org/bluesummit*

BlanX Whitening Toothpaste is Europe's number one-selling whitening toothpaste and the only tooth whitener that whitens via Arctic moss and without abrasives or bleaches, which actually make teeth more prone to future staining. Choose the natural formula. Jason Oral Comfort Toothpaste contains powerfully antimicrobial grapefruit seed extract, aloe, proven decay-inhibitor xylitol, tissue-healer MSM and gum-healer CoQ10. Dentarome Ultra Toothpaste and Thieve's Mouthwash from Young Living Essential Oils incorporates a powerful essential oil blend including

BATHROOM CABINET PRODUCTS

cinnamon, rosemary, lemon, wintergreen, and eucalyptus oils. Sweetened with xylitol for added dental protection and great taste.

Sleep Products from Herbs, Etc., Silent Snore, and Essence of Vali

www.herbsetc.com • www.silentsnore.com • www.essenceofvali.com

Deep Sleep by Herbs, Etc., is a very effective combination of the most effective sleep herbs in their most potent form. Silent Snore, sprayed to the back of the throat and then swallowed, stopped or reduced snoring in 90 percent of people tested in a clinical trial. Similar products work by reducing swelling and blockage in the back of the throat. Essence of Vali's Sleep Bedtime Balm, featuring essential oils, such as lavender, has demonstrated sedative effects in several studies. Balms are applied directly to the upper lip. This award-winning balm is formulated to reduce anxiety and can be used conveniently and portably at any time, unlike diffusers.

See also:"Mail-Order Sources" for Gaiam, where you can purchase dust-mite barrier bedding.

Antimicrobials from North American Herb and Spice, Nutribiotic, Sovereign Silver, and Spry

www.xlear.com • www.vitaminshoppe.com

Nutribiotic's Grapefruit Seed Extract (GSE) products come in liquid, capsules, ear drops, foot sprays, deodorants, and dental products; these products feature GSE's powerful antimicrobial action. Oregano oil products from North American Herb and Spice, such as Oreganol, were shown to kill strep and Candida albicans in test-tube studies. Work with your doctor if you're fighting an illness. Sovereign Silver's silver hydrosol is the gold standard for effective and safe colloidal silver. Xlear Nasal Wash, shown to inhibit oral, nasal, and middle-ear infections, is a valuable staple.

Immune Enhancers from Zand, EpiCor, American BioSciences, and Sambucol

www.zand.com • www.swansonvitamins.com

Zand's Echinacea and Goldenseal Tincture is one of the favorite bathroom cabinet staples for those who are very informed. Boosts immunity and fights infection. EpiCore has been hailed a revolutionary immunogen-based, powerful immune booster. Ave was the NutrAward "best new product of the year" at the largest natural products trade show in 2006. The level of research for Ave is topped only by the degree of hope this product gives people who have chronic immune imbalances. Sambucol is the standout when it comes to flu season, as its key ingredient, elderberry, has been shown to shorten the duration and lessen the symptoms of flu.

HOME APPLIANCES

Multi-Pure Water Filters

800-622-9206
One of the best water purifiers out there.

Nikken Water Filters

212-222-9972 • *www.mynikken.net/bluesummit*
This is the tap water filter I use. Order from any Nikken distributor or from our above Informed Beauty affiliate. These are the magnetized and alkalizing sink, shower, and portable, high-end, water filters that increase water absorption and alkalize the body. More expensive than standard filters.

Shower Filter by Sprite Water

800-327-9137 • *www.totaltransformationstore.com*
This is the shower filter I use. Slimline Universal and Handheld Chrome trim shower filters, both with KDF and Chlorgon filtering media, offer high-quality filtration for the broadest temperature range and remove at least 95 percent of chlorine, lead, iron oxides (which ruin hair color!), odors, and sediment. Dramatically reduces toxic fumes. Mention Kat James to get 20 percent off retail and free shipping from our source.

Vita-Mix Super 5000

800-VITAMIX • *www.vitamix.com*
Without question the most used kitchen tool I own, this is the only machine that makes lower-glycemic, higher-fiber, and nutrient "whole juice" with a minimum of produce and labor. I use it to make my Beauty Detox Elixirs for my Total Transformation® Programs. Equally impressive, it makes instant ice creams and sorbets from rock-hard frozen fruit. It also liberates nutrients from seeds and even makes tahini from sesame seeds (a blender can't). For free shipping, use our Informed Beauty code: 06-001126.

MAIL-ORDER AND ONLINE CATALOGS AND SERVICES

Gaiam

877-989-6321 • *www.gaiam.com*

A holistic lifestyle source for personal care products, organic clothing and bedding, unbleached paper and feminine hygiene products, nontoxic household cleaners, yoga and fitness products, mind/body/spirit books, solar-powered products, water and air purifiers, and great gifts.

Cutting Edge Catalog

800-497-9516 • *www.cutcat.com*

This catalog has water and air purifiers, full-spectrum lighting, Chromalux lightbulbs, electromagnetic field (EMF) computer and cell phone shields, and therapeutic light boxes.

Life Extension Magazine

800-544-4440 • *www.lef.org*

This stellar publication put out by the nonprofit Life Extension Foundation is educational and a mail-order resource for some of the best supplements available—and for learning which studies have been done on them. You can even order personal blood testing.

Nikken

212-222-9972 • *www.mynikken.net/bluesummit*

This company revolutionized magnet and infrared technology apparel and products (like the mattress pad and quilt I highly recommend), making them a favorite of Olympic athletes. It also features some of the most advanced water filtration systems (including the one with the ceramic, alkalizing attachment I use), high-end supplements, and much more.

Swanson Health Products

800-437-4148 • *www.swansonvitamins.com*

This company offers affordable and harder-to-find supplements.

The Vitamin Shoppe

800-223-1216 • *www.vitaminshoppe.com*

Offers an endless array of most of the reputable brand-name supplements, natural personal care products, and specialty teas and foods. Its website and most stores offer an easy-to-use Healthnotes database to look up specific supplements, health issues, and published research.

Health Testing Services
ALCAT Delayed Food Allergy Testing
800-881-2685, ext. 107 • *www.alcat.com*
Considered to be the most accurate and sensitive test for food sensitivities.

Blood Testing Services Through Life Extension Foundation
800-544-4440 • *www.lef.org*
State-of-the-art testing is offered directly to consumers from top labs all over the country. Have your DHEA, hormone levels, homocysteine, and other health issues tested.

ORGANIZATIONS, EDUCATIONAL RESOURCES, AND SERVICES

American Association of Naturopathic Physicians (AANP)
www.naturopathic.org
An organization of physicians dedicated to promoting the effective use of natural therapies. It offers an online directory of member physicians.

The American Botanical Council (ABC)
www.herbalgram.org
ABC publishes information on the safe and effective use of medicinal plants. ABC members may access an online version of the German Commission E Monographs—Therapeutic Guide to Herbal Medicines.

Broda O. Barnes, MD, Research Foundation, Inc.
203-261-2101 • *www.brodabarnes.org*
A key source for thyroid diagnosis and treatment information.

Co-op America
www.coopamerica.org
Find out which corporations are benefiting people, which ones are harming people and the environment, and how to buy and invest in harmony with your values.

Environmental Working Group's Skin Deep Database

www.ewg.org/reports/skindeep/

Similar to glycemic index charts, once you're using very natural products, there'll be little need to research chemical names with this site's helpful tools, but occasionally there's a natural ingredient that reads like a chemical. You can quickly get a rating on it here. I also appreciate its listing of companies using nanotechnologies. Very helpful for formulators and store buyers needing quick evaluations of product safety.

Informed Beauty

www.informedbeauty.com

Since 1998, this website has been my information and science-focused resource for beauty-oriented health and lifestyle information, where you can subscribe to my free periodic newsletters and program updates. My online Total Transformation store is a tool for finding many of my recommended products in one place.

HealthWorld Online

www.healthy.net

This virtual health village provides a wide range of information, products, and services to help consumers create and manage a wellness-based lifestyle. Click on "Find a Professional" to find a complementary physician near you.

Herb Research Foundation

www.herbs.org

A great resource for information on herbs and their proven effects. The Herb Research Foundation's custom research service provides affordable searches for literature on herbs.

Life Extension Foundation (LEF)

800-544-4440 • *www.lef.org*

One of the best professional and consumer-friendly sources for information on combining conventional and proven alternative therapies. It has historically broken medical news many years before the mainstream. Visit its Consumer Alerts often.

Local Harvest

www.localharvest.org

Use this site to find an organic farmer's market and resources near you.

The National Eating Disorders Association (NEDA)

www.nationaleatingdisorders.org

Among eating disorder professionals in general, a brain-chemistry-supportive, strategic nutritional (natural) approach has been tragically overlooked in favor of aggressive drug therapies. I am encouraged by NEDA's interest in expanding its educational offerings to include more holistic and nutritional approaches such as mine. Let them know of your interest in these if you contact them.

The New Zealand Dermatological Society

www.dermnetnz.org

This award-winning website offers graphic pictures and details about any skin disorder to help you identify mysterious skin problems and rashes.

www.Omega-Research.com

This is the authoritative clearinghouse for published research on the many benefits of omega-3 fatty acids and fish oil.

Organic Consumers Association (OCA)

www.organicconsumers.org

The OCA is one of the best mailing lists to get on, and one of the best sites to frequent to stay up to date on what is really happening that will affect your health.

PubMed on Medline

www.pubmed.org

This is the database your doctor relies on, though it is unlikely that he searches or views much of its information on natural therapies. There is some key research missing from it, including the thirty-six years of research represented in the respected *Journal of Orthomolecular Medicine.* Hopefully, this will change.

Safe Harbor International Guide to Alternative Mental Health

www.alternativementalhealth.com

This is the largest international online directory for articles and practitioners dealing in nondrug mental health approaches.

Total Transformation® Programs

877-54-TOTAL • *www.informedbeauty.com*

Kat James's land- and sea-based experiential programs, where participants experience the dawn-to-dusk principles and results of the process of shedding.

ORGANIZATIONS, EDUCATIONAL RESOURCES, AND SERVICES

NEWSLETTERS AND PERIODICALS

These newsletters, which are also very popular with doctors, can help one stay five or more years ahead of the curve without plowing through medical journals.

Dr. David Williams's *Alternatives*

800-527-3044 • *www.drdavidwilliams.com*

You'll learn many facts in this newsletter years before they hit mainstream.

American Botanical Council's *HerbalGram*

www.herbalgram.org

A top educational resource on herbs published by the American Botanical Council for its members. Worth joining.

Dr. Julian Whitaker's *Health and Healing*

800-539-8219 • *www.drwhitaker.com*

Dr. Whitaker is not only a medical pioneer, but also a health freedom hero.

The Health Sciences Institute Members Alert

800-981-7157 • *www.hsibaltimore.com*

A cutting-edge newsletter put out by a stellar editorial board of top medical experts. Here you will learn many facts before you hear them anywhere else.

Life Extension Magazine

800-544-4440 • *www.lef.org*

This exciting publication of the Life Extension Foundation (LEF) features breaking, integrative health news to use and to show your doctor. LEF saves untold lives and fights to preserve our medical freedom.

Dr. Joseph Mercola's Newsletter

www.mercola.com

One of the most read and respected natural health e-newsletters, from the most visited natural health website on the Internet. Get it for free.

Dr. Jonathan V. Wright's *Nutrition and Healing*

800-851-7100 • *www.wrightnewsletter.com*

Dr. Wright is one of the most peer-respected pioneers and authorities on alternatives.

Total Health Magazine

888-316-6051 • *www.totalhealthmagazine.com*

Always offers the knowledge of a variety of the most informed experts. I highly recommend this magazine.

VitaSearch Clinical Pearls Weekly Updates

www.vitasearch.com

The most amazing, free weekly e-mail summarizes the bulk of just-published studies on vitamins and herbs and disease. User-friendly and lifesaving.

SUGGESTED READING

The most valuable health resources for you and your family are those that will resonate with your doctor via peer-reviewed, published studies, but which at the same time are presented in a way that laymen can easily use and understand. The following resources meet these tough criteria and will put you light years ahead of the general public in terms of usable quality-of-life choices. I highly recommend that you use several of them the next time you or a loved one has a health concern. And you may want to offer a second copy as a gift to the skeptical conventional physician in your life. Most of these books can be ordered from www.informedbeauty.com.

Balch, James F., MD, and Phyllis A. Balch, CNC. *Prescription for Nutritional Healing*, 4th ed. New York: Avery, 2006.

Blaylock, Russell L., MD. *Excitotoxins: The Taste That Kills*. Santa Fe, N. Mex.: Health Press, 1997.

Blumenthal, Mark, Josef Brinckman, and Alicia Goldberg. *Herbal Medicine: Expanded Commission E Monographs*. Boston: Integrative Medicine Communication, 2000.

Bradshaw, John. *Bradshaw on the Family: A New Way of Creating Self-Esteem*. Deerfield Beach, Fla.: Health Communications, 1996.

Brand-Miller, Jennie, Thomas M.S. Wolever, MD, Kaye Foster-Powell, and Stephen Colagiuri, MD. *The Glycemic Revolution*. New York: Marlowe & Co., 1996, 1998, 1999, 2002, 2003.

Diamond, John W., MD, and W. Lee Cowden, MD, eds. *The Definitive Guide to Cancer*. Tiburon, Calif.: Future Medicine Publishing, Inc., 1997.

Duke, James A., and Michael Castleman. *The Green Pharmacy Anti-Aging Prescriptions: Herbs, Foods, and Natural Formulas to Keep You Young: The Ultimate Compendium of Natural Remedies from the World's Foremost Authority on Healing Herbs*. Emmaus, Pa.: Rodale Press, 2001.

Epstein, Samuel, and David Steinman. *The Breast Cancer Prevention Program*. New York: Macmillan, 1997.

Erasmus, Udo. *Fats That Heal, Fats That Kill: The Complete Guide to Fats, Oils, Cholesterol, and Human Health*. Burnaby, B.C., Canada: Alive Books, 1993.

Fife, Bruce, ND. *Cooking with Coconut Flour: A Low-Carb, Gluten-Free Alternative to Wheat*. Colorado Springs: Piccadilly Books, Ltd., 2005.

Garcia, Oz. *Look and Feel Fabulous Forever*. New York: Regan Books, 2002.

Glenmullen, Joseph. *Prozac Backlash*. New York: Touchstone Books, 2001.

Hampton, Aubrey, and Susan Hussey. T*he Take Charge Beauty Book: The Ultimate Guide to Beautiful Hair and Skin*. Tampa, Fla.: Organica Press, 1999.

Jeffers, Susan. *Feel the Fear and Do it Anyway*. San Diego: Harcourt Brace Jovanovich, 1987.

Larson, Joan Matthews. *Seven Weeks to Sobriety*. New York: Fawcett Books, 1997.

Lee, John R., with Virginia Hopkins. *What Your Doctor May Not Tell You About Menopause*. New York: Warner Books, 1996.

Miller, Philip L., MD with Monica Reinagel. *The Life Extension Revolution: The New Science of Growing Older Without Aging*. New York: Bantam Books, 2006.

Northrup, Christiane. *The Wisdom of Menopause: Creating Physical and Emotional Health and Healing During the Change*. New York: Bantam Books, 2001.

Perricone, Nicholas, MD. *The Perricone Prescription*. New York: HarperCollins, 2002.

Raichur, Pratima, and Marian Raichur Cohn. *Absolute Beauty: Radiant Skin and Inner Harmony Through the Ancient Secrets of Ayurveda*. New York: HarperCollins, 1997.

Reaven, Gerald M., Terry Kristen Strom, and Barry Fox. *Syndrome X, the Silent Killer: The New Heart Disease Risk*. New York: Fireside Books, 2001.

Rivera, Rudy, and Roger D. Deutsch. *Your Hidden Food Allergies Are Making You Fat: The ALCAT Food Sensitivities Weight Loss Breakthrough*, 2nd ed. Roseville, Calif.: Prima Publishing, 2002.

Rosedale, Ron, MD. *The Rosedale Diet*. New York: HarperCollins, 2004.

Sears, Barry, and Bill Lawren. *The Zone: A Dietary Road Map to Lose Weight Permanently, Reset Your Genetic Code, Prevent Disease, Achieve Maximum Physical Performance.* New York: Regan Books, 1995.

Schachter, Michael B., MD and Deborah Mitchell. *What Your Doctor May Not Tell You About Depression.* New York: Warner Wellness, 2006.

Steinman, David, and R. Michael Wisner. *Living Healthy in a Toxic World: Simple Steps to Protect You and Your Family from Everyday Chemicals, Poisons, and Pollution.* New York: Berkley Publishing Group, 1996.

Vanderhaeghe, Lorna R. *Healthy Immunity: Scientifically Proven Treatments for Conditions from A-Z.* New York: John Wiley & Sons, 2003.

Wetherall, Charles F. *Quit: Read This Book and Stop Smoking.* Philadelphia, Pa.: Running Press, 2001.

Winter, Ruth. *A Consumers Dictionary of Cosmetic Ingredients,* 5th ed. New York: Three Rivers Press, 1999.

BIBLIOGRAPHY

Chapter 3

Adler, S.R., and J.R.Fosket. "Disclosing Complementary and Alternative Medicine Use in the Medical Encounter: A Qualitative Study in Women with Breast Cancer." *Journal of Family Practice* 48, no. 6 (June 1999): 453–58.

Adlercreutz, H., Y. Mousavi, J. Clark, K. Hockerstedt, E. Hamalainen, K. Wahala, T. Makela, and T. Hase. "Dietary Phytoestrogens and Cancer: In Vitro and In Vivo Studies." *Journal of Steroid Biochemistry and Molecular Biology* 41, no. 3–8 (March 1992): 331–37.

Arliss, R.M., and C.A. Biermann. "Do Soy Isoflavones Lower Cholesterol, Inhibit Atherosclerosis, and Play a Role in Cancer Prevention?" *Holistic Nursing Practice* 16, no. 5 (October 2002): 40–48.

Associated Press. "Canada Rejects P&G's Olestra." *Cincinnati Post*, 23 June 2000.

Challem, Jack. "Natural vs. Synthetic Vitamin E." *Nutrition Science News*, November 2001.

Cover, C.M., et al. "Indole-3-carbinol and Tamoxifen Cooperate to Arrest the Cell Cycle of MCF-7 Human Breast Cancer Cells." *Cancer Research* 59 (1999): 1244–51.

De Pinieux, G., P. Chariot, M. Ammi-Said, F. Louarn, J.L. Lejonc, A. Astier, B. Jacotot, and R. Gherardi. "Lipid-lowering Drugs and Mitochondrial Function: Effects of HMG-CoA Reductase Inhibitors on Serum Ubiquinone and Blood Lactate/Pyruvate Ratio." *British Journal of Clinical Pharmacology* 42, no. 3 (September 1996): 333–37.

Erasmus, Udo. *Fats That Heal, Fats That Kill*. Burnaby, B.C., Canada: Alive Books, 1983, 1993.

Erickson, Kim. *Drop Dead Gorgeous*. New York, N.Y.: Contemporary Books, 2002.

"FDA: Authority over Cosmetics." U.S. Food and Drug Administration Center for Food Safety and Applied Nutrition, Office of Cosmetics and Colors, 3 February 1995.

Grady, Denise. "Risks of Hormone Therapy Exceed Benefits, Panel Says." *New York Times*, 17 October 2002.

Horwitz, Ralph I., MD, Lawrence M. Brass, MD, Walter N. Kernan, MD, and Catherine M. Viscoli, PhD. "Phenylpropanolamine and Risk of Hemorrhagic Stroke: Final Report of the Hemorrhagic Stroke Project." FDA submission, 10 May 2000.

Kolpin, Dana W., et al. "Pharmaceuticals, Hormones, and Other Organic Wastewater Contaminants in U.S. Streams, 1999–2000: A National Reconnaissance." *Environmental Science and Technology* 36 (2002): 1202–11.

Linde, K., et al. "St. John's Wort for Depression—an Overview and Meta-analysis of Randomised Clinical Trials." *British Medical Journal* 313, no. 7052 (3 August 1996): 253–58.

Morrow, Michele G., DO. "A Celebration of First Amendment Victories Against the FDA." *Life Extension Magazine*, April 2002, p. 27.

Mulvihill, Keith. "Tobacco Company Influenced Nicotine Gum, Patch Ads." *Reuters Health*, 14 August 2002.

Peterson, Melody. "Heartfelt Advice, Hefty Fees." *New York Times*, 11 August 2002.

Poole, K. "Mechanisms of Bacterial Biocide and Antibiotic Resistance." *Journal of Applied Microbiology* 92, supplement (2002): 55S–64S.

Salaman, Maureen K., and Jonathan V. Wright. "Would You Buy a Used Car from FDA? Distorting the 'Pure Food' (and Other) Laws Since 1906." *Townsend Letter for Doctors* 133: 968–71.

Smeh, Nikolaus J. *Health Risks in Today's Cosmetics*. Garrison, Va.: Alliance Publishing, 1994, p. 14.

Stolberg, Sheryl Gay. "F.D.A. Ban Sought on Chemical Used for Cold Remedies." *New York Times*, 20 October 2000.

Uehling, Mark D. "Free Drugs from Your Faucet." *Salon* 25 (October 2002).

U.S. Preventive Services Task Force. "Postmenopausal Hormone Replacement Therapy for Primary Prevention of Chronic Conditions: Recommendations and Rationale." *Annals of Internal Medicine* 137 (2002): 834–39.

Verrengia, Joseph B. "America's Waterways Contaminated by Medications, Personal Care Products." Associated Press, 13 March 2002. Environmental News Network Website: www.enn.com/news.

Chapter 4

Aviram, M., L. Dornfeld, M. Rosenblat, et al. "Pomegranate Juice Consumption Reduces Oxidative Stress, Atherogenic Modifications to LDL, and Platelet Aggregation: Studies in Humans and in Atherosclerotic Apolipoprotein E-deficient Mice." *American Journal of Clinical Nutrition* 71 (2000): 1062–76.

Borghouts, L.B., and H.A. Keizer. "Exercise and Insulin Sensitivity: A Review." *International Journal of Sports Medicine* 21 (2000): 1–12 [review].

Cherniske, Stephen, MS. *Caffeine Blues*. New York: Warner Books, 1998.

Curi, R., M. Alvarez, R.B. Bazotte, et al. "Effect of Stevia Rebaudiana on Glucose Tolerance in Normal Adult Humans." *Brazilian Journal of Medical and Biological Research* 19 (1986): 771–74.

Dulloo, A.G., J. Sevdoux, L. Girardier, et al. "Green Tea and Thermogenesis: Interactions Between Catechin-polyphenols, Caffeine and Sympathetic Activity." *International Journal of Obesity and Related Metabolic Disorders* 24, no. 2 (February 2000): 252–58.

Eliasson, B., S. Attvall, M.R. Taskinen, and U. Smith. "Smoking Cessation Improves Insulin Sensitivity in Healthy Middle-aged Men." *European Journal of Clinical Investigation* 27 (1997): 450–56.

Garland, E.M., and S.M. Cohen. "Saccharin-induced Bladder Cancer in Rats." *Progress in Clinical Biological Research* 391 (1995): 237–43 [review].

Geleijnse, J.M., L.J. Launer, D.A. Van der Kuip, A. Hofman, and J.C. Witteman. "Inverse Association of Tea and Flavonoid Intakes with Incident Myocardial Infarction: The Rotterdam Study." *American Journal of Clinical Nutrition* 75, no. 5 (May 2002): 880–86.

Gutshall, D.M., G.D. Pitcher, and A.E. Langley. "Mechanism of the Serum Thyroid Hormone Lowering Effect of Perflouro-n-decanoic Acid (PDFA) in Rats." *Journal of Toxicology and Environmental Health* (1989): 28(1): 58-65.

Heinrich, U., K. Neukam, et al. "Long-term Ingestion of High Flavenol Cocoa Provides Photoprotection Against UV-induced Erythema and Improves Skin Condition in Women." *Journal of Nutrition* (2006): 136(6): 1565-9.

Hoie, L.H., A. Sjoholm, M. Guldstrand, H.J. Zunft, W. Leuder, H.J. Graubaum, and J. Gruenwald. "Ultra heat treatment destroys cholesterol-lowering effect of soy protein." *International Journal of Food Sciences and Nutrition*, Vol. 57, Nos. 7–8, –8/November–December 2006, pp. 512–519(8)

Jenkins, D.J., M. Axelsen, C.W. Kendall, et al. "Dietary Fibre, Lente Carbohydrates and the Insulin-resistant Diseases." *British Journal of Nutrition* 83 (2000): S157–63 [review].

Keijzers, G.B., B.E. De Galan, C.J. Tack, and P. Smits. "Caffeine Can Decrease Insulin Sensitivity in Humans." *Diabetes Care* 25, no. 2 (February 2002): 364–69.

Kozlovsky, A., et al. "Effects of Diets High in Simple Sugars on Urinary Chromium Losses." *Metabolism* 35 (June 1986): 515–18.

Lien, L., N. Lien, S. Heyerdahl, M. Thoreson, and E. Bjertness. "Consumption of Soft Drinks and Hyperactivity, Mental Distress and Conduct Problem Among Adolescents in Oslo, Norway." *American Journal of Public Health* (October 2006): 96(10): 1815-20.

Lingelbach, L.B., A.E. Mitchell, R.B. Rucker, and R.B. McDonald. "Accumulation of Advanced Glycation Endproducts in Aging Male Fischer 344 Rats during Long-term Feeding of Various Dietary Carbohydrates." *Journal of Nutrition* 130, no. 5 (May 2000): 1247–55.

Nakachi, K., K. Suemasu, K. Suga, T. Takeo, K. Imai, and Y. Higashi. "Influence of Drinking Green Tea on Breast Cancer Malignancy among Japanese Patients." *Japanese Journal of Cancer Research* 89, no. 3 (1998): 254–61.

Pawlak, D.B., J.M. Bryson, G.S. Denyer, and J.C. Brand-Miller. "High Glycemic Index Starch Promotes Hypersecretion of Insulin and Higher Body Fat in Rats without Affecting Insulin Sensitivity." *Journal of Nutrition* 131, no. 1 (January 2001): 99–104.

Smith-Warner, S.A., D. Spiegelman, S.S. Yaun, P.A. van den Brandt, A.R. Folsom, R.A. Goldbohm, S. Graham, L. Holmberg, G.R. Howe, J.R.Marshall, A.B. Miller, J.D. Potter, F.E. Speizer, W.C. Willett, A. Wolk, and D.J. Hunter. "Alcohol and Breast Cancer in Women: A Pooled Analysis of Cohort Studies." *Journal of the American Medical Association* 279, no. 7 (18 February 1998): 535–40.

Stellman, S., and L. Garfinkel. "Short Report: Artificial Sweetener Use and Weight Changes among Women." *Preventive Medicine* 15 (1986): 195–202.

Uehara, M., J. Sugiura, and K. Sakurai. "A Trial of Oolong Tea in the Management of Recalcitrant Atopic Dermatitis." *Archives of Dermatology* 137 (2001): 42–43.

U.S. Food and Drug Administration. "Final Rule" for Sucralose, 21 CFR Part 172, Docket No. 87F-0086.

Warner, Jennifer. "Broccoli Pill Prevents Breast Cancer." *WebMD Medical News,* 19 August 2002.

White, J.R., Jr., J. Kramer, R.K. Campbell, and R. Bernstein. "Oral Use of a Topical Preparation Containing an Extract of Stevia Rebaudiana and the Chrysanthemum Flower in the Management of Hyperglycemia." *Diabetes Care* 17 (1994): 940.

Wilkison, W., K.H. Golding, P.K. Robinson, et al. "Mercury Removed by Immobilized Algae in Batch Culture Systems." *Journal of Applied Phycology* 2 (1990): 223–30.

Wolever, T.M. "Dietary Carbohydrates and Insulin Action in Humans." *British Journal of Nutrition* 83 (2000): S97–102 [review].

Woods, D. "U.S. Scientists Challenge Approval of Sweetener." *British Medical Journal* 313, no. 7054 (17 August 1996): 386.

Wu, C.H., Y.C. Yang, W.J. Yao, F.H. Lu, J.S. Wu, and C.J. Chang. "Epidemiological Evidence of Increased Bone Mineral Density in Habitual Tea Drinkers." *Archives of Internal Medicine* 162, no. 9 (13 May 2002): 1001–6.

Xiangyang, Q., et al. "Effect of Siraitia Grosvenori Extract Containing Mogrosides on the Cellular Immune System of Type I Diabetes Mellitus Mice." *Molecular Nutrition Food & Research* (November–December, 2006): 57(7): 512-9: 45646 (March 2007).

Zaizen, Y., et al. "Antitumor Effects of Soybean Hypocotyls and Soybeans on the Mammary Tumor Induction by N-methyl-n-nitrosourea in F344 Rats." *Anti-cancer Research* 20, no. 3A (2000): 1439–44.

Chapter 5

Burton, C. "Low-fat Diets Are Associated With Increased Rates of Depression, Psychological Problems, Fatigue, Violence and Suicide." *The Lancet* (March 21, 1993): 339.

Cross, A.J., U. Peters, et al. "Prospective Study of Meat and Meat Mutagens and Prostate Cancer Risk." *Cancer Research* (2005): 65(24): 11,779-84.

De Lorgeril, M., and P. Salen. "Modified Cretan Mediterranean Diet in the Prevention of Coronary Heart Disease and Cancer." *World Review of Nutrition and Dietetics* (2007): 97: 1-32.

Fallon, S., and M. Enig. "Tripping Lightly Down the Prostaglandin Pathways." *Price Pottenger Nutrition Foundation Journal* (1998): 20: 3.

Felton, C.V., et al. "Dietary Polyunsaturated Fatty Acids and Composition of Human Aortic Plaques." *Lancet* (1994): 344(8931): 1195-6.

Gardner, C., et al. "Carbohydrate Intake and Weight Loss In Women." *Journal of the American Medical Association* (2007): 297: 921.

Hodgson, J.M., V. Burke, et al. "Partial Substitution of Carbohydrate Intake With Protein Intake From Lean Red Meat Lowers Blood Pressure in Hypertensive Persons." *American Journal of Clinical Nutrition*, 83, 4 (2006): 780-7.

Howard, B.V., L. Van Horn, et al. "Low-fat Dietary Pattern and Risk of Cardiovascular Disease: The Women's Health Initiative Randomized Controlled Dietary Modification Trial." *Journal of the American Medical Association* 295, 6 (2006): 693-5.

Hu, F.B., et al. "A Propective Study of Egg Consumption and Risk of Cardiovascular Disease in Men and Women." *Journal of the American Medical Association* (1999): 281(15): 1387-94.

Layman, D.K., R.A. Boileau, and D.J. Erickson, et al. "A reduced ratio of dietary carbohydrate to protein improves body composition and blood lipid profiles during weight loss in adult women." *J Nutr* 2003;133:411–7.

National Heart and Lung Institute. "Multiple Risk Factor Intervention Trial: Risk Factor Changes and Mortality Results." *Journal of the American Medical Association* (1982): 248(12): 1465.

Schmidt M., MD. "Smart Fats: How Dietary Fats and Oils Affect Mental, Physical and Emotional Intelligence." *Price Pottenger Nutrition Foundation Journal* (1997): 20: 3.

Schupf, N., R. Costa, J. Luchsinger, M. Tang, J. Lee, and R.J. Mayeux. "Relationship Between Plasma Lipids and All-Cause Mortality in Nondemented Elderly." *Journal of the American Geriatrics Society* (February 2005): 53: 219: doi:10.1111/j.1532-5415.2005.53106.x.

Sondike, S.B., N. Copperman, and M.S. Jacobson. "Effects of a low-carbohydrate diet on weight loss and cardiovascular risk factor in overweight adolescents." *Journal of Pediatric Psychology* 2003;142:253–8.

Tholstrup, T., C. Hoy, L. Normann-Andersen, D. Robin, B. Sandstrom, and C. Sandstrom. "Does Fat in Milk, Butter and Cheese Affect Blood Lipids and Cholesterol Differently?" *Journal of the American College Nutrition* (2003): 22:6.

Willett, W.C. "Is Dietary Fat a Major Determinant of Body Fat?" *American Journal of Clinical Nutrition* 67 (1998): 556–62.

Wolk, A., et al. "A Prospective Study of the Association of Monounsaturated Fat and Other Types of Fat With Risk of Breast Cancer." *Archives of Internal Medicine* (1998): 158(41).

Chapter 6

Aga, M., K. Iwaki, Y. Ueda, S. Ushio, N. Masaki, S. Fukuda, T. Kimoto, M. Ikeda, and M. Kurimoto. "Preventive Effect of Coriandrum Sativum (Chinese Parsley) on Localized Lead Deposition in ICR Mice." *Journal of Ethnopharmacology* 77 (2001): 203–8.

Ammon, H.P., et al. "Mechanism of Anti-inflammatory Actions of Curcumin and Boswellic Acids." *Journal of Ethnopharmacology* 38 (1993): 113.

Amodio, M.L., et al. "A Comparative Study of Composition and Postharvest Performance of Organically and Conventionally Grown Kiwifruits." *Journal of the Science of Food and Agriculture* (2007): 87(7): 1228–1236.

Benbrook, Charles. "Evidence of the Magnitude and Consequences of the Roundup Ready Soybean Yield Drag from University-Based Varietal Trials in 1998." Ag BioTech InfoNet Technical Paper Number 1, 13 July 1999.

Berkson, D. Lindsey. *Hormone Deception*. Lincolnwood, Ill.: Contemporary Books, 2000.

Birnbaum, L. "Addition of Conjugated Linoleic Acid to a Herbal Anticellulite Pill." *Advances in Therapy* 18, no. 5 (September–October 2001): 225–29.

Blaylock, Russell L., MD. *Excitotoxins: The Taste That Kills*. Santa Fe, N.M.: Health Press, 1997.

Booth, Sarah L. "Vitamin K: Another Reason to Eat Your Greens." *Agricultural Research Magazine* 48, no. 1 (January 2000): 16–17.

Cass, H., MD. "Author confirms cranberry oil's powerful properties: absorbed easily through the skin, acts as a superb moisturizer, and helps to relieve itchy, scaly, irritated skin." *8 Weeks to Vibrant Health*. New York: McGraw-Hill, 2005.

Chang, S.T., P.F. Chen, and S.C. Chang. "Antibacterial Activity of Leaf Essential Oils and Their Constituents from Cinnamomum Osmophloeum." *Journal of Ethnopharmacology* 77 (2001): 123–27.

Chen, H.L., et al. "Konjac Supplement Alleviated Hypercholesterolemia and Hyperglycemia in Type 2 Diabetic Subjects—A Randomized Double-blind Trial." *Journal of the American College of Nutrition* (2003): 22(1): 36–42.

Chavarro, J.E., J.W. Rich-Edwards, B. Rosner, and W.C. Willett. "A Prospective Study of Dairy Foods Intake and Anovultory Infertility." *Human Reproduction* (2007): doi: 10.1093/humrep/dem019.

Dannenberger, D., et al. "Effect of Pasture Versus Concentrate Diet on CLA Isomer Distribution in Different Tissue Lipids of Beef Cattle." *Lipids* (2005): 40(6): 589–598.

Dashwood, R.H., et al. "Cancer Chemopreventive Mechanisms of Tea against Heterocyclic Amine Mutagens from Cooked Meat." *Proceedings of the Society for Experimental Biology and Medicine* 220 (1999): 239–43.

David, J.A., Cyril Jenkins, W.C. Kendall, and Vladimir Vuksan. "Inulin, Oligofructose and Intestinal Function." *Journal of Nutrition* 129 (1999): 1431S–33S.

Dhiman, T.R., et al. "Conjugated Linoleic Acid Content of Milk from Cows Fed Different Diets." *Journal of Dairy Science* 82, no. 10 (October 1999): 2146–56.

Editorial. "The Goji Berry, The Wolfberry, The Fruit of Lycium Barbarum." *The Healing Journal* (February/March 2007): www.thehealingjournal.com/prev_issues/feb_march07_goji.htm.

Environmental Protection Agency. "National Sewage Sludge Survey: Availability of Information and Data, and Anticipated Impacts on Proposed Regulation." 40 CFR Part 503 (FRL-3857-2). *Federal Register* 55, no. 218 (9 November 1990): 47210.

Erasmus, Udo. *Fats That Heal, Fats That Kill.* Burnaby, B.C., Canada: Alive Books, 1993.

Ernst, E. "Cardioprotection and Garlic." *Lancet* 349 (1997): 131.

Friedman, M., ed. *Nutritional and Toxicological Consequences of Food Processing.* New York: Plenum Press, 1991.

Gaby, Alan R., MD. "Eat Nuts for a Healthy Heart." *Healthnotes Newswire*, 1 August 2002.

Garcia-Segovia, P., and A. Sanchez-Villegas, et al. "Olive Oil Consumption and the Risk of Breast Cancer in the Canary Islands: A Population-based Case-control Study." *Public Health Nutrition* 9, 1A (2006): 163–7.

Gijsbers, B.L., K.S. Jie, and C. Vermeer. "Effect of Food Composition on Vitamin K Absorption in Human Volunteers." *British Journal of Nutrition* 76, no. 2 (August 1996): 223–29.

Gilbert, Susan. "Fears Over Milk, Long Dismissed, Still Simmer." *New York Times*, 19 January 1999.

Glinsmann, W., H. Irausquin, and K. Youngmee. "Evaluation of Health Aspects of Sugar Contained in Carbohydrate Sweeteners." FDA Report of Sugars Task Force 39 (1986): 36–38.

"GM Crop DNA Found in Human Gut Bugs." *NewScientist.com* 12:10, 18 July 2002.

Guh, J.H., et al. "Antiplatelet Effect of Gingerol Isolated from Zingiber officinale." *Journal of Pharmacy and Pharmacology* 47 (1995): 329–32.

Healthnotes, Inc. "Cayenne as an herbal remedy." 2002. www.mycostompak.com/healthnotes/herb/cayenne.htm.

Horowitz, B.J., S. Edelstein, and L. Lippman. "Sugar Chromatography Studies in Recurrent Candida Vulvovaginitis." *Journal of Reproductive Medicine* 29 (1984): 441–43.

Josse, A.R., C.W. Kendall, et al. "Almonds and Post-prandial Glycemia—A Dose-Response Study." *Metabolism* 56, 3 (2007): 400–4.

Justi, K.C., et al. "Nutritional Composition and Vitamin C Stability in Stored Camu-camu (Myrciaria Dubia) Pulp." *Archives of Latinoam Nutrition* (2000): 50(4): 405–8.

Kaur, N., and A.K. Gupta. "Applications of Inulin and Oligofructose in Health." *Journal of Bioscience* 27, 7 (December 2002): 703–14.

Kekwick, A., and G.L.S. Pawan. "Calorie Intake in the Relation to Body Weight Changes in the Obese." *Lancet* 2 (1956): 155–61.

Lee, D.H., et al. "Association Between Serum Concentrations of Persistent Organic Pollutants and Insulin Resistance Among Nondiabetic Adults." *Diabetes Care* (2007): 30: 622–8.

Li, W., S.Z. Dai, W. Ma, and L. Gao. "Effects of oral Administration of Wolfberry on Blood Superoxide Dismutase (SOD), Hemoglobin (Hb) and Lipid Peroxide (LPO) Levels in Old People." *Chinese Traditional and Herbal Drugs* (1991) (22): 251,268.

Lingelbach, L.B., A.E. Mitchell, R.B. Rucker, and R.B. McDonald. "Accumulation of Advanced Glycation Endproducts in Aging Male Fischer 344 Rats during Long-term Feeding of Various Dietary Carbohydrates." *Journal of Nutrition* 130, no. 5 (May 2000): 1247–55.

Lu, C., K. Toepel, et al. "Organic Diets Significantly Lower Children's Dietary Exposure to Organophosphorus Pesticides." *Environmental Health Perspective* 114, 2 (2006): 260–3.

Mang, B., M. Wolters, et al. "Effects of a Cinnamon Extract on Plasma Glucose, HbA, and Serum Lipids in Diabetes Mellitus Type 2." *European Journal of Clinical Investigation* 36, 5 (2006): 340-4.

Matthäus, B., and J. Agric. "Antioxidant Activity of Extracts Obtained from Residues of Different Oilseeds. *Food Chemistry* 2002: 50(12): 3444 – 52: DOI: 10.1021/jf011440s.

Mellon, Margaret, Charles Benbrook, and Karen Lutz Benbrook. "Hogging It: Estimates of Antimicrobial Abuse in Livestock." Cambridge, Mass.: Union of Concerned Scientists, 2001, p. xiii.

Morganti P., MD. "Clinical Evidence for Lutein and Zeaxanthin in Skin Health, Part 1: Comparison of Placebo, Oral, Topical and Combined Oral/Topical Xanthophyll Treatments." Beyond Beauty Paris Conference, Paris, France September 12, 2006.

Moschos, S.J., and C.S. Mantzoros. "The Role of the IGF System in Cancer: From Basic to Clinical Studies and Clinical Applications." *Oncology* 63, no. 4 (2002): 317–32 [review].

Nair, M.G., MD. "Natural Painkillers and Strong Antioxidants Found in Tart Cherries" *Journal of Natural Products* (January 28, 1999).

Nerurkar, P.V., et al. "Effects of Marinating with Asian Marinades or Western Barbecue Sauce on PhIP and MeIQx Formation in Barbecued Beef." *Nutrition and Cancer* 34 (1999): 147–52.

Organic Consumers Association Website: www.organicconsumers.org.

Palomboa, P. et al. "Beneficial Long-Term Effects of Combined Oral/Topical Antioxidant Treatment with the Carotenoids Lutein and Zeaxanthin on Human Skin: A Double-Blind, Placebo-Controlled Study." *Skin Pharmacology and Physiology* (2007): 20: 199–210.

Perricone, Nicholas, MD. *The Perricone Prescription.* New York: HarperCollins, 2002, p. 34.

Ponnampalam, E.N., et al. (2006) "Effect of Feeding Systems on Omega-3 Fatty Acids, Conjugated Linoleic Acid and Trans Fatty Acids in Australian Beef Cuts: Potential Impact on Human Health." *Asia Pacific Journal of Clinical Nutrition* (2006): 15(1): 21–9.

Prineas, R.J., G. Grandits, P.M. Rautaharju, J.D. Cohen, Z.M. Zhang, and R.S. Crow. "Long-term Prognostic Significance of Isolated Minor Electrocardiographic T-wave Abnormalities in Middle-aged Men Free of Clinical Cardiovascular Disease (The Multiple Risk Factor Intervention Trial [MRFIT])." *American Journal of Cardiology* 90 (2002): 1391–95.

Rauha, J.-P., S. Remes, et al. "Antimicrobial Effects of Finnish Plant Extracts Containing Flavonoids and Other Phenolic Compounds." *International Journal of Food Microbiology* (May 25, 2000): 56(1): 3–12.

Reddy, B.S., H. Newmark, N. Suh, A.M. Rimando, and C.V. Rao. "Novel Approaches for Colon Cancer Prevention by Types of Dietary Fat, Pterostilbene and Other

Food Components." *233rd National Meeting of the American Chemical Society.* (March 25, 2007): Abstract: AGFC 009.

Sanchez, A., et al. "Role of Sugars in Human Neutrophilic Phagocytosis." *American Journal of Clinical Nutrition* 261 (1973): 1180–84.

Scanto, S., and J. Yudkin. "The Effect of Dietary Sucrose on Blood Lipids, Serum Insulin, Platelet Adhesiveness and Body Weight in Human Volunteers." *Post-graduate Medicine Journal* 45 (1969): 602–7.

Sears, Barry, PhD. *The Zone.* New York: Regan Books, 1995, p. 21.

Séralini, G.E., et al. "New analysis of a rat feeding study with a genetically modified maize reveals signs of hepatorenal toxicity." *Archives of Environmental Contamination and Toxicology* (October 2007) Published online ahead of print, doi: 10.1007/s00244-006-0149-5.

Spears, Tom. "GE Canola Superweeds Spread Across Canada." *The Ottawa Citizen,* 6 February 2001.

Talcott, S., S. Percival, D. Del Pozo-Insfran, S. Mertens-Talcott, et al. "Brazilian Berry Destroys Cancer Cells in Lab." UF study shows *Journal of Agricultural and Food Chemistry* (February 22, 2006): 54(22).

Thomas, B J., R.J. Jarrett, H. Keen, and H.J. Ruskin. "Relation of Habitual Diet to Fasting Plasma Insulin Concentration and the Insulin Response to Oral Glucose." *Human Nutrition Clinical Nutrition* 36C, no. 1 (1982): 49–56.

Vutyavanich, T., T. Kraisarin, and R. Ruangsri. "Ginger for Nausea and Vomiting in Pregnancy: Randomized, Double-masked, Placebo-controlled Trial." *Obstetrics and Gynecology* 97 (2001): 577–82.

Zambon, D., J. Sabate, S. Munoz, B. Campero, E. Casals, M. Merlos, J.C. Laguna, and E. Ros. "Substituting Walnuts for Monounsaturated Fat Improves the Serum Lipid Profile of Hypercholesterolemic Men and Women: A Randomized Crossover Trial." *Annals of Internal Medicine* 132, no. 7 (2000): 538–46.

Chapter 8

Bernstein, J., et al. "Depression of Lymphosyte Transformation Following Oral Glucose Ingestion." *American Journal of Clinical Nutrition* 30 (1997): 613.

Engs, R.C. *Alcohol and Other Drugs: Self-Responsibility.* Bloomington, IN: Tichenor, 1987.

Juneja, L.R., D.C. Chu, and T. Okubo, et al. "L-Theanine – A Unique Amino Acid of Green Tea and Its Relaxation Effect in Humans." *Trends Food Science Technology* 10 (1999): 199–204.

Mischoulon, D., and M. Fava. "Docosahexanoic Acid and Omega 3 Fatty Acids in Depression." *Psychiatric Clinics of North America* 23 (2000): 785–94.

Sandyk, Reuven. "L-Tryptophan in Neuropsychiatric Disorders: A Review." *International Journal of Neuroscience* 67 (1992): 127-44.

Su. K., S. Huang, C. Chiu, et al. "Omega-3 Fatty Acids in Major Depressive Disorder. A Preliminary Double-Blind, Placebo-Controlled Trial." *European Neuropsychopharmacology* 2003: 13(4): 267–71.

Chapter 9

Aguillera, A.A., G.H. Diaz, et al. "Induction of Cd36 Expression Elicited by Fish Oil PUFA in Spontaneously Hypertensive Rats." *Journal of Nutritional Biochemistry* 17, 11 (1992): 760–5.

Anderson, R.A. "Chromium, Glucose Intolerance and Diabetes." *Journal of the American College of Nutrition* 17 (1998): 548–55.

Baskaran, K., et al. "Antidiabetic Effect of a Leaf Extract from Gymnema Sylvestre in Non-insulin-dependent Diabetes Mellitus Patients." *Journal of Ethnopharmacology* 30, no. 3 (October 1990): 295–300.

Baur, J.A., K.J. Pearson, et al. "Resveratol Improves Health and Survival of Mice on a High-calorie Diet." *Nature* 444, 7117 (2006): 337–42.

Bjørneboe, A., E. Søyland, G.E. Bjørneboe, et al. "Effect of Dietary Supplementation with Eicosapentaenoic Acid in the Treatment of Atopic Dermatitis." *British Journal of Dermatology* 117 (1987): 463–69.

Bjørneboe, A., E. Søyland, G.E. Bjørneboe, et al. "Effect of n-3 Fatty Acid Supplement to Patients with Atopic Dermatitis." *Journal of Internal Medicine: Supplement* 225 (1989): 233–36.

Blask, D.E., L.A. Sauer, and R.T. Dauchy. "Melatonin as a Chronobiotic/Anticancer Agent: Cellular, Biochemical, and Molecular Mechanisms of Action and Their Implications for Circadian-based Cancer Therapy." *Current Topics in Medical Chemistry* 2, no. 2 (February 2002): 113–32 [review].

Boldyrev, A., R. Song, D. Lawrence, et al. "Carnosine Protects against Excitotoxic Cell Death Independently of Effects on Reactive Oxygen Species." *Neuroscience* 94 (1999): 571–77.

Boldyrev, A., S.L. Stvolinsky, O.V. Tyulina, et al. "Biochemical and Physiological Evidence that Carnosine Is an Endogenous Neuroprotector against Free Radicals." *Cellular and Molecular Neurobiology* 17, no. 2 (1997): 259–71.

Brownson, C., and A.R. Hipkiss. "Carnosine Reacts with a Glycated Protein." *Free Radical Biology and Medicine* 28, no. 10 (2000): 1564–70.

Bunce, C.E. "Nutrition and Eye Disease of the Elderly." *Journal of Nutritional Biochemistry* 5 (February 1994): 66–76.

Calder, P.C., and S. Kew. "The Immune System: A Target for Functional Foods?" *British Journal of Nutrition* 88, supplement 2 (2002): S165–77.

Caruso, I., et al. "Double-blind Study of 5htp Versus Placebo in the Treatment of Primary Fibromyalgia Syndrome." *Journal of International Medical Research* 18 (May–June 1990): 201–9.

Ceconi, C., S. Curello, A. Cargnoni, et al. "The Role of Glutathione Status in the Protection against Ischaemic and Reperfusion Damage: Effects of N-acetyl cysteine." *Journal of Molecular and Cellular Cardiology* 20 (1988): 5–13.

Chernomorsky, S.A., and A.B. Segelman. "Biological Activities of Chlorophyll Derivatives." *New Jersey Medicine* 85 (1988): 669–73.

Chou, F.P., Y.D. Chu, J.D. Hsu, H.C. Chiang, and C.J. Wang. "Specific Induction of Glutathione S-transferase GSTM2 Subunit Expression by Epigallocatechin Gallate in Rat Liver." *Biochemical Pharmacology* 60, no. 5 (1 September 2000): 643–50.

Clark, L.C., G.F. Combs, Jr., B.W. Turnbull, et al. "Effects of Selenium Supplementation for Cancer Prevention in Patients with Carcinoma of the Skin: A Randomized Controlled Trial." Nutritional Prevention of Cancer Study Group. *Journal of the American Medical Association* 276 (1996): 1957–63.

Cover, C.M., et al. "Indole-3-carbinol Inhibits the Expression of Cyclin-dependent Kinase-6 and Induces a G1 Cell Cycle Arrest of Human Breast Cancer Cells Independent of Estrogen Receptor Signaling." *Journal of Biological Chemistry* 273 (1998): 3838–47.

Diehm, C., H.J. Trampisch, S. Lange, and C. Schmidt. "Comparison of Leg Compression Stocking and Oral Horse-chestnut Seed Extract Therapy in Patients with Chronic Venous Insufficiency." *Lancet* 347, no. 8997 (1996): 292–94.

Diehm, C., D. Vollbrecht, K. Amendt, and H.U. Comberg. "Medical Edema Protection—Clinical Benefit in Patients with Chronic Deep Vein Incompetence: A Placebo-control Double-blind Study." *Vasa* 21, no. 2 (1992): 188–92.

Dulloo, A.G., C. Duret, D. Rohrer, L. Girardier, N. Mensi, M. Fathi, P. Chantre, and J. Vandermander. "Efficacy of a Green Tea Extract Rich in Catechin Polyphenols and Caffeine in Increasing 24-h Energy Expenditure and Fat Oxidation in Humans." *American Journal of Clinical Nutrition* 70, no. 6 (December 1999): 1040–45.

Eliaz, I., Rode, D. "The Effect of Modified Citrus Pectin on Urinary Excretion of Toxic Elements." *Fifth Annual Conference of Environmental Health Scientists.* Nutritional Toxicology and Metabolomics, University of California, Davis.

Enstrom, J.E., et al. "Vitamin C Intake and Mortality Among a Sample of the United States Population." *Epidemiology* 3 (1992): 194–202.

Fischer, Tobias W., Trevor W. Sweatman, Igor Semak, Robert M. Sayre, Jacobo Wortsman, and Andrzej Slominsk. "Constitutive and UV-induced Metabolism of Melatonin in Keratinocytes and Cell-free Systems." *The Journal of the Federation of American Societies for Experimental Biology* 20 (2006): 1564–1566.

Fogarty, A., and J. Britton. "The Role of Diet in the Aetiology of Asthma." *Clinical & Experimental Allergy* 30 (2000): 615–627.

Foster, Harold D., PhD. "Selenium and Cancer: A Geographical Perspective." *The Journal of Orthomolecular Medicine* 13, 1 (1998): 8–10.

Fuchs, C.S., et al. "The Influence of Folate and Multivitamin Use on the Familial Risk of Colon Cancer in Women." *Cancer Epidemiology, Biomarkers, and Prevention* 11 (2002): 227–34.

Fuchs, Nan Catherine. "Q & A." *Women's Health Letter* 8 (January 1999), p. 8.

Fujita, T., Y. Fujii, B. Goto, A. Miyauchi, and Y. Takagi. "Peripheral Computed Tomography (pQCT) Detected Short-term Effect of AAACa (Heated Oyster Shell with Heated Algal Ingredient HAI): A Double-blind Comparison with CaCO3 and Placebo." *Journal of Bone and Mineral Metabolism* 18 (2000): 212–15.

Gaby, A.R. "The Role of Coenzyme Q10 in Clinical Medicine: Part II. Cardiovascular Disease, Hypertension, Diabetes Mellitus and Infertility." *Alternative Medicine Review* 1 (1996): 168–75.

Ganguli, S., et al. "Effects of Maternal Vanadate Treatment of Fetal Development." *Life Sciences* 55, no. 16 (1994): 1267–76.

Garland, C.F., Gorham, E.D., et al. "Vitamin D and Prevention of Breast Cancer: Pooled Analysis." *The Journal of Steriod Biochemistry and Molecular Biology* 103, 3-5 (2007): 708–11.

Green P., I. Gispan-Herman, and G. Yadid. "Increased arachidonic acid concentration in the brain of Flinders Sensitive Line rats, an animal model of depression." *Journal of Lipid Res*, 2005; 46:1093–1096.

Greul, A.K., J.U. Grundmann, F. Heinrich, et al. "Photoprotection of UV-irradiated Human Skin: An Antioxidative Combination of Vitamins E and C, Carotenoids, Selenium and Proanthocyanidins." *Skin Pharmacology and Applied Skin Physiology* 15 (2002): 307–315.

Gruskin, B. "Chlorophyll—Its Therapeutic Place in Acute and Suppurative Disease." *American Journal of Surgery* 49 (1940): 49–56.

Hagen, T.M., et al. "Feeding Acetyl-L-carnitine and Lipoic Acid to Old Rats Significantly Improves Metabolic Function while Decreasing Oxidative Stress." *Proceedings of the National Academy of Sciences* 99, no. 4 (19 February 2002): 1870–75.

Hagino, N., and S. Ichimura. "Effects of Chlorella on Fecal and Urinary Cadmium Excretion in 'Itai-itai.'" *Japanese Journal of Hygiene* 30, no. 1 (1975): 77.

Hammes, H.P., X. Du, D. Edelstein, T. Taguchi, T. Matsumura, Q. Je, J. Lin, A. Bierhaus, P. Nawroth, D. Hannak, M. Neumaier, T. Bergfeld, I. Giardino, and M. Brownlee. "Benfotiamine blocks three major pathways of hyperglycemic damage and prevents experimental diabetic retinopathy." *Natural Medicine* 3 (9 Mar, 2003): 294–299.

Heaney, R.P. "The Vitamin D Requirement in Health and Disease." *Journal of Steroid Biochemistry and Molecular Biology* 97, 1-2 (2005): 13–19.

Heerdt, A.S., et al. "Calcium Glucarate as a Chemopreventive Agent in Breast Cancer." *Journal of Medical Sciences* (Israel) 31, nos. 2–3 (1995): 101–5.

Heinrich, U., H. Tronnier, et al. "Antioxidant Supplements Improve Parameters Rekated to Skin Structure in Humans." *Skin Pharmacology and Physiology* 19, 4 (2006): 224–31.

Hitti, M. "Study: Brown Seaweed May Burn Fat." CBSNews.com www.cbsnews.com/stories/2006/09/11/health/webmd/main1998080.shtml

Hoeger, W.W., C. Harris, E.M. Long, and D.R. Hopkins. "Four-week Supplementation with a Natural Dietary Compound Produces Favorable Changes in Body Composition." *Advances in Therapy* 15, no. 5 (September–October 1998): 305–14.

Holick, M.F. "Sunlight and Vitamin D for Bone Health and Prevention of Autoimmune Diseases, Cancers, and Cardiovascular Disease." *The Journal of Clinical Nutrition* 80, 1 (2004): (supplement): 678S–88S.

Horrobin, D.F. "The Importance of Gamma-linolenic Acid and Prostaglandin E1 in Human Nutrition and Medicine." *Journal of Holistic Medicine* 3 (1981): 118–39.

Ingels, Darin. "Diglyceride-Rich Foods May Promote Weight Loss." *Healthnotes Newswire*, 23 January 2003.

Interview. "Pumping Immunity." *Nutrition Action Health Letter* (April 1993): 5–7.

Iwamoto, J., T. Takeda, S. Ichimura, and M. Uzawa. "Effects of Five-year Treatment with Elcatonin and Alfacalcidol on Lumbar Bone Mineral Density and the Incidence of Vertebral Fractures in Postmenopausal Women with Osteoporosis: A Retrospective Study." *Journal of Orthopaedic Science* 7 (2002): 637–43.

Jain, S.K. "Should High-Dose Vitamin E Supplementation Be Recommended to Diabetic Patients?" *Diabetes Care* 22, 8 (Aug 1999): 1242–44.

Jordan, Karin G., MD. "Can Silibinin Arrest Cancer Cells Growth?" *Life Extension Magazine*, June 2000, p. 27.

Jordan, Karin G., MD. "Nature's Pluripotent Life Extension Agent." *Life Extension Magazine*, January 2001, p. 27.

Kaats, G., K. Blum, D. Pullin, et al. "A Randomized, Double-masked, Placebo-controlled Study of the Effects of Chromium Picolinate Supplementation on Body Composition: A Replication and Extension of a Previous Study." *Current Therapeutic Research* 59 (1998): 379–88.

Kagan, V., S. Khan, C. Swanson, et al. "Antioxidant Action of Thioctic Acid and Dihydrolipoic Acid." *Free Radical Biology and Medicine* 9S (1990): 15.

Kamenova, P. "Improvement of Insulin Sensitivity in Patients with Type 2 Diabetes Mellitus After Oral Administration of Alpha-Lipoic Acid." *Hormones* (Athens), 2006; 5(4): 251–8.

Kramer, J.M. "N-3 Fatty Acid Supplements in Rheumatoid Arthritis." *American Journal of Clinical Nutrition* 71, supplement 1 (2000): 349S–51S.

Kotsopoulos, J., and S.A. Narod. "Toward a Dietary Prevention of Hereditary Breast Cancer." *Cancer Causes Control* 16 (2005): 16: 125–38.

Kuriyama, K., T. Shimizu, T. Horiguchi, M. Watabe, and Y. Abe. "Vitamin E Ointment at High Dose Levels Suppresses Contact Dermatitis in Rats by Stabilizing Keratinocytes." *Inflammation Research* 51, no. 10 (October 2002): 483–89.

Kuriyan, R., et al. "Effect of Caralluma Fimbriata Extract on Appetite, Food Intake and Anthropometry in Adult Indian Men and Women." *Appetite* (2006): doi: 10.1016/j.appet. 2006.09.013.

Landi, G. "Oral Administration of Borage Oil in Atopic Dermatitis." *Journal of Applied Cosmetology* 11 (1993): 115–20.

Limpens, J., F.H. Schroder, et al. "Combined Lycopene and Vitamin E Treatment Suppresses the Growth of PC-346-C Human Prostate Cancer Cells in Nude Mice." *The Journal of Nutrition* 136, 5 (2006): 1287–93.

Lin, F.Y., N.A. Monteiro-Riviere, J.M. Grichnik, J.E. Zielinski, and S.R. Pinnell. "A Topical Antioxidant Solution Containing Vitamin C, Vitamin E, and Ferulic Acid Prevents Ultraviolet-radiation-induced Caspase-3 Induction in Skin." *Journal of American Academy of Dermatology* 52 (2005): 158.

Lockwood, K., et al. "Progress on Therapy of Breast Cancer with Vitamin Q10 and the Regression of Metastases." *Biochemical and Biophysical Research Communications* 212 (1995): 172–77.

Mahoney, Sarah. "A new wave of ocean-based beauty products extols the virtues of algae, but is the power in the ingredient or in the marketing?" *Spa Finder Global Spa Resource* January/February 2005.

Majamaa, H. "Probiotics: A Novel Approach in the Management of Food Allergy." *Journal of Allergy and Clinical Immunology* 99, no. 2 (1997): 179–85.

Mancini, M., F. Rengo, M. Lingetti, et al. "Controlled Study on the Therapeutic Efficacy of Propionyl-L-carnitine in Patients with Congestive Heart Failure." *Arzneimittelforschung* 42 (1992): 1101–4.

Meletis, C.D., ND, and Ben Bramwell. "Natural Approaches to the Prevention and Management of Diabetes." *Alternative & Complementary Therapies* 7, 3 (June 2001): 132–7.

Melnikova, V.M., N.M. Gracheva, G.P. Belikov, et al. "The Chemoprophylaxis and Chemotherapy of Opportunistic Infections." *Antibiotiki i Khimioterapiia* 38 (1993): 44–48.

Mori, H., K. Niwa, Q. Zheng, Y. Yamada, K. Sakata, and N. Yoshimi. "Cell Proliferation in Cancer Prevention: Effects of Preventive Agents on Estrogen-related Endometrial Carcinogenesis Model and on an In Vitro Model in Human Colorectal Cells." *Mutation Research* 480–81 (1 September 2001): 201–7.

Mortensen, S.A., A. Leth, E. Agner, and M. Rohde. "Dose-related Decrease of Serum Coenzyme Q10 during Treatment with HMG-CoA Reductase Inhibitors." *Molecular Aspects of Medicine* 18, supplement (1997): S137–44.

Muzzarelli, R.A. "Clinical and Biochemical Evaluation of Chitosan for Hypercholesterolemia and Overweight Control." *Experientia Supplementa* (EXS) 87 (1999): 293–304.

Nakachi, K., K. Suemasu, K. Suga, T. Takeo, K. Imai, and Y. Higashi. "Influence of Drinking Green Tea on Breast Cancer Malignancy among Japanese Patients." *Japanese Journal of Cancer Research* 89, no. 3 (1998): 254–61.

Nelson, S., A. Swapan, K. Bose, G. Grunwald, P. Myhill, and J. McCord. "The Induction of Human Superoxide Dismutase and Catalase in Vivo: A Fundamental New Approach to Antioxidant Therapy." *Free Radical Biology & Medicine* 40 (2006): 341–347.

Nesaretnam, K., R. Stephen, R. Dils, and P. Darbre. "Tocotrienols Inhibit the Growth of Human Breast Cancer Cells Irrespective of Estrogen Receptor Status." *Lipids* 33 (1998): 461–69.

Newberne. P.M. "Lipotropic Factors and Oncogenesis." *Advances in Experimental Medicine and Biology* 206 (1986): 223–51.

Nusgens, B.V., P. Humbert, A. Rougier, et al. "Stimulation of Collagen Biosynthesis by Topically Applied Vitamin C." *European Journal of Dermatology* 12 (2002): xxxii–xxxiv.

Ohia, S.E., C.A. Opere, A.M. LeDay, et al. "Safety and Mechanism of Appetite Suppression by a Novel Hydroxycitric Acid Extract (HCA-SX)." *Molecular and Cellular Biochemistry* 238 (2002): 89–103.

Olson, P.E., et al. "Oral Vitamin E for Refractory Hand Dermatitus." *Lancet* 343 (March 12, 1994): 672–3.

Paneerselvam, K.S., and S. Kumaran. "L-carnitine and Alpha-lipoic Acid Improves Mitochondrial Function During Ageing Process." *Clinical Nutrition* (May 9, 2006).

Perricone, Nicholas, MD. *The Perricone Prescription*. New York: HarperCollins, 2002, p. 129.

Pinnell, S.R. "Cutaneous Photodamage, Oxidative Stress, and Topical Antioxidant Protection." *Journal of the American Academy of Dermatology* 48, no. 1 (January 2003): 1–19.

Psasad, A.S., F.W.J. Beck, B. Bao, D.C. Fitzgerald, D.C. Snell, J.D. Steinberg, and L.J. Cardozo. "Zinc Supplementation Decreases Incidence of Infections in the Elderly: Effect of Zinc on Generation of Cytokines and Oxidative Stress." *American Journal of Clinical Nutrition* 85, 3 (2007): 837–44.

Rimm, Eric, et al. "Vitamin E and Heart Disease Incidence in the Health Professionals Study." *American Heart Association Annual Meeting*, New Orleans (Nov 18, 1992).

Ringsdorf, W.M., Jr., and E. Cheraskin. "Vitamin C and Human Wound Healing." *Oral Surgery* 14, 2 (March 1982): 124–136.

Riserus, U., L. Berglund, and B. Vessby. "Conjugated Linoleic Acid (CLA) Reduced Abdominal Adipose Tissue in Obese Middle-aged Men with Signs of the Metabolic Syndrome: A Randomised Controlled Trial." *International Journal of Obesity and Related Metabolic Disorders* 25, no. 8 (August 2001): 1129–35.

Rose, D.P., and J.M. Conolley. "Omega-3 Fatty Acids as Cancer Chemopreventive Agents." *Pharmacology and Therapeutics* 83 (1999): 217–44.

Sajithlal, G.B., P. Chithra, and G. Chandrakasan. "Advanced Glycation End Products Induce Cross-linking of Collagen In Vitro." *Biochimica Biophysica Acta* 1407 (1998): 215–24.

Saliou, C., G. Rimbach, H. Moini, et al. "Solar Ultraviolet-induced Erythema in Human Skin and Nuclear Factor-kappa-B-dependent Gene Expression in Keratinocytes are Modulated by a French Maritime Pine Bark Extract." *Free Radical Biology and Medicine* 30 (2001): 154-160.

Sardi, W. "Is High Dose Vitamin C Risky?" *Epidemiology* 11: 440–5.

Scambia, G., et al. "Antiproliferative Effect of Silybin on Gynaecological Malignancies: Synergism with Cisplatin and Doxorubicin." *European Journal of Cancer* 32A (1996): 877–82.

Schellenberg, R. "Treatment for the Premenstrual Syndrome with Agnus Castus Fruit Extract: Prospective, Randomized, Placebo Controlled Study." *British Medical Journal* 20 (2001): 134–37.

Schnyder, G., et al. "Decreased Rate of Coronary Restenosis after Lowering of Plasma Homocysteine Levels." *New England Journal of Medicine* 345 (2001): 1593–600.

Schrauzer, G.N., et al. "Cancer Mortality Correlation Studies—III: Statistical Associations with Dietary Selenium Intakes." *Bioinorganic Chemistry* 7 (1977): 23–31.

Shanmugasundaram, E.R., et al. "Use of Gymnema Sylvestre Leaf Extract in the Control of Blood Glucose in Insulin-dependent Diabetes Mellitus." *Journal of Ethnopharmacology* 30, no. 3 (October 1990): 281–94.

Shao, Z.M., Z.Z. Shen, C.H. Liu, M.R. Sartippour, V.L. Go, D. Heber, and M. Nguyen. "Curcumin Exerts Multiple Suppressive Effects on Human Breast Carcinoma Cells." *International Journal of Cancer* 98, no. 2 (10 March 2002): 234–40.

Shixian, Q., B. VanCrey, et al. "Thermogenesis-induced Weight Loss by Epigallocatechin Gallate Inhibition of Catechol-O-methyltransferase." *Journal of Medicinal Food* 9, 4 (Winter 2006): 451–8.

Singer, Sydney Ross, and Soma Grismaijer. *Dressed to Kill: The Link between Breast Cancer and Bras.* Pahoa, Hawaii: ISCD Press, 1995.

"Slendesta Potato Extract Promotes Satiety & Weight Loss: A recent study at Iowa State University." *Nutritional Outlook* (November 1, 2006).

Søyland, E., G. Rajka, A. Bjørneboe, et al. "The Effect of Eicosapentaenoic Acid in the Treatment of Atopic Dermatitis: A Clinical Study." *Acta Dermato-Venereologica* (Stockholm) 144, supplement (1989): 139.

Stampfer, Meir, Walter Willett, et al. "Vitamin E and Heart Incidence in the Nurses Health Study." *American Heart Association Annual Meeting*, New Orleans (Nov 18, 1992).

St-Onge, M.P., C. Bourque, P.J. Jones, R. Ross, and W.E. Parsons. "Medium- versus Long-chain Triglycerides for Twenty-seven Days Increases Fat Oxidation and Energy Expenditure without Resulting in Changes in Body Composition in Overweight Women." *International Journal of Obesity and Related Metabolic Disorders* 27, no. 1 (January 2003): 95–102.

Sullivan, A.C., J.G. Hamilton, O.N. Miller, et al. "Inhibition of Lipogenesis in Rat Liver by (-)-hydroxycitrate." *Archives of Biochemistry and Biophysics* 150 (1972): 183–90.

Tan, Sharon. "The Bra Connection to Breast Cancer." Frost & Sullivan, August 2002. www.frost.com.

Thomson, M. "Molecular and Cellular Mechanisms Used in the Acute Phase of Stimulated Steroidogeneisis." *Hormone and Metabolic Research* 1 (Jan 30, 1998): 16–28.

Theriault, A., J.T. Chao, Q. Wang, et al. "Tocotrienol: A Review of Its Therapeutic Potential." *Clinical Biochemistry* 32 (1999): 309–19 [review].

Thiel, F.J. "Natural Vitamins May Be Superior to Synthetic Ones." *Medical Hypotheses* 55, no. 6 (December 2000): 461–69.

Touillard, M.S., F. Clavel-Chapelon, et al. "Dietary Lignan Intake and Post-menopausal Breast Cancer Risk by Estrogen and Progesterone Receptor Status." *Journal of the National Cancer Institute* 99, 6 (2007): 475-86.

Valenzuela, A., and A. Garrido. "Biochemical Bases of the Pharmacological Action of the Flavonoid Silymarin and of Its Structural Isomer Silibinin." *Biological Research* 27 (1994): 105–12.

"Vegetables Without Vitamins." *Life Extension Magazine*, March 2001, p. 28.

Wagner, H., H. Nörr, and H. Winterhoff. "Plant Adaptogens." *Phytomedicine* 1 (1994): 63–76 [review].

Wang, M., E. Fox, B. Stoecker, et al. "Serum Cholesterol of Adults Supplemented with Brewer's Yeast or Chromium Chloride." *Nutrition Research* 9 (1989): 989–98.

Wasserman, M., et al. "Organochlorine Compounds in Neoplastic and Adjacent Apparently Normal Breast Tissue." *Bulletin of Environmental Contaminants and Toxicology* 15 (1976): 478–84.

Weber, C., T.S. Jakobsen, S.A. Mortensen, et al. "Antioxidative Effect of Dietary Coenzyme Q10 in Human Blood Plasma." *International Journal for Vitamin and Nutrition Research* 64 (1994): 311–15.

Westin, J., and E. Richter. "Israeli Breast Cancer Anomaly." *Annals of the New York Academy of Sciences* 609 (1990): 269–79.

Whitaker, Julian, MD. *Health and Healing*. Potamac, Md.: Phillips Publishing, 2002.

Wilkinson, I.B., I.L. Megson, H. MacCallum, et al. "Oral Vitamin C Reduces Arterial Stiffness and Platelet Aggregation in Humans." *Journal of Cardiovascular Pharmacology* 34 (1999): 690–93.

Wilkinson, S.C., K.H. Goulding, P.K. Robinson. "Mercury Removal by Immobilized Algae in Batch Culture Systems." *Journal of Applied Phycology* 2 (1990): 223–30.

Yan, J., K. Jujjii, J. Yao, et al. "Reduced Coenzyme Q10 Supplementation Decelerates Senescence in SAMP1 Mice." *Exp Gerontol* 41, 2 (February 2006): 130–40.

Yim, C.Y., J.B. Hibbs, Jr., J.R. McGregor, et al. "Use of N-acetyl Cysteine to Increase Intracellular Glutathione during the Induction of Antitumor Responses by IL-2." *Journal of Immunology* 152 (1994): 5796–805.

Yuneva, M.O., E.R. Bulygina, S.C. Gallant, et al. "Effect of Carnosine on Age-induced Changes in Senescence-accelerated Mice." *Journal of Anti-Aging Medicine* 2, no. 4 (1999): 337–42.

Zhao, J., and R. Agarwal. "Tissue Distribution of Silibinin, the Major Active Constituent of Silymarin: Implications in Cancer Chemoprevention." *Carcinogenesis* (1999): 2101–8.

Zhu, Z.R., J.A.S. Mannisto, P. Pietinene, et al. "Fatty Acid Composition of Breast Adipose Tissue in Breast Cancer Patients and Patients with Benign Breast Disease." *Nutrition and Cancer* 24 (1995): 151–60.

Zi, X., D.K. Feyes, and R. Agarwal. "Anticarcinogenic Effect of a Flavonoid Antioxidant, Silymarin, in Human Breast Cancer Cells MDA-MB 468: Induction of G1 Arrest through an Increase in Cip1/p21 Concomitant with a Decrease in Kinase Activity of Cyclin-dependent Kinases and Associated Cyclins." *Clinical Cancer Research* 4, no. 4 (April 1998): 1055–64.

Ziboh, V.A., C.C. Miller, and Y. Cho. "Metabolism of Polyunsaturated Fatty Acids by Skin Epidermal Enzymes: Generation of Anti-inflammatory and Antiproliferative

Metabolites." *American Journal of Clinical Nutrition* 71, supplement 1 (2000): 361S–66S [review].

Zurier, R.B., et al. "Gamma-Linolenic Acid Treatment of Rheumatoid Arthritis: A Randomized, Placebo-controlled Trial." *Arthritis and Rheumatism* 39 (1996): 1808–17.

Chapter 11

Erasmus, Udo. *Fats That Heal, Fats That Kill.* Burnaby, B.C., Canada: Alive Books, 1986, 1993, pp. 58–59.

Frost, Phillip, MD, and Steven Horwitz, MD. *Principles of Cosmetics for the Dermatologist.* St. Louis, Mo.: The C. V. Mosby Company, 1982.

Kligman, A.M., and O.H. Mills. "Acne Cosmetica." *Archives of Dermatology* 106 (1972): 843–50.

Lewis, Carol. "Sunning for Science: The Effects of Common Substances on Sun-exposed Skin." *FDA Consumer magazine*, November–December 2002. www.fda.gov/fdac/602_toc.html.

Morris, Robert, et al. "Chlorination, Chlorination By-products, and Cancer: A Meta-analysis." *American Journal of Public Health* 82, no. 7 (July 1992): 955–63.

Poole, K. "Mechanisms of Bacterial Biocide and Antibiotic Resistance." *Journal of Applied Microbiology* 92, supplement (2002): 55S–64S.

Prottey, C. "The Molecular Basis of Skin Irritation." *Cosmetic Science*, 1978.

Roeding, J., and M. Ghyczy. "Control of Skin Humidity with Liposomes: Stabilization of Skin Care Oils and Lipophillic Active Substances with Liposomes." *Seifen-Ole-Fette-Wachse (S...FW)* 10 (1991): 378.

Vance, Judi. *Beauty to Die For.* San Jose, Calif.: To Excel, 1999, p. 19.

Yow, Elizabeth. "Acid Washed Face: Are AHAs and Glycolics Damaging Your Skin?" *Fashion Wire Daily*, 17 November 1999. www.fashionwiredaily.com.

Chapter 12

Berkson, D. Lindsey. *Hormone Deception.* Lincolnwood, Ill.: Contemporary Books, 2000.

Blout, B., et al. "Levels of Seven Urinary Phthalate Metabolites in a Human Reference Population." *Environmental Health Perspectives* 108 (2000): 972–82.

Bradbard, Laura. "On the Teen Scene: Cosmetics and Reality." *FDA Consumer*, November 1993, Publication No. (FDA) 94-5015.

The Cancer Prevention Coalition Website: www.preventcancer.com.

"Chemicals in the Environment: Toluene." Office of Pollution Prevention and Toxics, U.S. Environmental Protection Agency, August 1994. www.epa.gov/chemfact/f_toluen.txt.

Colon, I., et al. "Identification of Phthalate Esters in the Serum of Young Puerto Rican Girls with Premature Breast Development." *Environmental Health Perspectives* 108 (2000): 895–900.

"Cosmetic Product-Related Regulatory Requirements and Health Hazard Issue." In *Cosmetic Handbook*. U.S. Food and Drug Administration Center for Food Safety and Applied Nutrition FDA/Industry Activities Staff Booklet, 1992. www.cfsan.fda.gov/~dms/cos-hdb3.html.

De Fazio, Angel. "How Environmentally Aware Are You?" *Holistic Times* 6, no. 3 (1999).

Epstein, Samuel, MD, and Amy Marsh. "Perfume: Cupid's Arrow or Poison Dart?" Joint press release issued by the Cancer Prevention Coalition and the Environmental Health Network, 7 February 2002.

Epstein, Samuel S., and David R. Obey. *The Politics of Cancer Revisited*. Hankins, N.Y.: East Ridge Press, 1998.

Erickson, Kim. *Drop Dead Gorgeous*. New York: McGraw-Hill, Contemporary Books, 2002, p. 120.

Gago-Dominguez, M., J.E. Castelao, J.M. Yuan, M.C. Yu, and R.K. Ross. "Use of Permanent Hair Dyes and Bladder-cancer Risk." *International Journal of Cancer* 91, no. 4 (15 February 2001): 575–79.

Guidotti, Sylvana, William E. Wright, John Peters, MD, et al. "Multiple Myeloma in Cosmetologists." *American Journal of Industrial Medicine* 3, no. 2 (September 1982): 169–71.

Harte, John, Cheryl Holdren, Richard Schneider, and Christine Shirley. *Toxics A to Z: A Guide to Everyday Pollution Hazards*. Berkeley and Los Angeles: University of California Press, 1991.

"Hypoallergenic Cosmetics." FDA Office of Cosmetics and Colors Fact Sheet. U.S. Food and Drug Administration. 19 December 1994, revised 18 October 2000. www.cfsan.fda.gov/~dms/cos-224.html.

Kirkland, D.J., MD, et al. "Hair Dye Genotoxicity." *American Heart Journal* 98, no. 6 (December 1979): 814.

Kligman, A.M., and O. Mills. "Acne Cosmetica." *Archives of Dermatology* 106 (1972): 843–50.

National Research Council. *Toxicity Testing: Strategies to Determine Needs and Priorities*. Washington, D.C.: National Academy Press, 1984.

Paustenbach, D.J. "The U.S. EPA Science Advisory Board Evaluation (2001) of the EPA Dioxin Reassessment." *Regulatory Toxicology and Pharmacology* 36, no. 2 (October 2002): 211–19.

"Public Health Statement for Toluene." U.S. Department of Health and Human Services Agency for Toxic Substances and Disease Registry. May 1994. *www.atsdr.cdc.gov/toxprofiles/phs56.html*.

"Report on the Consensus Workshop on Formaldehyde." *Environmental Health Perspectives* 58 (December 1984): 323–81.

Rogers, J.M., and M.S. Denison. "Analysis of the Antiestrogenic Activity of 2,3,7,8-tetra-chlorodibenzo-p-dioxin in Human Ovarian Carcinoma BG-1 Cells." *Molecular Pharmacology* 61, no. 6 (June 2002): 1393–403.

Routledge, E.J., J. Parker, J. Odum, J. Ashby, and J.P. Sumpter. "Some Alkyl Hydroxy Benzoate Preservatives (Parabens) Are Estrogenic." *Toxicology and Applied Pharmacology* 153, no. 1 (November 1998): 12–19.

Schafer, T., E. Bohler, S. Ruhdorfer, L. Weigl, D. Wessner, B. Filipiak, H.E. Wichmann, and J. Ring. "Epidemiology of Contact Allergy in Adults." *Allergy* 56, no. 12 (December 2001): 1192–96.

Scheinman, P.L. "Prevalence of Fragrance Allergy." *Dermatology* 205, no. 1 (2002): 98–102.

Schlumpf, Margaret, Beata Cotton, Marianne Conscience, Vreni Haller, Beate Steinmann, and Walter Lichtensteiger. "In Vitro and In Vivo Estrogenicity of UV Screens." *Environmental Health Perspectives* 109 (March 2001): 239–44.

Smeh, Nicholas J. *Health Risks in Today's Cosmetics*. Garrisonville, Va.: Alliance Publishing Company, 1994, p. 1.

Steinmann, David, and Samuel Epstein. *The Safe Shopper's Bible*. New York: Macmillan, 1995.

Thun, Michael J., Sean F. Alterkruse, Mohan M. Namboodiri, Eugenia E. Calle, Dena G. Meyers, and Clark W. Heath, Jr. "Hair Dye Use and Risk of Fatal Cancers in U.S. Women." *Journal of the National Cancer Institute* 86 (1994): 210–15.

U.S. Department of Health and Human Services. Cosmetics Handbook. U.S. Food and Drug Administration Center for Food Safety and Applied Nutrition FDA/Industry Activities Staff Booklet. Washington, D.C.: U.S. Government Printing Office, 1992.

Winter, Ruth. *A Consumer's Dictionary of Cosmetic Ingredients.* New York: Crown, 1989, p. 9.

Yu, M.C., P.L. Skipper, S.R. Tannenbaum, K.K. Chan, and R.K. Ross. "Arylamine Exposures and Bladder Cancer Risk." *Mutation Research* 506–7 (30 September 2002): 21–28 [review].

Chapter 13

Abels, D.J., T. Rose, and J.E. Bearman. "Treatment of Psoriasis at a Dead Sea Dermatology Clinic." *International Journal of Dermatology* 34, no. 2 (February 1995): 134–37.

Aertgeerts, P., et al. "Comparative Testing of Kamillosan Cream and Steroidal (0.25% Hydrocortisone, 0.75% Fluocortin Butyl Ester) and Non-steroidal (5% Bufexamac) Dermatologic Agents in Maintenance Therapy of Eczematous Diseases" (in German). *Zeitschrift für Hautkrankheiten* 60, no. 3 (1985): 270–77.

Aesoph, Lauri. *Your Natural Health Makeover.* Upper Saddle River, N.J.: Prentice-Hall, 1998.

Allison, J.R. "The Relation of Hydrochloric Acid and Vitamin B Complex Deficiency in Certain Skin Diseases." *Southern Medical Journal* 38 (1945): 235–41.

Almas, K. "Antimicrobial Effects of Extracts of Azadirachta Indica (Neem) and Salvadora Persica (Arak) Chewing Sticks." *Indian Journal of Dental Research* 10 (January–March 1999): 23–26.

Angermeier, M. C. "Treatment of Facial Vascular Lesions with Intense Pulsed Light." *Journal of Cutaneous Laser Therapy* 1, no. 2 (April 1999): 95–100.

Armugam, M.Q., W. Bonfield, R.A. Brooks, N. Rushton, et al. "Orthosilic Acid Increases Collagen Type I mRNA Expression in Human Bone-Derived Osteoblasts in Vitro." *Cambridge University School of Clinical Medicine* 0-87849-932-6.

"Azelaic Acid—A New Topical Treatment for Acne." *Drug and Therapy Bulletin* 31 (1993): 50–52.

Benoit, I., L. Danoux, V. Gillon, P. Moussou, and G. Pauly. "Oligopeptides from Hibiscus esculentus seeds to smooth expression lines." *Skin Care Forum* (39).

Berbis, P., S. Hesse, and Y. Privat. "Essential Fatty Acids and the Skin." *Allergie et Immunologie* (Paris) 22, no. 6 (June 1990): 225–31.

Bernstein, J.E., L.C. Parish, M. Rapaport, M.M. Rosenbaum, and H.H. Roenigk, Jr. "Effects of Topically Applied Capsaicin on Moderate and Severe Psoriasis Vulgaris."

Journal of the American Academy of Dermatology 15, no. 3 (September 1986): 504–7.

Bierhaus, A., et al. "Advanced Glycation End Product-induced Activation of NF-kappaB Is Suppressed by Alpha-lipoic Acid in Cultured Endothelial Cells." *Diabetes* 46, no. 9 (September 1997): 1481–90.

Blumenthal, Mark, Alicia Goldberg, and Josef Brinckmann. Herbal Medicine: Expanded Commission E Monographs. Newton, Mass.: *Integrative Medicine Communications*, 2000.

Boelsma, E., H.F. Hendriks, and L. Roza. "Nutritional Skin Care: Health Effects of Micronutrients and Fatty Acids." *American Journal of Clinical Nutrition* 73, no. 5 (May 2001): 853–64.

Brown, A., et al. "Medical Nutrition Therapy as a Potential Complementary Treatment for Psoriasis—Five Case Reports." *Alternative Medicine Review* 9, 3 (2004): 297–307.

Brownstein, Arlen, MS, ND, and Donna Schoemaker, CN. *Rosacea: Your Self-Help Guide*. Oakland, Calif.: New Harbinger Publications, 2001.

Buffalo, Jody. "The Science of Cellulite" (Pentapeptides). *Shape* (May 2004).

Chang, P., J. Wiseman, T. Jacoby, A.V. Salisbury, and R.A. Esrek. "Non-invasive Mechanical Body Contouring: (Endermologie) a One-year Clinical Outcome Study Update." *Aesthetic Plastic Surgery* 22, 2 (Mar-Apr 1998): 145-53.

Chithra, P., et al. "Influence of Aloe Vera on Collagen Characteristics in Healing Dermal Wounds in Rats." *Molecular and Cellular Biochemistry* 181, nos. 1–2 (April 1998): 71–76.

Cordain, L., S. Lindeberg, M. Hurtado, K. Hill, S.B. Eaton, and J. Brand-Miller. "Acne Vulgaris: A Disease of Western Civilization." *Archives of Dermatology* 138, no. 12 (December 2002): 1584–90.

Deutch, C.H., "Cosmetics Break the Skin Barrier (GABA relaxes muslces and wrinkles)." *New York Times* January 8, 2005.

Diehm C., D. Vollbrecht, K. Amendt, and H.U. Comberg. "Medical Edema Protection—Clinical Benefit in Patients with Chronic Deep Vein Incompetence: A Placebo-controlled Double-blind Study." *Vasa* 21, no. 2 (1992): 188–92.

Dreno, B., D. Moyse, M. Alirezai, P. Amblard, N. Auffret, C. Beylot, I. Bodokh, M. Chivot, F. Daniel, P. Humbert, J. Meynadier, and F. Poli. "Multicenter Randomized Comparative Double-blind Controlled Clinical Trial of the Safety and Efficacy of Zinc Gluconate versus Minocycline Hydrochloride in the Treatment of Inflammatory Acne Vulgaris." *Dermatology* 203, no. 2 (2001): 135–40.

Ebbett, V., K. Rule, and P. Vikesland. "Formation of Chloroform and Chlorinated Organics by Free-Chlorine-Medicated Oxidation of Triclosan." *Environmental Science & Technology* (2005): 39(9): 3,176–85.

El-Akawi, Z., N. Abdel-Latif, et al. "Does the Plasma Level of Vitamins A and E Affect Acne Condition?" *Clin Exp Dermatol* 31, 3 (2006): 430-3.

Ellis, C.N., et al. "A Double-blind Evaluation of Topical Capsaicin in Pruritic Psoriasis." *Journal of the American Academy of Dermatology* 29, no. 3 (September 1993): 438–42.

Evans, F.Q. "The Rational Use of Glycyrrhetinic Acid in Dermatology." *British Journal of Clinical Practice* 12 (1958): 269–79.

Fitton, A., and K.L. Goa. "Azelaic Acid: A Review of Its Pharmacological Properties and Therapeutic Efficacy in Acne and Hyperpigmentary Skin Disorders." *Drugs* 41 (1991): 780–98.

Fitzpatrick, R.E., and E.F. Rostan. "Double-blind, Half-face Study Comparing Topical Vitamin C and Vehicle for Rejuvenation of Photodamage." *Dermatologic Surgery* 28, no. 3 (March 2002): 231–36.

Fluhr, J.W., J. Kao, M. Jain, S.K. Ahn, K.R. Feingold, and P.M. Elias. "Generation of Free Fatty Acids from Phospholipids Regulates Stratum Corneum Acidification and Integrity." *Journal of Investigative Dermatology* 117, no. 1 (July 2001): 44–51.

Frost, Phillip, MD, and Steven N. Horwitz. *Principles of Cosmetics for the Dermatologist.* St. Louis, Mo.: The C. V. Mosby Company, 1982.

Fu, M.X., J.R. Requena, A.J. Jenkins, T.J. Lyons, J.W. Baynes, and S.R. Thorpe. "The Advanced Glycation End-product, Ne-(carboxymethyl)lysine, Is a Product of Both Lipid Peroxidation and Glycoxidation Reactions." *Journal of Biological Chemistry* 271 (1996): 9982–86.

Futoryan, T., and B.E. Gilchrest. "Retinoids and the Skin." *Nutrition Review* 52 (1994): 299–310.

Gieler, U., A. von der Weth, and M. Heger. "Mahonia Aquifolium—a New Type of Topical Treatment for Psoriasis." *Journal of Dermatological Treatment* 6, no. 1 (March 1995): 31–34.

Gollnick, H.P., and A. Krautheim. "Topical Treatment in Acne: Current Status and Future Aspects." *Dermatology* 206, no. 1 (2003): 29–36.

Grimm, T., Z. Chovanova, et al. "Inhibition of NF-KappaB Activation and MMP-9 Secrection by Plasma of Human Volunteers After Ingestion of Maritime Pine Bark Extract (Pycnogenol)." *Journal of Inflammation* 3, 1 (2006).

Hahn, G.S. "Strontium Is a Potent and Selective Inhibitor of Sensory Irritation." *Dermatologic Surgery* 25, no. 9 (September 1999): 689–94.

Horrobin, D.F. "The Importance of Gamma-linolenic Acid and Prostaglandin E1 in Human Nutrition and Medicine." *Journal of Holistic Medicine* 3 (1981): 118–39.

Imaizumi A., MD, M. Kashima, MD, T. Kawakami, MD, M. Mizoguchi, MD, Y. Soma, MD, and H. Takahama, MD. "Moisturizing Effects of Topical Nicotinamide on Atopic Dry Skin." *International Journal of Dermatology* (2005): 44, 3: 197–202.

Jugdaohsingh, R., K.L. Tucker, D.P. Kiel, N. Qiao, and J.J. Powell. "Silicon Uptake is a Major Dietary Determinant of Bone Mineral Density (BMD) in Man and Premenopausal Women of the Framingham Offspring Cohort." *Bone* (May 2003): 32: S192.

Katiyar, S.K., B.M. Bergamo, P.K. Vyalil, and C.A. Elmets. "Green Tea Polyphenols: DNA Photodamage and Photoimmunology." *Journal of Photochemistry and Photobiology* 65, nos. 2–3 (31 December 2001): 109–14.

Kimball, MD, A., et al. "New! Arthritis, UV-Damage Treatment in One?" *Health & Aging* (July 19, 2006).

Kumagai, A., M. Nanaboshi, Y. Asanuma, et al. "Effects of Glycyrrhizin on Thy-molytic and Immunosuppressive Action of Cortisone." *Endocrinologia Japonica* 14 (1967): 39–42.

Kunt, T., et al. "Alpha-lipoic Acid Reduces Expression of Vascular Cell Adhesion Molecule-1 and Endothelial Adhesion of Human Monocytes after Stimulation with Advanced Glycation End Products." *Clinical Science* (London) 96, no. 1 (January 1999): 75–82.

Lautenschlager, H., J. Roeding, and M. Ghyczy. "The Use of Liposomes from Soy-bean Phospholipids in Cosmetics." *Seifen-Ole-Fette-Wachse (S...FW)* 14, no. 88: 531–34.

Letawe, C., M. Boone, and G.E. Pierard. "Digital Image Analysis of the Effect of Topically Applied Linoleic Acid on Acne Microcomedones." *Clinical Experimental Dermatology* 23, no. 2 (March 1998): 56–58.

Leung, Lit-Hung, MD. "Pantothenic Acid in the Treatment of Acne Vulgaris: A Medical Hypothesis." *Orthomolecular Medicine* 12, 2 (1997): rev. 1998.

Liao, S. "Androgen Action: Molecular Mechanism and Medical Application." *Journal of the Formosan Medical Association* 93, no. 9 (September 1994): 741–51.

Maurice, P.D.L., B.R. Allen, A.S.J. Barkley, et al. "The Effects of Dietary Supplementation with Fish Oil in Patients with Psoriasis." *British Journal of Dermatology* 1117 (1987): 599–606.

McFarland, G.A., and R. Holliday. "Retardation of the Senescence of Cultured Human Diploid Fibroblasts by Carnosine." *Experimental Cell Research* 212, no. 2 (1994): 167–75.

Micans, P. "Aminoguanidine: AGE Inhibitor" www.smart_drugs.net/ias-aminoguanidine.htm.

Morrissey, Stephen. "Incurable No Longer: An Extract from the Oregon Grape Eliminates Psoriasis Suffering." *Health Sciences Member Alert*, December 1999, p. 5.

Mrowietz, et al. "Treatment of Severe Psoriasis With Fumeric Acid Esters: Scientific Background and Guidelines for Therapeutic Use. The German Fumaric Acid Concensus Conference." *The British Journal of Dermatology* 141, 3 (Sept 1999): 424–9.

Murray, Michael T., ND. *Natural Alternatives to Over-the-Counter and Prescription Drugs*. New York: William Morrow, 1994.

Nagabhushana, N.R., and K.S. Kulkarni. "Clinical Efficacy of Tablet and Ointment in Eczematous Skin Disorders." *The Indian Practitioner* 54, (November 2001): 807–813.

Nguyen, Q.H., and T.P. Bui. "Azelaic Acid: Pharmacokinetic and Pharmacodynamic Properties and Its Therapeutic Role in Hyperpigmentary Disorders and Acne." *International Journal of Dermatology* 34 (1995): 75–84.

Parsad, D., R. Pandhi, and A. Juneja. "Effectiveness of Oral Ginkgo Biloba in Treating Limited Slow Spreading Vitilgo." *Clinical Exp Dermatology* 28, 3 (May 2003): 285–7.

Perricone, Nicholas, MD. *The Perricone Prescription*. New York: HarperCollins: 2002.

Putzier, E. "Dermatomycoses and an Antifungal Diet." *Wiener Medizinische Wochenschrift* 139, nos. 15–16 (31 August 1989): 379–80.

Reffitt, D.M., N. Ogston, R. Jugdaohsingh, H.F. Cheung, B.A. Evans, R.P. Thoimpson, J.J. Powell, and G.N. Hampson. "Orthosilicic Acid Stimulates Collagen Type 1 Synthesis and Osteoblastic Differentiation in Human Osteoblast-like Cells in Vitro." *Bone* (February 2003): 32(2): 127–35.

Reynolds, T., et al. "Aloe Vera Leaf Gel: A Review Update." *Journal of Ethnopharmacology* 68, nos. 1–3 (December 1999): 3–37.

Roan, S. "Worship Your Skin." *Argus Leader*, 30 July 1996.

Schultz Jr., E., et al. "Neem: A Tree for Solving Global Problems." *National Academy Press* (1992).

Seki, T., and M. Morohashi. "Effect of Some Alkaloids, Flavinoids, and Triterpenoids, Contents of Japanese-Chinese and Traditional Herbal Medicines, on the Lipogenesis of Sabeceous Glands." *Skin Pharmacol* 6, 1 (1993): 56–60.

Sharquie K.E., R.A. Najim, et al. "Oral Zinc Sulfate in Treatment of Roseacea: A Double-blind, Placebo Controlled Study." *International Journal of Dermatology* 45, 7 (2006): 857–61.

Siddiqui, A.H., L.M. Stolk, R. Bjagge, et al. "L-Phenylalanine and UVA Irradiation in the Treatment of Vitiligo." *Dermatology* 188 (1994): 215–8.

Smeh, Nicholas J. *Health Risks in Today's Cosmetics.* Garrisonville, Va.: Alliance Publishing Company, 1994, p. 33.

Sudel, K.M., K. Venzke, H. Mielke, U. Breitenbach, C. Mundt, S. Jaspers, U. Koop,, K. Sauermann, E. Knussman-Hartig, I. Moll, G. Gercken, A.R. Young, F. Stab, H. Wenck, and S. Gallinat. "Novel Aspects of Intrinsic and Extrinsic Aging of Human Skin: Beneficial Effects of Soy Extract." *Photochemisty Photobiology* 81,3 (May–June 2005): 581–7.

Traber, M.G., et al. "Diet Derived Topically Applied Tocotrienols Accumulate in Skin and Protect the Tissue against UV Light-induced Oxidative Stress." *Asia Pacific Journal of Clinical Nutrition* 6 (1997): 63–67.

Trowell, H., D. Burkitt, and K. Heaton. "Dietary Fiber, Fiber-Depleted Foods and Disease." *London: Academic Press*, 1985.

Walker, M. "Astonishing Healing of Psoriasis Using the Euro-import." *Townsend Letter,* January 1997, pp. 58–64.

Warner, R.R., J.R. Schwartz, Y. Boissy, and T.L. Dawson, Jr. "Dandruff Has an Altered Stratum Corneum Ultrastructure That Is Improved with Zinc Pyrithione Shampoo." *Journal of the American Academy of Dermatology* 45, no. 6 (December 2001): 897–903.

Ziboh, V.A. "Prostaglandins, Leukotrienes, and Hydroxy Fatty Acids in Epidermis." *Seminars in Dermatology* 11, no. 2 (June 1992): 114–20.

Ziboh, V.A., and C.C. Miller. "Essential Fatty Acids and Polyunsaturated Fatty Acids: Significance in Cutaneous Biology." *Annual Review of Nutrition* 10 (1990): 433–50.

Chapter 14

Abou-Donia, M. "Use Caution When Using DEET." Duke Health Note, July 2002. www.dukehealth.org/news/healthtip_ julyo2.asp.

Allen, P. "Tea Tree Oil: The Science Behind the Antimicrobial Hype." *Journal of Antimicrobial Chemotherapy* 48 (2001): 450.

Aridogan, B.C., H. Baydar, S. Kaya, M. Demirci, D. Ozbasar, and E. Mumcu. "Antimicrobial Activity and Chemical Composition of Some Essential Oils." *Archives of Pharmacal Research* 25, no. 6 (December 2002): 860–64.

Balch, James F., MD, and Phyllis A. Balch, CNC. *Prescription for Nutritional Healing*, 3rd ed. New York: Avery, 2000.

Bauer, V.R., K. Jurcic, J. Puhlmann, et al. "Immunologic In Vivo and In Vitro Studies on Echinacea Extracts." *Arzneimittelforschung* 38, no. 2 (February 1988): 276–81.

Bronner, C., and Y. Landry. "Kinetics of the Inhibitory Effect of Flavonoids on Histamine Secretion from Mast Cells." *Agents Actions* 16 (1985): 147–51.

Buck, D.S., D.M. Nidorf, and J.G. Addino. "Comparison of Two Topical Preparations for the Treatment of Onychomycosis: Melaleuca Alternifolia (Tea Tree) Oil and Clotrimazole." *Journal of Family Practice* 38, no. 6 (June 1994): 601–5.

Caelli, M., J. Porteous, C.F. Carson, R. Heller, and T.V. Riley. "Tea Tree Oil as an Alternative Topical Decolonization Agent for Methicillin-resistant Staphylococcus Aureus." *Journal of Hospital Infection* 46, no. 3 (November 2000): 236–37.

Carson, C.F., B.J. Mee, and T.V. Riley. "Mechanism of Action of Melaleuca Alternifolia (Tea Tree) Oil on Staphylococcus Aureus Determined by Time-kill, Lysis, Leakage, and Salt Tolerance Assays and Electron Microscopy." *Antimicrobial Agents and Chemotherapy* 46, no. 6 (June 2002): 1914–20.

Cramer, Daniel W., et al. "Ovarian Cancer and Talc: A Case-Control Study." *Cancer* 50 (15 July 1982): 372–76.

Guin, J.D., and R. Reynolds. "Jewelweed Treatment of Poison Ivy Dermatitis." *Contact Dermatitis* (1980) 6(4): 287–288.

Hay, I.C., M. Jamieson, and A.D. Ormerod. "Randomized Trial of Aromatherapy: Successful Treatment for Alopecia Areata." *Archives of Dermatology* 134, no. 11 (November 1998): 1349–52.

Heggers, J.P., J. Cottingham, J. Gusman, L. Reagor, L. McCoy, E. Carino, R. Cox, J.G. Zhao, and L. Reagor. "The Effectiveness of Processed Grapefruit-seed Extract as an Antibacterial Agent: II. Mechanism of Action and In Vitro Toxicity." *Journal of Alternative and Complementary Medicine* 8, no. 3 (June 2002): 333–40.

Lassus, A., et al. "A Comparative Study of a New Food Supplement, Viviscal, with Fish Extract for the Treatment of Hereditary Androgenic Alopecia in Young Males." *The Journal of International Medical Research* 20 (1992): 445–53.

Lassus, A., J. Santalahti, and M. Sellmann. "Treatment of Hereditary Androgenic Alopecia in Middle-aged Males by Combined Oral and Topical Administration of Special

Marine Extract-Compound (Viviscal)." *Les Nouvelles Dermatologiques* 13 (1994): 254–55.

Luettig, B., et al. "Macrophage Activation by the Polysaccharide Arabinogalactan Isolated from Plant Cell Cultures of Echinacea Purpurea." *Journal of the American Cancer Institute* 81, no. 9 (1989): 669–75.

Manohar, V., C. Ingram, J. Gray, N.A. Talpur, B.W. Echard, D. Bagchi, and H.G. Preuss. "Antifungal Activities of Origanum Oil against Candida Albicans." *Molecular and Cellular Biochemistry* 228, nos. 1–2 (December 2001): 111–17.

Mercola, Joseph M., DO. "Oregano, Other Essential Oils Destroy Strep Pneumonia Cells." *Townsend Letter*, August/September 1998.

Mittman, P. "Randomized, Double-blind Study of Freeze-dried Urtica Dioica in the Treatment of Allergic Rhinitis." *Planta Medica* 56 (1990): 44–47.

Ooshima, T., T. Minami, W. Aono, et al. "Reduction of Dental Plaque Deposition in Humans by Oolong Tea Extract." *Caries Research* 28 (1994): 146–49.

Oyedele, A.O., A.A. Gbolade, M.B. Sosan, F.B. Adewoyin, O.L. Soyelu, and O.O. Orafidya. "Formulation of an Effective Mosquito-repellant Topical Product from Lemongrass Oil." *Phytomedicine* 9, no. 3 (April 2002): 259–62.

Peterson, C., W. Rowley, and J. Coats. "Catnip Essential Oil as a Mosquito Repellent." *American Chemical Society's 222nd National Meeting* (2001) Chicago.

Prager, N., K. Bickett, N. French, and G. Marcovici. "A Randomized, Double-blind, Placebo-controlled Trial to Determine the Effectiveness of Botanically Derived Inhibitors of 5-alpha-reductase in the Treatment of Androgenetic Alopecia." *Journal of Alternative and Complementary Medicine* 8, no. 2 (April 2002): 143–52.

Rabbani, G.H., et al. "Randomized Controlled Trial of Berberine Sulfate Therapy for Diarrhea Due to Enterotoxigenic Escherichia Coli and Vibrio Cholerae." *The Journal of Infectious Diseases* 155, no. 5 (1987): 979–84.

Ratner, P.H., P.M. Ehrlich, S.M. Fineman, E.O. Meltzer, and D.P. Skoner. "Use of Intranasal Cromolyn Sodium for Allergic Rhinitis." *Mayo Clinic: Proceedings* 77, no. 4 (April 2002): 350–54.

Reagor, L., J. Gusman, L. McCoy, E. Carino, and J.P. Heggers. "The Effectiveness of Processed Grapefruit-seed Extract as an Antibacterial Agent: I. An In Vitro Agar Assay." *Journal of Alternative and Complementary Medicine* 8, no. 3 (June 2002): 325–32.

Reid, G. "The Role of Cranberry and Probiotics in Intestinal and Urogenital Tract Health." *Critical Reviews in Food Science and Nutrition* 42, supplement 3 (2002): 293–300.

Roesler, J., A. Emmendorffer, C. Steinmuller, et al. "Application of Purified Polysaccharides from Cell Cultures of the Plant Echinacea purpurea to Test Subjects Mediates Activation of the Phagocyte System." *International Journal of Immunopharmacology* 13, no. 7 (1991): 931–41.

"The Safety of Sporanox Capsules and Lamisil Tablets for the Treatment of Onychomycosis." FDA Public Health Advisory, 9 May 2001. www.fda.gov/cder/drug/advisory/sporanox-lamisil/advisory.htm.

Schlumpf, Margaret, Beata Cotton, Marianne Conscience, Vreni Haller, Beate Steinmann, and Walter Lichtensteiger. "In Vitro and In Vivo Estrogenicity of UV Screens." *Environmental Health Perspectives* 109 (March 2001): 239–44.

Thompson, K.D. "Antiviral Activity of Viracea against Acyclovir Susceptible and Acyclovir Resistant Strains of Herpes Simplex Virus." *Antiviral Research* 39, no. 1 (July 1998): 55–61.

Uhari, M., et al. "Xylitol in Preventing Acute Otitis Media." *Vaccine* 19, supplement 1 (2000): S144–47.

U.S. Food and Drug Administration, Center for Drug Evaluation and Research Approval Letter. Nasalcrom. Application No. 20-463/S-002, 27 March 2001.

Winn, D.M., W.J. Blot, J.K. McLaughlin, D.F. Austin, R.S. Greenberg, S. Preston-Martin, J.B. Schoenberg, and J.F. Fraumeni, Jr. "Mouthwash Use and Oral Conditions in the Risk of Oral and Pharyngeal Cancer." *Cancer Research* 51, no. 11 (1 June 1991): 3044–47.

Xiong, H., Y. Li, M.F. Slavik, and J. Walker. "Spraying Chicken Skin with Selected Chemicals to Reduce Attached Salmonella Typhimurium." *Journal of Food Protection* 61 (1998): 272–75.

Zabner, J., et al. "The Osmolyte Xylitol Reduces the Salt Concentration of Airway Surface Liquid and May Enhance Bacterial Killing." *Proceedings of the National Academy of Sciences* (USA) 97 (10 October 2000): 11614–19.

Chapter 15

Barregård, L., G. Lindstedt, A. Schütz, and G. Sällsten. "Endocrine function in mercury exposed chloralkali workers." *Occup Envir Med.* 1994; 51: 536–40.

Bouic, P.J.D., P.P. van Jaarsveld, A. Clark, J.H. Lamprecht, M. Freestone, and R.W. Liebenberg. "The Effects of B-sitosterol (BSS) and B-sitosterol Glucoside (BSSG) Mixture on Selected Immune Parameters of Marathon Runners: Inhibition of Post Marathon Immune Suppression and Inflammation." *International Journal of Sports Medicine* 20 (1999): 258–62.

Brown, David. "Women Taking Another Look at Ways to Treat Menopause Problems with Hormone Therapy May Boost Other Remedies." *The Washington Post*, 29 August 2002, p. A03.

Bunevicius, Robertas, G. Kazanavicius, R. Zalinkevicius, A.J. Prange, Jr. "Effects of Thyroxine as Compared with Thyroxine Plus Triiodothyronine in Patients with Hypothyroidism." *New England Journal of Medicine* 340, no. 6 (11 February 1999): 424–29.

Cherniske, Stephen. *Caffeine Blues.* New York: Warner Books, 1998.

Duker, E.M., L. Kopanski, H. Jarry, and W. Wuttke. "Effects of Extracts from Cimicifuga Racemosa on Gonadotropin Release in Menopausal Women and Ovariectomized Rats." *Planta Medica* 57 (1991): 420–24.

Ferri, J. "Under Pressure." *Tampa Tribune-Times*, 27 April 1997.

Gaby, A.R. "Treatment with Thyroid Hormone." *Journal of the American Medical Association* 262, no. 13 (6 October 1989): 1774–75.

Khatri, Parinda, James A. Blumenthal, Michael A. Babyak, W. Edward Craighead, Steve Herman, Teri Baldewicz, David J. Madden, Murali Doraiswamy, Robert Waugh, and K. Ranga Krishnan. "Effects of Exercise Training on Cognitive Functioning Among Depressed Older Men and Women." *Journal of Aging and Physical Activity* 9, no. 1 (2001): 43.

Kolata, Gina. "Citing Risks, U.S. Will Halt Study of Drugs for Hormones." *The New York Times*, 9 June 2002.

Lark, Susan M. "Research Corner: Coffee Increases Estrogen Levels." *The Lark Letter* 9, no. 3 (March 2000) (Phillips Health, LLC, Potomac, Maryland).

Lark, Susan M. "Research on HRT, Soy, and Vitamin C." *The Lark Letter* 9, no. 4 (April 2000).

Lark, Susan M. "Undoing Estrogen Dominance." *The Lark Letter* 9, no. 3 (March 2000).

Lazarou, J., B.H. Pomeranz, and P.N. Corey. "Incidence of Adverse Drug Reactions in Hospitalized Patients: A Meta-analysis of Prospective Studies." *Journal of the American Medical Association* 279, no. 15 (15 April 1998): 1200–1205.

Lehmann-Willenbrock, E., and H.-H. Riedel. "Clinical and Endocrinologic Examination Concerning Therapy of Climacteric Symptoms Following Hysterectomy with Remaining Ovaries." *Zentralblatt Gynäkologie* 110 (1988): 611–18.

Lucero, J., B.L. Harlow, R.L. Barbieri, P. Sluss, and D.W. Cramer. "Early Follicular Phase Hormone Levels in Relation to Patterns of Alcohol, Tobacco, and Coffee Use." *Fertility and Sterility* 76, no. 4 (October 2001): 723–29.

Ray, Paul H., and Sherry Ruth Anderson. *The Cultural Creatives: How Fifty Million People Are Changing the World.* New York: Harmony Books, 2000.

Rosignol, Annette MacKay. "Caffeine-containing Beverages and Premenstrual Syndrome in Young Women." *American Journal of Public Health* 75 (1985): 1335–37.

Stoll, W. "Phytopharmacon Influences Atrophic Vaginal Epithelium: Double Blind Study—Cimicifuga vs. Estrogenic Substances." *Therapeuticum* 1 (1987): 23–31.

Warnecke, G. "Influencing Menopausal Symptoms with a Phytotherapeutic Agent: Successful Therapy with Cimicifuga Mono-extract." *Medizinische Welt* 36 (1985): 871–74.

INDEX

Note: **s** indicates a sidebar, **c** indicates a chart.